Hand and Wrist Injuries in Baseball

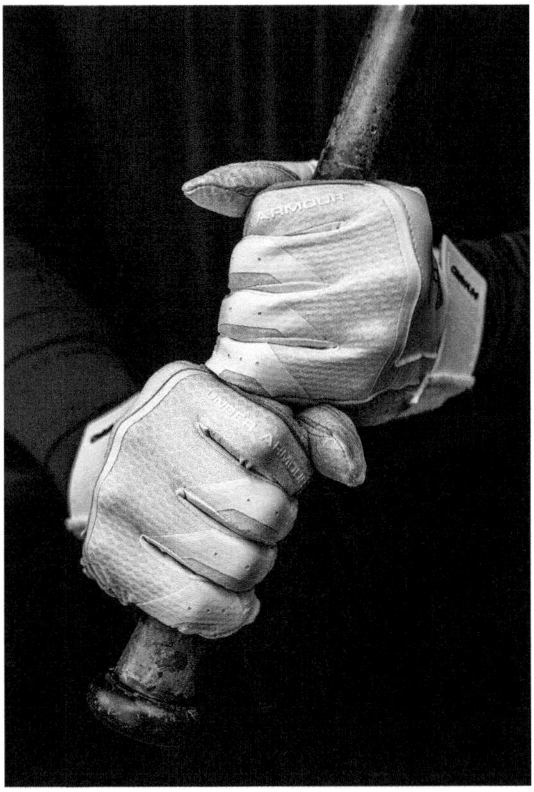

Freddie Freeman Atlanta Braves. (Photo Courtesy of Kevin D. Liles)

Gary M. Lourie
Editor

Hand and Wrist Injuries in Baseball

A Clinical Guide

Springer

Editor
Gary M. Lourie
The Hand and Upper Extremity Center of Georgia
Atlanta, GA
USA

ISBN 978-3-030-81658-2 ISBN 978-3-030-81659-9 (eBook)
https://doi.org/10.1007/978-3-030-81659-9

This Springer imprint is published by the registered company Springer Nature Switzerland AG
The registered company address is: Gewerbestrasse 11, 6330 Cham, Switzerland

Foreword

When we discuss the importance of this specific book, nothing serves the orthopaedic surgeon involved in baseball medicine better than a single source for baseball injuries to the hand and wrist.

As sports medicine has become large and a more complicated part of orthopaedic surgery, it has also become more sports specific. It is so specific that it has now been broken down into certain individual positions of a particular sport.

Baseball is no exception to this phenomenon. As seen in this book on hand and wrist injuries in baseball, it can even be specific for individual positions such as the pitcher, catcher, and position players.

As discussed in Dr. Lourie's introduction: a recent review of Major League Baseball injuries had hand and wrist injuries as the number three most common. This was only secondary behind shoulder and elbow injuries. Even more important is the likelihood of significant time on the disabled list with a hand or wrist injury because of its importance to both throwing and fielding a ball, as well as batting.

The lead author has had significant experience with baseball, especially hand and wrist. As a lead orthopaedic consultant to a professional baseball team, a high-level college baseball team, and experience with a large number of high school youth teams, he has put together a most comprehensive book on baseball hand and wrist injuries! He has also included a who's who list of expert co-authors for individual chapters that have a world of experience.

This book addresses in order from the mundane to the more complex injuries seen in the baseball hand and wrist. This includes from fractures to ligaments to tendon and nerve injuries, and contains special topics such as the injuries seen in the youth hand and wrist. It also includes the cumulative knowledge as seen through the eyes of some very prominent baseball athletic trainers who are on the front lines.

For those of us with a keen interest in all injuries seen in baseball (called baseball medicine) we cannot thank Dr. Lourie and his contributors enough for sharing their experience and expertise with us!

Enough said except for a thought to the interested surgeon: "there is no better source of direction and guidance than this all-encompassing text."

Andrews Institute
Gulf Breeze, FL, USA

James R. Andrews

Introduction

Baseball remains America's pastime and has truly captured a worldwide audience. With a jump in participation has come an escalating incidence of injury. A recent MLB review of hand and wrist injuries found its incidence third in frequency, closely behind the elbow and shoulder. Further, time on the injured list can frequently surpass the elbow and shoulder. Youth baseball may have an even more profound effect due to the underestimation of the injury and delay in diagnosis and treatment. The position played, the need to bat and field, along with the inability to play with protective splints make management of these injuries a task for the clinician. The goal remains early return to play with minimal risk; however, the literature is deficient with specific recommendations in managing these injuries specific to baseball. The goal of this book is to provide a comprehensive review of soft tissue, bone, ligament, nerve, and vascular injury particular to baseball. Well-recognized team physicians and surgeons along with athletic trainers serve as authors holding to a consistent outline of pertinent clinical anatomy, diagnosis, treatment, and recommendations for return to play. I want to thank my head athletic trainers, specifically Jeff Porter and George Poulis of the Atlanta Braves and Joe B. Chandler, MD, our emeritus team physician, for their friendship, guidance, and mentoring throughout the years. Many thanks to my nurse Brittany Logan who took such great care of my patients allowing me more time to work on the book. In addition, special gratefulness to my children Jackson, Wesleigh, and Allie along with my wife Yvette for understanding the time necessary to complete this project.

Hand and Upper Extremity Surgeon Atlanta Braves
Head Team Physician Georgia Tech Baseball
Atlanta, GA, USA
May 2021

Gary M. Lourie

Contents

Contributors

Jacob W. Brubacher, MD Department of Orthopedic Surgery, The University of Kansas Medical Center, Kansas City, KS, USA

Douglas Carlan, MD Eaton Orthopaedics, LLC, St. Petersburg, FL, USA

Michelle G. Carlson, MD Hospital for Special Surgery, New York, NY, USA

George A. Cibulas II, PharmD, MD Department of Orthopedic Surgery, New York Presbyterian/Columbia University Irving Medical Center, New York, NY, USA

Randall W. Culp, MD Orthopedic Surgery, Thomas Jefferson University, Philadelphia, PA, USA

Matthew C. DeWolf, MD Philadelphia Hand to Shoulder Center and Thomas Jefferson University, Philadelphia, PA, USA

Jake S. Enos, BS, MD Department of Orthopedic Surgery, The University of Kansas Medical Center, Kansas City, KS, USA

Michael B. Frostad, ATC, CAT(C) Atlanta Braves Baseball Club, Atlanta, GA, USA

R. Glenn Gaston, MD OrthoCarolina Hand Center, Charlotte, NC, USA

Charles A. Goldfarb, MD Department of Orthopaedic Surgery, Washington University School of Medicine, Barnes Jewish Hospital, Saint Louis, MO, USA

Thomas J. Graham, MD Ohio Hand at Kettering Health, Dayton, OH, USA

Department of Orthopedic Surgery, NYU Langone Health, New York, NY, USA

A. Jordan Grier, MD OrthoCarolina Hand Center, Charlotte, NC, USA

Timothy B. Griffith, MD Peachtree Orthopedic Clinic, Atlanta, GA, USA

Elizabeth A. Helsper, MD Department of Orthopaedic Surgery, University of Kansas School of Medicine-Wichita, Wichita, KS, USA

Caroline H. Hu, MD Department of Orthopaedic Surgery, University of Minnesota, Minneapolis, MN, USA

Jeffrey B. Husband, MD Hand Surgery, TRIA Orthopedic Center, Minneapolis, MN, USA

Joseph T. Labrum IV, MD Department of Orthopaedic Surgery, Vanderbilt Medical Center, Nashville, TN, USA

Fraser J. Leversedge, MD Department of Orthopedic Surgery, University of Colorado, Aurora, CO, USA

Gary M. Lourie, MD The Hand and Upper Extremity Center of Georgia, Atlanta, GA, USA

Michael J. Moses, MD Department of Orthopedic Surgery, NYU Langone Health, New York, NY, USA

Jeffrey A. O'Donnell, MD Department of Orthopaedic Surgery, Duke University Medical Center, Durham, NC, USA

Dimitrios V. Papadopoulos, MD, PhD University of Pittsburgh School of Medicine – UPMC, Pittsburgh, PA, USA

Loukia K. Papatheodorou, MD, PhD Department of Orthopaedic Surgery, University of Pittsburgh School of Medicine – UPMC, Pittsburgh, PA, USA

Allan E. Peljovich, MD, MPH The Hand & Upper Extremity Center of Georgia, Atlanta, GA, USA

The Hand & Upper Extremity Program, Children's Healthcare of Atlanta, Atlanta, GA, USA

WellStar Atlanta Medical Center Orthopaedic Surgery Residency Program, Atlanta, GA, USA

The Hand & Upper Extremity Program, The Shepherd Center, Atlanta, GA, USA

George C. Poulis, MA, ATC Atlanta Braves Baseball Club, Atlanta, GA, USA

Mia M. Qin, MD Department of Orthopaedic Surgery, Northwestern University Feinberg School of Medicine, Chicago, IL, USA

Marc Richard, MD Department of Orthopaedic Surgery, Duke University Medical Center, Durham, NC, USA

Melvin P. Rosenwasser, MD Department of Orthopedic Surgery, New York Presbyterian/Columbia University Irving Medical Center, New York, NY, USA

David S. Ruch, MD Department of Orthopaedic Surgery, Duke University Medical Center, Durham, NC, USA

Chirag M. Shah, MD Department of Orthopaedic Surgery, Northwestern University Feinberg School of Medicine, Chicago, IL, USA

Steven S. Shin, MD Department of Orthopaedic Surgery, Cedars-Sinai Medical Center, Los Angeles, CA, USA

T. Greg Sommerkamp, MD Cincinnati Hand Surgery Specialists, Department of Orthopedics, University of Cincinnati, Cincinnati, OH, USA

Dean G. Sotereanos, MD Department of Orthopaedic Surgery, University of Pittsburgh School of Medicine – UPMC, Pittsburgh, PA, USA

Jeffrey A. Stevenson, BS, ATC Atlanta Braves Baseball Club, Atlanta, GA, USA

Michael Sun, MD Department of Orthopaedic Surgery, Cedars-Sinai Medical Center, Los Angeles, CA, USA

E. Bruce Toby, MD Department of Orthopedic Surgery, The University of Kansas Medical Center, Kansas City, KS, USA

Adriana M. Urruela, MD Hospital for Special Surgery, New York, NY, USA

Douglas R. Weikert, MD Department of Orthopaedic Surgery, Vanderbilt Medical Center, Nashville, TN, USA

Keith G. Whitlock, MD Department of Orthopaedic Surgery, Duke University Medical Center, Durham, NC, USA

Thomas A. Wiedrich, MD Department of Orthopaedic Surgery, Northwestern University Feinberg School of Medicine, Chicago, IL, USA

Part I

Fractures of the Hand and Wrist

1 Distal Radius Fractures in Baseball

Jeffrey A. O'Donnell and Marc Richard

Define the Specific Injury Your Chapter Will Address

Distal radius fracture is a fracture of the distal metaphysis of the radius with or without articular involvement.

Discuss its overall incidence in sports in general and then give an estimate of its presence in baseball. In doing this, discuss how this injury may be unique to baseball.

Distal radius fractures are the most common fracture of the upper extremity and athletes are no exception. Injury can not only impact a player's competitiveness but also the longevity of their career [1]. The mechanism, evaluation, treatment, and rehabilitation strategies are similar among athletes with a few unique and important considerations.

Distal radius fractures occur in a bimodal distribution, peaking in youths and in adults over 65 [2, 3]. The increased prevalence in older adults is attributed to osteoporosis and postural instability leading to falls [4]. Fractures in youth occur commonly in sports-related settings with approximately 25% of all sports-related injuries involving the hand or wrist [5].

Upper extremity injuries are particularly common in baseball. From 2010 to 2016, there were 3512 injuries in Major League Baseball (MLB). Of these, 49% affected the upper extremity. On average, players were put on Injured Lists (IL) due to upper limb injuries for 71 ± 57 days [6].

A 2009 study assessing frequency of upper extremity fractures in the United States found the incidence of distal radius and ulna fractures to be the most common. Rates were 16.2 distal radius fractures per 10,000 persons [7]. This is in line with other epidemiological studies which estimate the incidence in the United States nearly 650,000 fractures annually [3].

Sport-related injuries represent the third most common cause of fracture [8]. Athletes represent a significant portion of the population sustaining distal radius fractures. In a 1-year sample of 1044 fractures treated at the Royal Infirmary of Edinburgh, 12.5% were related to sport [9]. This analysis did not include injuries from baseball and the incidence of distal radius fractures in baseball is not as clear. Fractures can occur through falls and collision or from direct ball-contact. Direct ball-contact causing fracture is exceedingly rare with only one radius fracture occurring within a 5-year period among collegiate baseball athletes [10].

J. A. O'Donnell (✉) · M. Richard
Department of Orthopaedic Surgery, Duke University Medical Center, Durham, NC, USA
e-mail: Jeffrey.odonnell@duke.edu

G. M. Lourie (ed.), *Hand and Wrist Injuries in Baseball*,
https://doi.org/10.1007/978-3-030-81659-9_1

Pertinent Anatomy of the Injury You Are Describing. Please Make It Clinical Anatomy

The distal radius is a platform for the carpus and has three independent articulating surfaces: the scaphoid fossa, the lunate fossa, and the sigmoid notch. These articulate with the scaphoid, lunate, and distal ulna, respectively. Ligamentous complexes provide stability to the articulations of the wrist. Extrinsic ligaments link the carpus to the distal radius. The distal radius and ulna, articulation with the carpus, and distal radioulnar joint (DRUJ) can be conceptualized into three distinct columns: (1) radial column, (2) intermediate column, and (3) ulnar column. The metadiaphysis of the distal radius functions as a supporting pillar of bone (Fig. 1.1) [11].

The radial column contains the radial styloid, scaphoid facet. The radial column does not have significant weight-bearing function, but rather it acts as a buttress for the carpus with radioulnar deviation with ligamentous attachments that prevent carpal translation. When disrupted from a fracture, the brachioradialis contractile force causes radial deviation, and loss of radial height and inclination [12].

The intermediate column of the distal radius is formed by the lunate facet and sigmoid notch. This column is responsible for load bearing through the lunate facet (Fig. 1.2). Ligamentous attachments prevent carpal translation. The robust ligaments of the lunate facet are necessarily strong that is why the carpus is virtually always displaced with the medial fragment of the fractured distal radius. The volar lunate facet fragment is at the distal, volar, and ulnar portion of the radius. This piece is critical because of its attachment to the volar radiocarpal and radioulnar ligaments. The fragment typically involves the sigmoid notch and can affect DRUJ stability [12]. Articular congruency and mechanical alignment of the intermediate column must be reestablished after a fracture given its weight-bearing function. The sigmoid notch acts as a saddle for the distal ulna to facilitate a combination of trans-

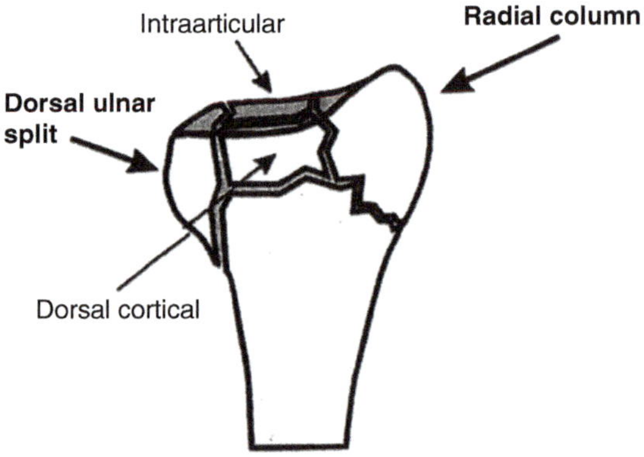

Fig. 1.2 Illustration depicting classification of fragments that may result from a multifragmentary distal radius fracture (He and Blazar [77])

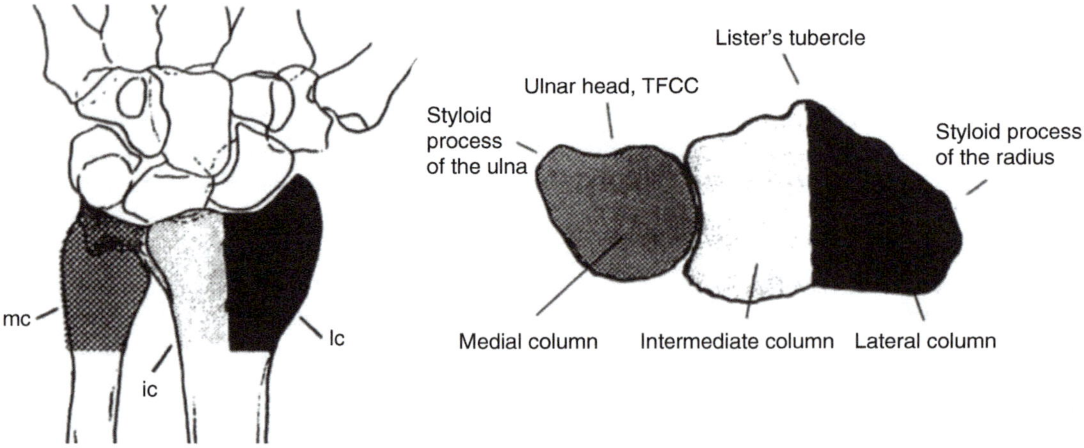

Fig. 1.1 Three-column model of distal radius fracture (He and Blazar [77])

lation and rotation. The ligament attachments between the radius and ulna stabilize the DRUJ in pronosupination [12].

The ulnar column is composed of the distal ulna and triangular fibrocartilage complex (TFCC). The volar and dorsal radioulnar ligaments are a component of the TFCC and are the primary stabilizers of the DRUJ. Together the ulnar column serves as a rotational axis for wrist pronation and supination. Loss of radial height with distal radius fractures can disrupt the TFCC and lead to loss of inclination and volar tilt [12].

The distal articular surface of the distal radius has a radial inclination averaging 22° (21–25°) and an average volar tilt of 11° (2–20°). The sigmoid notch angles distally and ulnarly an average of 22°. The average radial height is 12 mm with an ulnar variance of just under 1 mm negative with a large range [13]. With upper extremity use, the distal radius bears approximately 80% of the stress placed across the wrist joint with neutral ulnar variance. As positive ulnar variance increases, for instance, after a distal radius fracture resulting in shortening, there is increased stress placed across the distal ulna. This can lead to impaction of the ulna against the lunate and triquetrum, wrist pain, and ultimately degenerative changes in the carpus and TFCC [15].

The carpal tunnel is enclosed by carpal bones and by the flexor retinaculum with little room for expansion. The tunnel is narrow and allows passage of nine tendons and the median nerve and course volar with proximity to the distal radius. Acute carpal tunnel can occur after distal radius fractures and is characterized by pain and paresthesia due to increased carpal pressure within a non-expandable space. The etiology of this increased pressure can be due to fracture displacement and displaced fragments, hematoma, edema, anesthetic injection, and immobilization in excessive flexion [16].

The extensor pollicis longus (EPL) tendon is held against the dorsal surface of the distal radius wrapping around Lister tubercle. Injury can occur in fracture situations due to this close proximity to bone [17]. EPL rupture is a complication after distal radius fractures secondary to several distinct etiologies: laceration by a sharp fragment of bone, injury during reduction or fixation, injury or disturbance to the blood supply, and local adhesions [18]. Hirasawa et al. note that the third dorsal compartment narrows around Lister tubercle, and the tendon can become entrapped after a fracture leading to decreasing vascularity, nutrition, and eventually avascular necrosis and rupture [19].

The watershed line is a useful anatomic landmark for volar plating of distal radius fractures. The volar distal radius has a concave profile for the pronator fossa, and the distal ridge is the watershed line [20]. The mean distance between the distal margin of the pronator quadratus and the distal edge of the pronator fossa is 3.9 mm (Fig. 1.3) [21]. This is classically the distal margin for volar plating to mitigate flexor tendon irritation and possible rupture [22].

The pediatric patient with a distal radius fracture presents a unique set of challenges. Developmentally around 8 weeks of gestation, the primary ossification centers of the radius and ulna appear. The distal radial epiphysis becomes radiographically apparent between the ages of 8 and 18 months. The distal ulnar epiphysis ossifies at roughly 6 years of age [23]. The distal radial physis contributes approximately 75% of the longitudinal growth of the radius and for this reason can have significant remodeling potential in young children [24]. This will impact the treatment strategy for these fractures. It is thought that up to 10° of dorsal–volar angulation per year may remodel with continued growth [23]. Potential for remodeling depends on amount of growth remaining, distance from the adjacent physis, degree of angulation, and the direction of deformity. Fractures close to the physis in the plane of adjacent joint motion, in young patients, generally have the greatest potential for remodeling. The physis blood supply is primarily from the epiphysis and is rarely disrupted by a physeal fracture. Although most of these fractures heal without complication, some result in partial or complete physeal arrest which can have clinically impactful consequences given the growth potential of the distal radius [24].

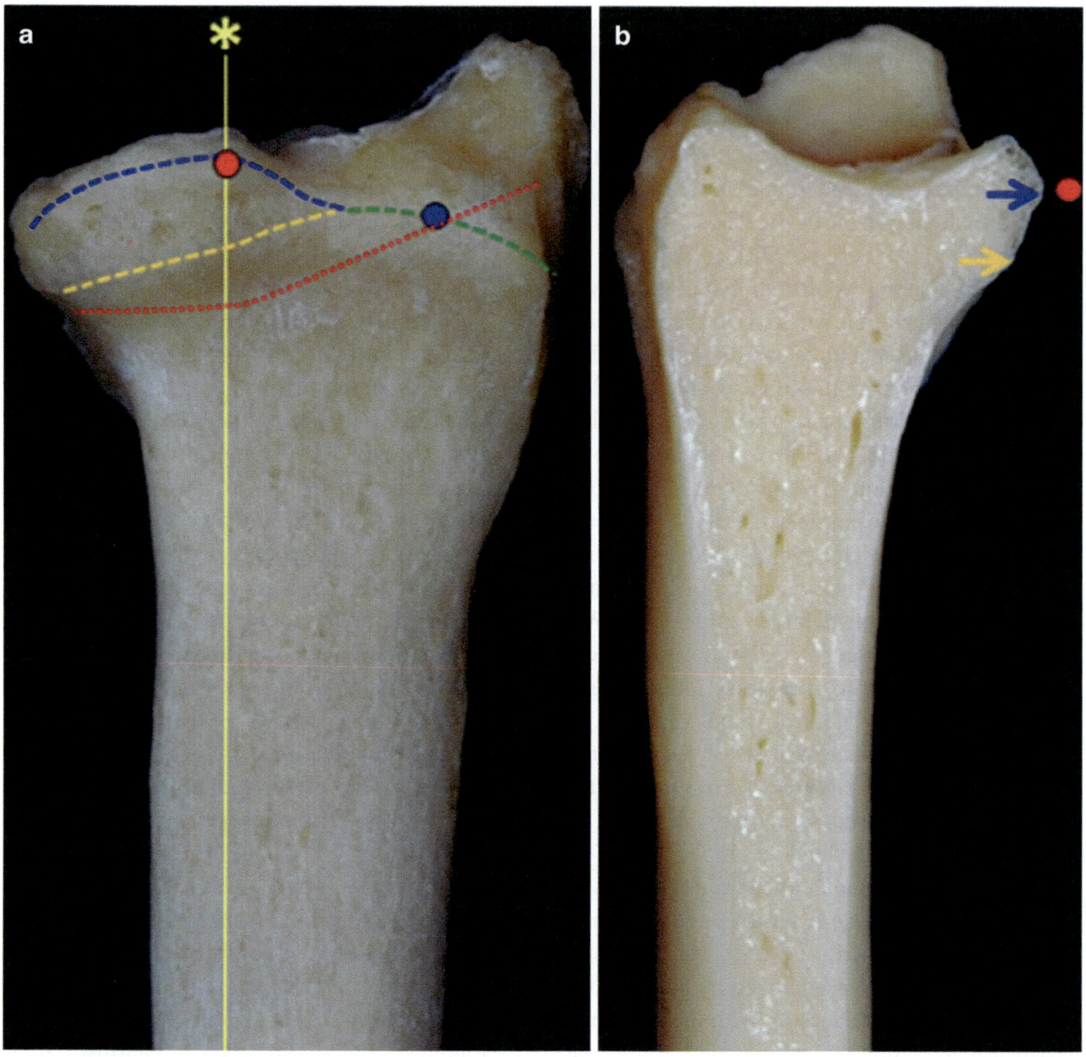

Fig. 1.3 (**a**) Radius from the volar aspect. The red dotted line indicates the distal margin of the pronator quadratus, and red and blue dots indicate the medial and lateral prominences, respectively. The blue dotted line indicates the connection of the distal bony demarcation points, and the orange dotted line indicates the connection of the proximal bony demarcation points. (**b**) Sagittal section of the radius, which is cut on the line that coincided with the yellow line indicated by an asterisk in (**a**). The red dot indicates the medial prominence. The blue arrow indicates the distal bony demarcation point, and the orange arrow indicates the proximal bony demarcation point (Imatani et al. [21])

Mechanism of Injury

The mechanism of injury of distal radius fractures in baseball is no different than in the community. In young athletes, distal radius fractures occur after collisions, falls, or direct impact injuries causing a compressive load to the distal radius. The most common mechanism of distal radius fracture is a fall onto an outstretched extended wrist. In this situation, the radius will fail in tension on the volar surface and progress dorsally where torsional, bending, compressive, and shear forces influence the injury pattern and articular involvement. Metaphyseal involvement can further affect the stability of the fracture [25, 26]. Often the scaphoid or lunate will impact into the distal radius which can create a "die-punch" fragment. There are several patterns of injury that depend on the violence of the injury as well as the position of the wrist during the contact. The ligamentous structures play an important role in the specific fracture pattern encountered.

History/Differential Dx

The presentation of a distal radius fracture is often clinically evident even prior to radiographic evidence has been obtained due to the associated wrist deformity seen. It is thus important to not fixate on the distal radius fracture, but rather perform a systematic history to avoid missing an occult or simultaneous injury. This is especially relevant in pediatric patients, in whom it can be more difficult to diagnose these injuries. History should focus on mechanism, duration, and quality of symptoms. Factors that may affect management include age, handedness, previous injuries, position and level of play in baseball, timing of the injury relative to season responsibilities, and comorbid conditions. Questioning should focus on location and character of pain, associated numbness, tingling, weakness, and discoloration [14]. The mechanism most commonly associated with a distal radius fracture, fall onto an extended outstretched hand, is associated with a number of other injuries, and the differential diagnoses for traumatic distal wrist pain are broad. Included on this list are other fractures, ligament injuries, instability patterns, and contusions. Fractures of the scaphoid, hamate, ulna, and other carpal bones should be ruled out. Injuries to the DRUJ, TFCC, scapholunate, and other ligamentous injuries are critical to identify. Ligament injuries can rarely present as lunate or perilunate dislocations or scapholunate dissociation. These injuries, although clinically distinct, can have similar presentations and may present simultaneously. Gathering a thorough but directed history can narrow this differential and guide future treatment strategy [27].

Directed Physical Exam

The clinician should begin a directed physical exam in the standard fashion with inspection, palpation, range of motion, strength, and special tests. Inspect the injured extremity for deformity, swelling, and any open fractures. Careful inspection is important to distinguish between an abrasion and a poke-hole open fracture. The typically location of skin breach of a poke-hole open fracture is at the volar, ulnar aspect of the distal radius. This area should be particularly scrutinized to avoid missing an open fracture.

A "dinner-fork" deformity can classically be seen with a dorsally displaced distal radius fracture, but any deformity should be noted. Palpation of the wrist can identify concomitant injuries as well. Anatomic snuffbox tenderness may be the only initial clue to identify a scaphoid fracture not initially visible on radiographic evaluation. Neurologic assessment including motor and sensory function of the median, radial, and ulnar nerves is essential. Acute carpal tunnel can occur with fractures of the distal radius and should not be missed. A vascular exam documenting radial pulse, capillary refill, and Allen testing is important especially prior to surgical intervention. Range of motion and evaluation of the DRUJ will be limited in the setting of a distal radius fracture due to the injury or discomfort. Finally, an examination of the ipsilateral shoulder, elbow, and hand should be completed as well.

Imaging Including Advanced Methods

Plain radiographs are often the first diagnostic imaging studies obtained when evaluating distal radius fractures. Radiographs can have an impact on how fractures are approached and treated. Computed tomography (CT) and magnetic resonance imaging (MRI) are adjuncts and can provide additional information in certain cases. CT yields anatomic details related to the fracture, articular reduction, and can be useful for surgical planning to reveal fracture fragment position. Data has shown that CT is more reliable for quantifying articular surface incongruity of the distal radius than plain radiographic measurements [28]. MRI is a helpful adjunct that can identify occult fractures, injuries to the TFCC, and intrinsic wrist ligaments.

Typically, standard posterior–anterior (PA), lateral, and oblique films are obtained and should be evaluated for changes in radiographic landmarks, parameters, and fragmentation pattern [14]. The PA should be acquired with the patient's elbow at 90° and the forearm in neutral rotation. When the lateral view is acquired correctly, the pisiform should be superimposed on the distal pole of the scaphoid. The lateral can be shot with a 10–20° inclined view directed from distal radial to proximal ulnar, for better assessment of tilt and articular congruence. A 45° pronated oblique view profiles the dorsal ulnar cortex that supports the dorsal lunate articular facet [29].

There are several measurements that can be made on a PA view including radial height, inclination, ulnar variance, and radial translation ratio. Radial height is measured as two perpendicular lines: one at the tip of the radial styloid and the other at the ulnar border of the distal radial articular surface (Fig. 1.4) [30]. The average radial height is 12 mm. Excessive shortening can be seen after fracture with associated TFCC injury [31]. Radial inclination is approximately 23° (range, 13–30°) and is formed from the angle between the radial articular surface and a line perpendicular to the longitudinal axis of the radius (Fig. 1.5) [14]. This is altered in fractures of the distal radius with styloid involvement as the brachioradialis tendon pulls and shortens this fragment. Ulnar variance is the distance between parallel lines drawn first at the level of the radial sigmoid notch and the second at the level of the lateral cortical margin of the distal ulna (Fig. 1.6) [30]. With radial shortening and positive ulnar variance, the stress

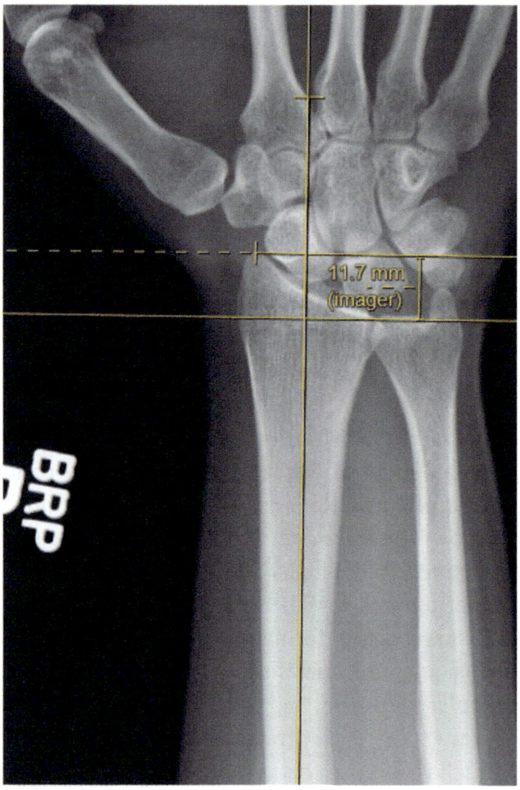

Fig. 1.4 Radial height – to obtain radial height, two lines are drawn perpendicular to a line that projects along long axis of the radius. One is at tip of radial styloid and the other at ulnar border of distal radial articular surface

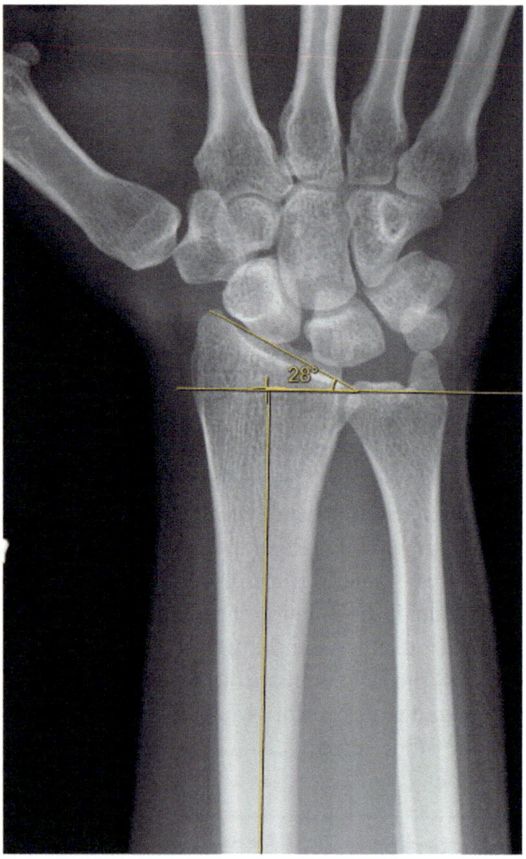

Fig. 1.5 Radial inclination – formed by a line perpendicular to long axis of radius and a line connecting radial and ulnar articular surface of distal radius

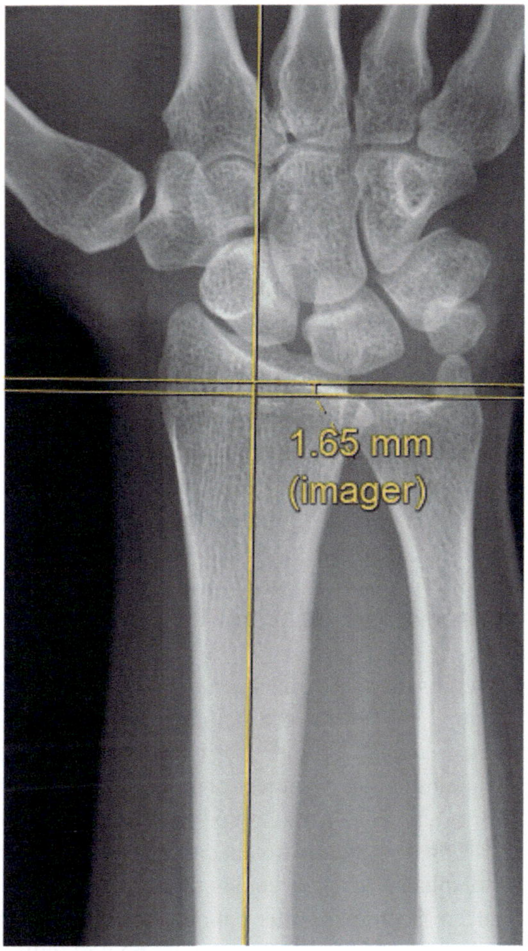

Fig. 1.6 Ulnar variance – the vertical distance between two tangential perpendicular to long axis of radius. One line is at the level of radial lunate fossa and the other is at the level of the lateral cortical margin of distal ulna

placed across the ulna increases. There is a wide range for "normal" variance and contralateral wrist radiographs can clue a clinician into what is normal for an individual. Radial translation ratio is measured as the fraction of the DRUJ gap relative to the radioulnar width of the proximal fracture fragment. The DRUJ gap is the distance between two longitudinal lines between the sigmoid notch and the adjacent ulnar head. This measurement has shown high diagnostic accuracy rate (90%) for predicting DRUJ instability with the relative risk of instability increasing by 50% with the ratio increasing by just 1% [31].

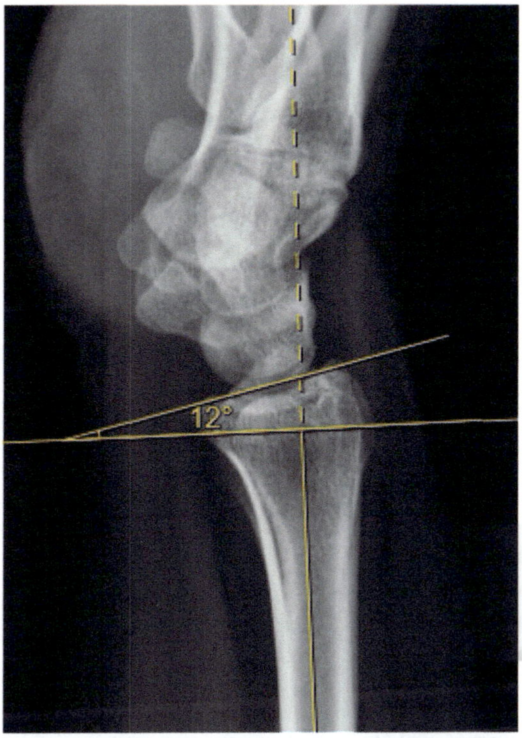

Fig. 1.7 Volar tilt – the angle between a line perpendicular to central axis of radius and a line connecting the dorsal and volar margins of the distal radius articular surface on a lateral view

Lateral radiographs can inform on volar tilt and teardrop angle. Volar tilt is measured from a line perpendicular to the longitudinal axis of the radius and one connecting the dorsal and volar articular surface of the distal radius [28]. Average volar tilt is roughly 11° (2–20°) (Fig. 1.7) [15]. Loss of this tilt can be seen with distal radius fractures. A teardrop angle can inform about articular incongruity. The volar rim of the lunate facet forms a teardrop shape at the distal, volar surface on the lateral view. A teardrop angle is measured by the angle made between the central axis of the radius and a line drawn through the lunate facet–teardrop. A normal teardrop angle is approximately 70° (Fig. 1.8) [14, 30].

The aim in measuring these radiographic parameters is to guide treatment strategy by clinicians and to predict fracture stability and critique reduction. The parameters for instability are poorly defined and vary with age and functional demands. In 1989, Lafontaine identified five fac-

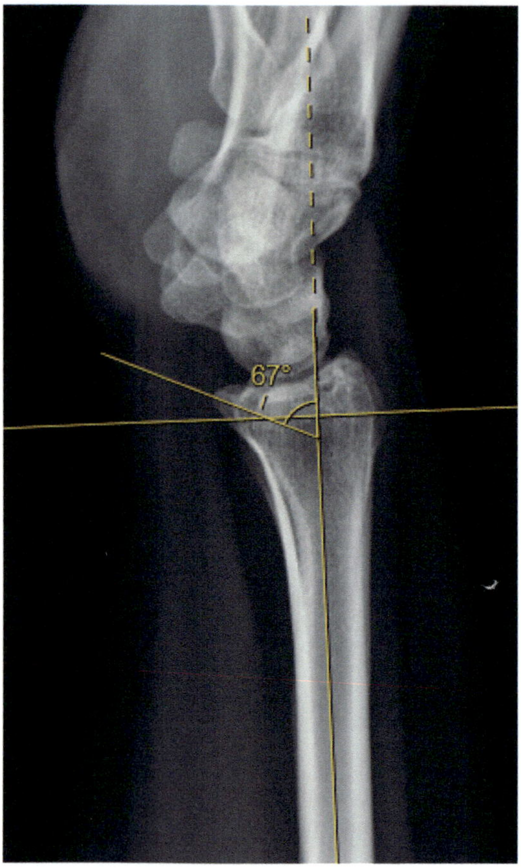

Fig. 1.8 Volar teardrop angle – formed by a line down long axis of radius that intersects a line drawn through center of lunate facet or teardrop

tors predictive of fracture instability including dorsal tilt exceeding 20°, dorsal comminution, fracture involvement of the radiocarpal joint, associated ulna fractures, and age over 60. A fracture was considered unstable if three or more of these variables were present [31]. This has evolved over the years with substantial effort made to identify predictors of secondary displacement. In the early 2000s, a fracture was thought to be inherently unstable with articular incongruity greater than 2 mm, dorsal tilt past neutral, radial inclination less than 15°, ulnar positive variance of greater than 4 mm, ulnar translation of the distal complex greater than 4 mm, and metaphyseal comminution of greater than 50% the PA dimension. In 2016, a systematic review of 27 studies found that the following radiographic parameters were predictive of secondary fracture displacement: shortening, volar comminution, loss of radial inclination, the presence of a volar hook, AO classification type 3 fractures, and Older's classification [32]. Interestingly, articular incongruity was not found to be predictive in this review. Although not predictive, the importance of a congruous reduction has been shown to prevent radiographic osteoarthrosis which has been found to be 100% in wrists with articular incongruity of 2 mm or more [33]. With articular displacement of just 1 mm, pain and stiffness can result [33, 34]. All of these factors can be described by plain radiographs, illustrating the unique and important role in their use after distal radius fractures.

Conservative Treatment

Closed or operative management of distal radius fractures seek to restore stability, motion, alignment, length, and articular congruity. Nonoperative management of a distal radius consists of a period of roughly 6 weeks in a splint or cast. Conservative treatment can be considered in nondisplaced, extra-articular fractures or stable, reduced fractures. If the patient presents with a nondisplaced fracture, they can be treated with 4 to 6 weeks of a short arm cast followed by a removable orthosis for comfort. If the fracture is displaced, a closed reduction prior to casting, or sugar-tong splinting, should be performed. This is followed by radiographs after reduction and weekly thereafter to assess for interval displacement. If no displacement after 1–2 weeks, the splint can be transitioned to a short arm cast to complete 6 weeks of immobilization [36].

The technique of closed reduction, briefly, relies on an understanding of the deforming forces and original mechanism of injury. For a typical distal radius fracture, this process involves recreation of the deformity through wrist extension, followed by traction, slight wrist flexion, volar carpal translation, and slight ulnar deviation with dorsal pressure on the fracture fragment. The traction can restore length and alignment through ligamentotaxis, while the volar carpal translation can assist with restoration of volar tilt and ulnar deviation combats the pull from the brachioradialis. Adjunct techniques like a local hematoma block and gentle hanging traction prior to a reduction can improve patient relaxation and fatigue forearm musculature to make reduction maneuvers easier to perform. It is important to place the patient in a sugar-tong splint with a three-point mold to hold the reduction and prevent rotation of the fracture fragments. Too much wrist flexion and ulnar deviation lead to acute carpal tunnel syndrome and stiffness. Radiographs are obtained to confirm an adequate reduction.

In order to pursue nonoperative management, several principles must be met. Enough stability is important to prevent secondary displacement, which prompts delayed surgical fixation. This can lead to prolonged time away from sport. Multiple studies have tried to predict the risk of secondary displacement, and factors suggested include age greater than 60, shortening, volar comminution, dorsal comminution, loss of radial inclination, the presence of a volar hook, AO type 3 fractures, associated ulna fractures, and intra-articular involvement. These factors are not absolute and serial clinical and radiographic evaluation has been recommended two to three times over the first 3 weeks after injury so that any displacement can be detected early and corrected prior to fracture union [37].

Articular fracture can lead to post-traumatic arthritis and stiffness in athletes if not properly reduced. A congruous reduction is critical to reduce cartilage wear and degenerative changes. Jupiter et al. showed that with just 2 mm or more of articular displacement on radiographs, wrists developed radiographic signs of arthrosis 100% of the time [33]. With articular displacement of just 1 mm, pain and stiffness can result [34, 35]. Near full range of motion is necessary for return to previous level of play, and any stiffness can adversely affect wrist kinematics and performance of an athlete. With limitations on motion, functional performance is decreased when wrist motion coupling is constrained with tasks like throwing [37]. Thus, before nonoperative treatment is pursued in an athlete, articular reduction must be critically analyzed with orthogonal radiographs or CT scan to improve future performance.

Nonoperative treatment in athletes with distal radius fractures can be a reasonable treatment option in sufficiently stable fractures, with articular congruity, normal radial length, alignment, and rotation. Initial nonoperative treatment or delayed surgical treatment can allow an athlete, who is late in a season, to effectively compete in a cast depending on the position they play. This is possible for athletes whose position can be performed with the use of one arm, and who are not limited by pain from the acute injury.

Surgical Treatment

In those who value a more rapid rehabilitation, those with unstable fractures, or those needing anatomic restoration, surgery is considered. There are many different options for fixation that primarily depend on fracture characteristics. Although it is widely accepted that surgical treatment results in a more anatomic restoration, there is no definite evidence to support one method of fixation over another [38–44]. More importantly is the recognition of the specific fracture pattern and the identification of a suitable fixation method. Fracture displacement is not uncommon, occurring in an average of one in eight people initially treated nonoperatively. It is critical to identify an unstable fracture to avoid lost reduction and prevent unnecessary time away from sport. The American Academy of Orthopaedic Surgeons practice guidelines on treatment of distal radius fractures suggest operative fixation for radial shortening greater than 3 mm, dorsal tilt greater than 10° from neutral, or intra-articular displacement of more than 2 mm.

The fixation options following a distal radius fracture include volar plating, dorsal plating, percutaneous pin fixation, fragment-specific fixation, external fixation, percutaneous Kirschner wires, and spanning plate fixation [27]. The surgical technique used depends on the location, number, and displacement of the fracture fragments. Of the options available, locked volar plating is performed most commonly. This evolved as a popular option in an attempt to decrease incidence of extensor tendon irritation. Clinical studies comparing dorsal and locked volar plating have shown mechanically equivalent, and potentially superior, outcomes with the latter [41, 42, 45, 46]. Fragment-specific fixation utilizes multiple small plates to address individual fracture fragments. Percutaneous pin fixation with supplemental casting can be an effective option in simple fractures. In cases of severe comminution, consideration is given to spanning plate fixation in order to regain normal length, alignment, and rotation (Fig. 1.9). Stiffness is common after placement of a dorsal spanning plate which can affect an athlete's performance. Fortunately, severe comminution is not typical in athletes due to excellent bone quality [46, 49].

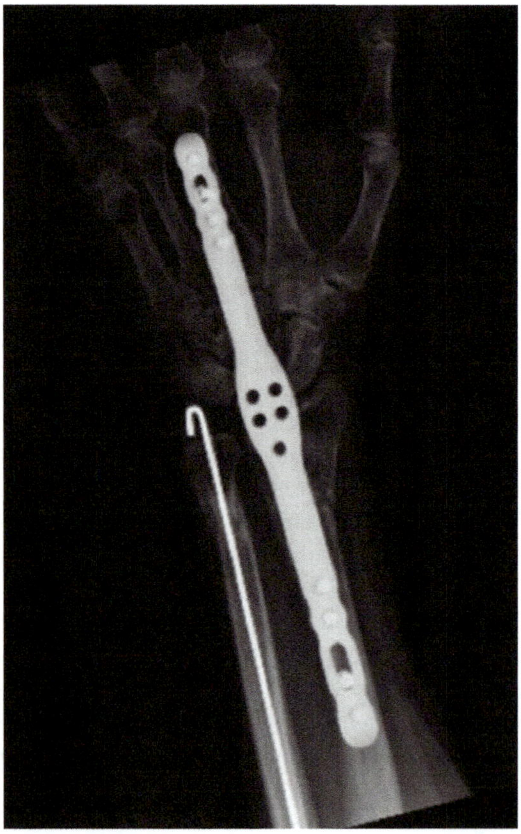

Fig. 1.9 Distal radius fracture treated with a dorsal spanning bridge plate (Brogan et al. [49])

Percutaneous pin fixation can be effective for reducible simple fracture patterns when supplemented by an external cast. Cast immobilization alone cannot adequately hold length and therefore, reduction can be lost. Percutaneous pinning can be less demanding, less invasive, and faster than open surgery. There are a variety of techniques that have been described and include radial styloid pins, crossed pins, dorsal–ulnar corner pins, intrafocal pinning, trans-ulnar oblique pinning, multifocal trans-ulnar to radius pins, and double intrafocal pinning [47]. Kapandji described the technique of double intrafocal wire fixation to buttress and reestablish the volar tilt. This procedure is performed after fluoroscopically confirmed closed reduction using Kirschner wires. A radial styloid pin is typically placed first to regain length and inclination. Careful attention to the anatomy and technique is important to avoid injury to the dorsal sensory nerves and extensor tendons. Further, wires may be added to increase the stability of the construct [48]. After wire insertion, the extensor tendons are checked by passive flexion of the digits and wrist tenodesis to ensure no tendons were tethered. Pins can be cut above or below the skin. A well-padded sugar-tong splint is applied for 2–3 weeks, followed by a short arm cast for an additional 3–4 weeks. Forearm rotation is allowed after 2 weeks. The pins are removed 5 to 6 weeks after reduction [27]. Of the surgery-related complications, infection requiring antibiotics and sometimes early wire removal occurred on average in 1 of 13 people who received percutaneous pinning for distal radius fractures [47]. This has the potential to delay return to sport in an athlete. Little data is available comparing percutaneous fixation to external immobilization in a cast.

Plate fixation is the most common means of internal fixation for surgical management. A dorsal approach is preferred in certain situations with more dorsal comminution because of improved articular visualization, or bone grafting. Attention to surgical technique and a subperiosteal elevation of the extensor compartments allows for periosteum interposition between the plate and extensor tendons. Indications for dorsal plating include comminuted dorsally displaced fractures, dorsal shear fractures, comminuted intra-articular fractures requiring direct visualization of the joint, and fractures associated with other carpal injuries requiring a dorsal approach (such as proximal pole scaphoid fractures) [51]. The dorsal aspect of the radius is convex and has little soft tissue between the plate, extensor tendons, and skin, thus risking complications including extensor tendon irritation and stiffness [42, 50, 51]. Volar plating through the flexor carpi radialis (FCR) approach allows for a soft tissue layer between the skin and the plate with less risk of tendon irritation.

Volar plating falls into four categories: buttress plates, tine or blade plates, fixed-angle locking plates, and polyaxial locking plates [42]. Buttress plating can be used in shear-type fractures, or those without comminution. Blade plates have tines incorporated into the plate. They have strength and stiffness to their construct, but the shape of the tines in the plate dictates the position it is placed in. Fixed-angle locking plates have gained popularity in patients with osteoporotic bone and are not limited to this patient population. They can engage target fracture fragments and lock into the plate. The design has been shown to be effective biomechanically and clinically. Polyaxial locking plates have similar advantages to locking plates but have more leeway for the trajectory of the screws with more fragment-specific fixation. Volar locking plates have led to a paradigm shift in the operative treatment of distal radius fractures. There is a lot of variety in these plates with multiple rows, screw holes, multiaxial screw projection, and custom drilling guides to make screw insertion easier. The main indications for use include volar shear fractures, radial shortening greater than 3 mm, dorsal tilt greater than 10° from neutral, or intra-articular displacement/step-off of more than 2 mm. With all of this interest, surgeons must remain aware that some highly comminuted and distal fractures may not be amenable to volar plate fixation, such as dorsal shear fractures and fractures involving the very distal volar ulnar corner [49].

Fragment-specific fixation allows a surgeon to independently stabilize fracture fragments using multiple implants. A combination of small implants is used to recreate the anatomy of the distal radius and increase rigidity with orthogonal plates (Fig. 1.10). These constructs have been shown to have equivalent or superior biomechanical properties when compared to augmented external fixation, dorsal internal fixation, and volar fixed-angle internal fixation. One disadvantage of fragment-specific fixation is higher rates of painful hardware in up to 10% of cases and subsequent surgery for its removal [52–59].

Ruch et al. described the classic approach to volar fixation, utilizing the interval between the FCR and radial artery [60]. Dissection is maintained on the radial aspect of the FCR tendon to avoid injury to the palmar branch of the median nerve. If a carpal tunnel release is necessary, a separate carpal tunnel incision is typically recommended to avoid damage to the palmar branch of the median nerve. The FCR tendon sheath is incised sharply in a longitudinal direction, and the FCR can be retracted ulnarly. The radial artery is identified within the radial flap of tissue so that its position can be referenced during the surgery. The floor of the FCR tendon sheath and the fascia overlying the flexor pollicis longus muscle are incised in line with the skin incision. The flexor pollicis longus muscle belly is swept ulnarly to expose the underlying pronator quadratus (PQ). Proximal to the PQ, the bare area of the radius is exposed. The pronator is sharply released with an inverted L-shaped incision, and then the muscle is elevated from the underlying periosteum. The radial attachment of the pronator tendon is preserved to cover the hardware at the completion of the surgery if desired.

The fracture site is exposed. Depending on the fracture type, the brachioradialis can be released from the radial styloid to aid with reduction, taking care to not injure the first dorsal compartment tendons. The brachioradialis tendon inserts on the radial column and can be a major deforming force. Volar periosteum is carefully elevated to expose the major fracture fragments with special attention to the volar lunate facet to the sigmoid notch. The fracture site can then be distracted and debrided of hematoma or callus.

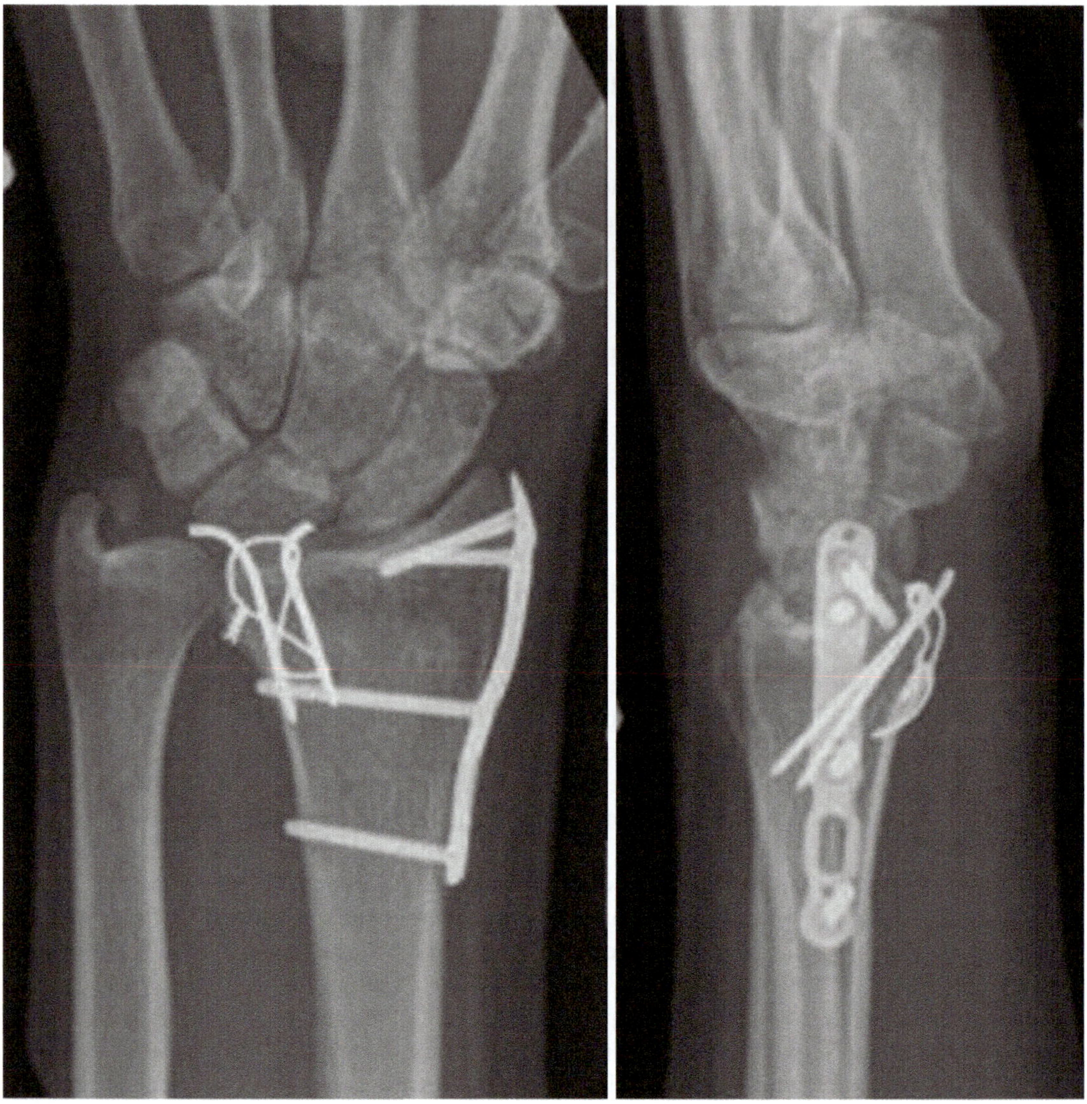

Fig. 1.10 Fragment-specific fixation (He and Blazar [77])

Fragmented intra-articular fractures can prove difficult to reduce. Our approach begins with the reduction of the volar lunate facet and moves progressively dorsally and radially. Restoration of the volar ulnar corner is crucial to reestablish the distal radioulnar joint. Restoration of the depressed lunate facet of the radius prevents the intra-articular step-off associated with the development of post-traumatic arthritis. To facilitate reduction and control of the proximal diaphysis, a serrated bone clamp is placed proximally on the radial shaft. Intra-articular depressions then can be elevated and reduced. A reduction is performed, typically by exaggerating the original deformity with extension, followed by axial traction, volar translation of the carpus, and ulnar deviation of the wrist. The reduction is constantly checked under fluoroscopy. A dental pick or freer elevator can be used to aid in positioning the volar lunate facet fragments to gain an anatomic reduction.

The volar locking plate of choice is obtained and positioned under fluoroscopic guidance while maintaining the reduction. Plates are typically pre-contoured and can be used as a template for anatomic reduction by bringing the fracture fragments to it. This is useful for restoration of volar tilt. Distal radius fractures tend to shorten, and distal screws inserted into subchondral bone can limit this.

First, the oval shaft screw hole is drilled, and a bicortical non-locking screw is placed. The position of the plate in the proximal-to-distal direction is assessed with the locking guide placed in the lunate facet screw hole to ensure that the trajectory of the screw will not violate the radiocarpal joint. The plate position is confirmed to be appropriate in the coronal plane with use of the sigmoid notch view. Once the proper plate position is attained, a second shaft screw is placed after the plate position is optimized.

The remaining fracture fragments are reduced to the plate with the use of a large pointed bone tenaculum, and the distal locking screws are placed from ulnar to radial. K-wires can be used to aid with the articular reduction. One or 2 K-wires can be placed through the radial styloid into the subchondral bone of the radiocarpal articulation, and another can be placed from the radial styloid into the proximal shaft. A 16-gauge needle is used as a soft tissue protector and wire guide to avoid injury to the superficial radial nerve or the radial artery.

After the plate and screw construct is complete, the stability of the distal radioulnar joint (DRUJ) is assessed using a shuck test with the forearm positioned in neutral, pronation, and then supination. If the DRUJ is unstable in pronation or neutral, but stable in supination, the patient is splinted in supination for 3 weeks. If the DRUJ is unstable in all positions of forearm rotation, then reduction and fixation of a large ulnar styloid fragment is performed. If no associated ulnar styloid fracture is present, then repair of the triangular fibrocartilage complex (TFCC) is performed. This can be achieved with either an open or arthroscopic technique.

With an armamentarium of fixation options available to surgeons, familiarity with the options and their specific advantages and indications is crucial to maximizing outcome for a patient. Given the heterogeneity of fracture patterns and factors specific to an individual, there is no universal treatment option when dealing with a distal radius fracture.

Post-treatment Rehab (There Will Be a Specific Chapter to General Guidelines)

Regardless of treatment modality, goals of rehabilitation after sustaining a distal radius fracture are to restore motion. Unique to a throwing athlete is the goal to restore wrist kinematics for throwing and pitching. Throwing motion occurs as a combination of movements in orthogonal planes: flexion/extension and radial/ulnar deviation. This motion is coupled to enhance force and accuracy. In post-traumatic situations, i.e., distal radius fractures, this coupling mechanism can be disrupted which can lead to altered mechanics and decreased performance [37].

An understanding of wrist kinematics can help guide rehabilitation goals after a wrist injury in a throwing athlete. The kinematics of the shoulder during pitching has been well-studied and is divided into phases. Motion at the wrist coincides with the coordinated actions of the shoulder. A study using a wrist goniometer and strain gauge to record flexion/extension and radial/ulnar deviation arcs in five professional pitchers during spring baseball training defined four stages of wrist motion during a pitch. The first phase of pitching is the cocking phase, where the wrist moves into maximal extension during late cocking phase. This is followed by an explosive phase with acceleration of the wrist which leads to ball propulsion, which coincides with shoulder acceleration. The ball is released leading to the third phase of wrist motion, deceleration. This occurs with a sharp decrease in wrist velocity as the wrist moves into maximal flexion and occurs with the early stages of shoulder follow-through. The final phase occurs as the wrist returns to neutral and has been termed the recovery phase [61].

Post-treatment rehabilitation in athletes includes a brief period of immobilization with a plaster splint or short arm cast typically for

14 days depending on the fracture stability, pattern, and patient age. This period is increased for some pediatric patients and for those treated nonoperatively. If there is doubt about stability, patient compliance, or interval callus formation, it is reasonable to delay the initiation of wrist motion. Calderon et al. showed that early range of motion exercises may speed early recovery but not necessarily change final range of motion [62]. With reliable fixation, the plaster splint or cast can be replaced with a removable orthosis typically between weeks 2 and 6 after the injury or surgery. At this time, early active motion can be initiated including wrist flexion, extension, radial–ulnar deviation, and forearm rotation for potentially faster recovery. After robust radiographic healing is seen, the removable orthosis can be weaned, and gentle strengthening is initiated with active and active-assisted motion [63].

Regaining finger motion in athletes is essential after a distal radius fracture. Those lacking ability to fully extend or flex their fingers can be severely limited, and active finger motion should be stressed and practiced by the patient. The majority of wrist motion after a distal radius fracture is regained within the first 3 months with more gradual improvements in strength and endurance. After 3 months, motion begins to plateau [64].

Complications/Adverse Results

Complications and adverse outcomes after distal radius fractures are relatively frequent and varied (Table 1.1) [21, 23, 39, 65–75]. Some of the complications can be performance altering for a baseball player. The complications are specific to the injury pattern itself and the modality of treatment. The rates of complication in the literature vary from 5% to 80% depending on how a complication is defined. Soft tissue injuries; compromised tendons, nerves, or blood vessels; and fracture displacement are the most common. Malunion or nonunion can occur with or without surgical fixation. If treated surgically, complications such as infection, hematoma, and wound dehiscence can occur as with any surgical procedure.

Table 1.1 Incidence of reported complication with distal radius fractures

Complication	Incidence
Loss of motion (marked deformity, decreased ROM, arthrofibrosis, Volkmann's ischemic contracture, finger stiffness)	0–31%
Delayed union/nonunion	0.7–4%
Nerve compression/neuritis	0–17%
Pain syndromes (RSD, shoulder–hand syndrome, persistent pain)	0.3–8%
Hardware complications	1.4–2.6%
Osteomyelitis	4–9%
Malunion	5%
Tendon (rupture, lag, trigger, tenosynovitis)	0–5%
Scar (keloids)	3%
Ligament damage	98%
Radioulnar (synostosis, disturbance)	0–1.3%
Bone graft hematoma	1%
Dupuytren's contracture (palmar fascia nodules/bands)	2–9%
Arthritis/arthrosis	7–65%
Unrecognized injury	2%

Turner et al. [78]

Abbreviations: ROM range of motion, *RSD* reflex sympathetic dystrophy

Complications related to nonoperative treatment of a distal radius can be related to the fracture or the method of immobilization. Casts may not accommodate swelling in the acute period, and patients should be warned about the potential of increased pain, nerve compression, and rarely, compartment syndrome. The cast should follow the metacarpal cascade and allow for full finger range of motion to prevent stiffness and decrease the risk of dystrophy [67]. A cast placed in too much flexion can predispose a patient to acute carpal tunnel syndrome. Additionally, a poorly applied cast or splint mold can lead to fracture displacement. There is a risk of EPL rupture following fractures treated nonoperatively as well. Engkvist and Lundborg postulated that the EPL tendon has poor intrinsic vascularity near Lister's tubercle, and hematoma formation can interfere with tendon nutrition, leading to tenosynovitis or delayed rupture [69].

Complications from surgery can be related to the approach, hardware, or technique and these can occur early or late. Postoperative infection is an ever-present risk after surgery. Pin-tract infection can be seen with percutaneous fixation or external fixators. Percutaneous pinning has a rate of superficial infection between 0% and 10% [70]. The rates of infection after open reduction internal fixation are much lower on the order of 0% to 3% [68].

Extensor tendon injuries occur in surgical treatment as well. Extensor tendon injury can occur with volar plating through drill penetration or screw prominence. Dorsal plating can cause extensor tendon rupture and tenosynovitis as well, especially with bulkier plates. Newer, ultralow-profile designs with recessed screw holes have reduced this complication. Percutaneous pinning can cause extensor tendon rupture as well with various trajectories with a rate of about 0.7% [72].

Flexor tendon injury is less common than extensor tendon injury. Orbay discussed the importance of the watershed line, along the volar edge of the distal radius marking the distal extent of where a plate should be placed. The flexor tendons are closest in proximity to the distal radius at the watershed line, and are thus at risk of flexor tendon irritation, resulting in tenosynovitis or rupture [21].

Nerve injury is not uncommon with an incidence ranging from around 2% to 8% after distal radius fracture [65]. Nerve injuries may be the result of direct injury from the fracture, hematoma/swelling, and over-distraction or iatrogenic during surgical fixation. Carpal tunnel syndrome can occur due to increased pressure in the carpal canal after a fracture. Several studies have identified the incidence of median neuropathy in nonoperative and operative groups with an incidence between 2.6% and 8.5% [60, 72, 73]. Carpal tunnel syndrome was found to be the complication with the highest incidence after volar plating of the distal radius in a systematic review [23]. The palmar cutaneous branch of the median nerve is at particular risk for injury during the volar approach and has been demonstrated to have a variable course in 18% of patients [74]. The superficial radial nerve is vulnerable during provisional fixation, percutaneous pinning, external fixator placement, and certain fragment-specific plates.

Complex regional pain syndrome is a major late complication causing pain and tenderness, stiffness, swelling, dystrophy, and vasomotor instability. The etiology is often unclear and can require months of physiotherapy. Rates range from 3% to 25% in the literature [49].

Malunion is a complication resulting from nonanatomic alignment either as a result of the injury or after treatment. It can occur with nonoperative or surgical treatment. It can have a range of clinical consequences and the degree of acceptable malalignment has not been established.

Post-traumatic arthritis can occur after a distal radius fracture regardless of treatment method. Jupiter showed radiographic prevalence of 65% after an intra-articular fracture, and other authors have found similarly high rates [34, 73, 75]. There is no clear evidence that this correlates with clinical outcome and a functional impact has not been shown.

Complications of volar plating of the distal radius include loss of fixation, injury to the palmar cutaneous branch of the median nerve, postoperative carpal tunnel syndrome, extensor tendon rupture, and postoperative loss of motion. Loss of fixation can occur catastrophically, particularly if care is not taken to reduce and capture the volar lunate facet fragment with the plate's more ulnar locking screws. If the mechanism of injury involves one of high energy, or if symptoms of carpal tunnel syndrome are present on preoperative physical exam by monofilament testing, a prophylactic carpal tunnel release should be performed. The lengths of the distal locking screws should be confirmed by depth gauge and fluoroscopy to avoid extensor tendon irritation and rupture.

Early Return to Play

Often the most difficult decision for an orthopedic surgeon is determination of when an athlete can return to play. Although not a contact sport, baseball carries a risk of reinjury through a collision or a fall. In some sports, a player can return in a well-padded cast prior to complete union;

however, that is not an option in baseball as every position requires the use of both hands in a functional position. Lawson reviewed 225 sports-related distal radius fractures. When surveyed at an average of 27 months from the injury, only 72.5% of patients returned to their original sport. This was dependent on the patient's age and level of competition [76].

The decision regarding return to play involves several factors including the type and severity of injury, fracture union, rehabilitation goals, age, sport, position, ability, and level of competition. Fracture healing typically takes 6 to 8 weeks. In patients treated operatively or nonoperatively, it is also important to restore wrist and finger range of motion and control swelling in order to prevent repeat injury or pain affecting performance. Additionally, intentionally guarding the wrist could lead to other injuries due to improper mechanics.

Wrist protectors, taping, and padding must be individualized for each athlete toward their involvement and position but should not be used as a substitute for complete healing and functional recovery. The question of when to return must be individualized for each player's injury, their position, and the specific demands required for them. Generally, requirements for return to play after a distal radius fracture include complete fracture union and completion of a graduated rehabilitation program resulting in near normal strength and painless functional motion. Return to sport would involve the ability to complete activities of daily living and then sport-specific tasks and practice, and finally return to sport when at least 80% strength has been regained with radiographic union [46].

References

1. Rugg CM, Wang D, Mayer EN, Sulzicki PL, Vail J, Hame SL. The impact of prior upper-extremity surgery on orthopedic injury and surgery in collegiate athletes. J Shoulder Elb Surg. 2019;28:1371–7.
2. Larsen CF, Lauritsen J. Epidemiology of acute wrist trauma. Int J Epidemiol. 1993;22:911–6.
3. Chung KC, Spilson SV. The frequency and epidemiology of hand and forearm fractures in the United States. J Hand Surg Am. 2001;26:908–15.
4. Louer CR, Boone SL, Guthrie AK, Motley JR, Calfee RP, Wall LB. Postural stability in older adults with a distal radial fracture. J Bone Joint Surg. 2016;98:1176–82.
5. Avery DM, Rodner CM, Edgar CM. Sports-related wrist and hand injuries: a review. J Orthop Surg Res. 2016;11:99.
6. Fares MY, Salhab HA, Khachfe HH, Kane L, Fares Y, Fares J, Abboud JA. Upper limb injuries in Major League Baseball. Phys Ther Sport. 2020;41:49–54.
7. Karl JW, Olson PR, Rosenwasser MP. The epidemiology of upper extremity fractures in the United States, 2009. J Orthop Trauma. 2015;29:242–4.
8. Court-Brown CM, Caesar B. Epidemiology of adult fractures: a review. Injury. 2006;37:691–7.
9. Court-Brown CM, Wood AM, Aitken S. The epidemiology of acute sports-related fractures in adults. Injury. 2008;39:1365–72.
10. Fraser MA, Grooms DR, Guskiewicz KM, Kerr ZY. Ball-contact injuries in 11 National Collegiate Athletic Association Sports: the injury surveillance program, 2009–2010 through 2014–2015. J Athl Train. 2017;52(7):698–707.
11. Rikli DA, Regazzoni P. Fractures of the distal end of the radius treated by internal fixation and early function. A preliminary report of 20 cases. J Bone Joint Surg Br. 1996;78-B:588–92.
12. Mauck BM, Swigler CW. Evidence-based review of distal radius fractures. Orthop Clin North Am. 2018;49(2):211–22.
13. Moore A, Dennison DG. Distal radius fractures and the volar lunate facet fragment: Kirschner wire fixation in addition to volar-locked plating. Hand (N Y). 2014;9(2):230–6.
14. Medoff RJ. Essential radiographic evaluation for distal radius fractures. Hand Clin. 2005;21:279–88.
15. Palmer AK, Werner FW. Biomechanics of the distal radioulnar joint. Clin Orthop Relat Res. 1984;187:26–35.
16. Pope D, Tang P. Carpal tunnel syndrome and distal radius fractures. Hand Clin. 2018;34(1):27–32.
17. Helal B, Chen SC, Iwegbu G. Rupture of the extensor pollicis longus tendon in undisplaced Colles' type of fracture. Hand. 1982;14:41–7.
18. Roth KM, Blazer PE, Earp BE, Han R, Leung A. Incidence of extensor pollicis longus tendon rupture after nondisplaced distal radius fractures. J Hand Surg Am. 2012;37A:942–7.
19. Hirasawa Y, Katsumi Y, Akiyoshi T, Tamai K, Tokioka T. Clinical and microangiographic studies on rupture of the E.P.L. tendon after distal radial fractures. J Hand Surg Br. 1990;15B:51–7.
20. Orbay JL, Touhami A. Current concepts in volar fixed-angle fixation of unstable distal radius fractures. Clin Orthop Relat Res. 2006;445:58–67.
21. Imatani J, Akita K, Yamaguchi K, Shimizu H, Kondou H, Ozaki T. An anatomical study of the watershed line on the volar distal aspect of the radius: implications for plate placement and avoidance of tendon ruptures.

J Hand Surg Am. 2012;37A:1550–4. https://doi.org/10.1016/j.jhsa.2012.05.011. PMID: 22835584.
22. Alter TH, Sandrowski K, Gallant G, Kwok M, Ilyas AM. Complications of volar plating of distal radius fractures: a systematic review. J Wrist Surg. 2019;8(3):255–62.
23. Bae DS, Waters PM. Pediatric distal radius fractures and triangular fibrocartilage complex injuries. Hand Clin. 2006;22:43–53.
24. Abzug JM, Little K, Kozin SH. Physeal arrest of the distal radius. J Am Acad Orthop Surg. 2014;22:381–9.
25. Meena S, Sharma P, Dawar A. Fractures of the distal radius: an overview. J Family Med Prim Care. 2014;3(4):325–32.
26. Koval KJ, Zuckerman JD, Kenneth E. Handbook of fractures. 2nd ed. Philadelphia: Lippincott Williams and Wilkins; 2002. p. 133–8.
27. Green DP, Wolfe SW. Green's operative hand surgery. New York: Churchill Livingstone; 2011.
28. Cole J, Binda RR, Evanoff BA, Gilula LA, Yamaguchi K, Gelberman RH. Radiographic evaluation of osseous displacement following intra-articular fractures of the distal radius: reliability of plain radiography versus computed tomography. J Hand Surg Am. 1997;22(5):792–800.
29. Henry MH. Distal radius fractures: current concepts. J Hand Surg Am. 2008;33:1215–27.
30. Porrino JA, Maloney E, Scherer K, Mulcahy H, Ha AS, Allan C. Fracture of the distal radius: epidemiology and premanagement radiographic characterization. AJR. 2014;203:551–9.
31. Fujitani R, Omokawa S, Akahane M, Iida A, Ono H, Tanaka Y. Predictors of distal radioulnar joint instability in distal radius fractures. J Hand Surg Am. 2011;36:1919–25.
32. Walenkamp MMJ, Aydin S, Mulders MA, Goslings JC, Schep NWL. Predictors of unstable distal radius fractures: a systematic review and meta-analysis. J Hand Surg Eur Vol. 2016;41(5):501–15.
33. Knirk J, Jupiter JB. Intra-articular fractures of the distal end of the radius in young adults. J Bone Joint Surg. 1986;68:647–59.
34. Trumble TE, Culp RW, Hanel DP, Geissler WB, Berger RA. Intra-articular fractures of the distal aspect of the radius. Instr Course Lect. 1999;48:465–80.
35. Fernandez DL, Geissler WB. Treatment of displaced articular fractures of the radius. J Hand Surg Am. 1991;16:375–84.
36. Beleckas C, Calfee R. Distal radius fractures in the athlete. Curr Rev Musculoskelet Med. 2017;10:62–71.
37. Garg R, Kraszewski AP, Stoecklein HH, Syrkin G, Hillstrom HJ, Backus S, Lenhoff ML, Wolff AL, Crisco JJ, Wolfe SW. Wrist kinematic coupling and performance during functional tasks: effects of constrained motion. J Hand Surg Am. 2014;39(4):634–42.
38. Chaudhry H, Kleinlugtenbelt YV, Mundi R, Ristevski B, Goslings JC, Bhandari M. Are volar locking plates superior to percutaneous K-wires for distal radius fractures? A meta-analysis. Clin Orthop Relat Res. 2015;473:3017–27.
39. Huang YY, Lin TY, Chen CH, Chou YC, Su CY. Surgical outcomes of elderly patients aged more than 80 years with distal radius fracture: comparison of external fixation and locking plate. BMC Musculoskelet Disord. 2020;21(1):91.
40. Jakubietz MG, Gruenert JG, Jakubietz RG. Palmar and dorsal fixed-angle plates in AO C-type fractures of the distal radius: is there an advantage of palmar plates in the long term? J Orthop Surg Res. 2012;7(1):8.
41. Ruch DS, Papadonikolakis A. Volar versus dorsal plating in the management of intra-articular distal radius fractures. J Hand Surg Am. 2006;31(1):9–16.
42. Martineau PA, Berry GK, Harvey EJ. Plating for distal radius fractures. Orthop Clin North Am. 2007;38(2):193–201.
43. Nana AD, Joshi A, Lichtman DM. Plating of the distal radius. J Am Acad Orthop Surg. 2005;13:159–71.
44. Yoshihiro A, Tokunaga S, Moriya T. Management of intra-articular distal radius fractures: volar or dorsal locking plate – which has fewer complications? Hand (N Y). 2017;12(6):561–7.
45. Kandemir U, Matityahu A, Desai R, et al. Does a volar locking plate provide equivalent stability as a dorsal nonlocking plate in a dorsally comminuted distal radius fracture?: a biomechanical study. J Orthop Trauma. 2008;22:605–10.
46. Henn CM, Wolfe SW. Distal radius fractures in athletes. Sports Med Arthrosc Rev. 2014;22:29–38.
47. Karantana A, Handoll HH, Sabouni A. Percutaneous pinning for treating distal radial fractures in adults. Cochrane Database Syst Rev. 2020;2(2):CD006080.
48. Rayhack JM, Langworthy JN, Belsole RJ. Transulnar percutaneous pinning of displaced distal radial fractures: a preliminary report. J Orthop Trauma. 1989;3(2):107–14.
49. Brogan DM, Richard MJ, Ruch DS, Kakar S. Management of severely comminuted distal radius fractures. J Hand Surg Am. 2015;40(9):1905–14. https://doi.org/10.1016/j.jhsa.2015.03.014. Epub 2015 Aug 1. PMID: 26243322.
50. Gliatis JD, Plessas SJ, Davis TR. Outcome of distal radial fractures in young adults. J Hand Surg (Br). 2000;25(6):535–43.
51. Cohen MS, Turner TM. Urban effects of implant material and plate design on tendon function and morphology. Clin Orthop Relat Res. 2006;445:81–90.
52. Gerostathopoulos N, Kalliakmanis A, Fandridis E, et al. Trimed fixation system for displaced fractures of the distal radius. J Trauma. 2007;62:913–8.
53. Dodds SD, Cornelissen S, Jossan S, et al. A biomechanical comparison of fragment-specific fixation and augmented external fixation for intra-articular distal radius fractures. J Hand Surg Am. 2002;27:953–64.
54. Benson LS, Minihane KP, Stern LD, et al. The outcome of intra-articular distal radius fractures treated with fragment specific fixation. J Hand Surg Am. 2006;31:1333–9.
55. Cooper EO, Segalman KA, Parks BG, et al. Biomechanical stability of a volar locking-screw

plate versus fragment-specific fixation in a distal radius fracture model. Am J Orthop (Belle Mead NJ). 2007;36:E46–9.
56. Schnall SB, Kim BJ, Abramo A, et al. Fixation of distal radius fractures using a fragment-specific system. Clin Orthop Relat Res. 2006;445:51–7.
57. Peine R, Rikli DA, Hoffmann R, et al. Comparison of three different plating techniques for the dorsum of the distal radius: a biomechanical study. J Hand Surg Am. 2000;25:29–33.
58. Taylor KF, Parks BG, Segalman KA. Biomechanical stability of a fixed-angle volar plate versus fragment-specific fixation system: cyclic testing in a C2-type distal radius cadaver fracture model. J Hand Surg Am. 2006;31:373–81.
59. Saw N, Roberts C, Cutbush K, et al. Early experience with the TriMed fragment-specific fracture fixation system in intraarticular distal radius fractures. J Hand Surg Eur Vol. 2008;33:53–8.
60. Protopsaltis TS, Ruch DS. Volar approach to distal radius fractures. J Hand Surg Am. 2008;33A:958–65.
61. Pappas AM, Morgan WJ, Schultz LA, Diana R. Wrist kinematics during pitching. A preliminary report. Am J Sports Med. 1995;23(3):312–5.
62. Lozano-Calderón SA, Souer S, Mudgal C, Jupiter JB, Ring D. Wrist mobilization following volar plate fixation of fractures of the distal part of the radius. J Bone Joint Surg Am. 2008;90:1297–304.
63. Abramo A, Kopylov P, Tägil M. Evaluation of a treatment protocol in distal radius fractures. Acta Orthop. 2008;79:376–85.
64. Dillingham C, Horodyski M, Struk AM, Wright T. Rate of improvement following volar plate open reduction and internal fixation of distal radius fractures. Adv Orthop. 2011;2011:1–4.
65. Seigerman D, Lutsky K, Fletcher D, Katt B, Kwok M, Mazur D, Sodha S, Beredijiklian PK. Complications in the management of distal radius fractures: how do we avoid them? Curr Rev Musculoskelet Med. 2019;12(2):204–12.
66. Lee DS, Weikert DR. Complications of distal radius fixation. Orthop Clin N Am. 2016;47:415–24.
67. Turner RG, Faber KJ, Athwal GS. Complications of distal radius fractures. Orthop Clin N Am. 2007;38:217–28.
68. McKay SD, MacDermid JC, Roth JH, et al. Assessment of complications of distal radius fractures and development of a complication checklist. J Hand Surg Am. 2001;26(5):916–22.
69. Engkvist O, Lundborg G. Rupture of the extensor pollicis longus tendon after fracture of the lower end of the radius–a clinical and microangiographic study. Hand. 1979;11(1):76–86.
70. Handoll HH, Vaghela MV, Madhok R. Percutaneous pinning for treating distal radial fractures in adults. Cochrane Database Syst Rev. 2007;(3):CD006080.
71. Arora R, Lutz M, Hennerbichler A, et al. Complications following internal fixation of unstable distal radius fracture with a palmar locking-plate. J Orthop Trauma. 2007;21(5):316–22.
72. Lutz K, Yeoh KM, MacDermid JC, et al. Complications associated with operative versus nonsurgical treatment of distal radius fractures in patients aged 65 years and older. J Hand Surg Am. 2014;39(7):1280–6.
73. Goldfarb CA, Rudzki JR, Catalano LW, et al. Fifteen year outcome of displaced intra-articular fractures of the distal radius. J Hand Surg Am. 2006;31(4):633–9.
74. Glickel SZ, Glynn SM, Chang AL, et al. Anomalous courses of the palmar cutaneous branch of the median nerve in relation to the flexor carpi radialis tendon for ORIF of distal radius fractures. Hand (N Y). 2020;15(4):521–5.
75. Trumble TE, Schmitt SR, Vedder NB. Factors affecting functional outcome of displaced intra-articular distal radius fractures. J Hand Surg Am. 1994;19(2):325–40.
76. Lawson GM, Hajducka C, McQueen MM. Sports fractures of the distal radius—epidemiology and outcome. Injury. 1995;26:33–6.
77. He JJ, Blazar P. Management of High Energy Distal Radius Injuries. Curr Rev Musculoskelet Med. 2019;12(3):379–85. https://doi.org/10.1007/s12178-019-09555-5. Epub ahead of print. PMID: 31302860; PMCID: PMC6684690.
78. Turner RG, Faber KJ, Athwal GS. Complications of distal radius fractures. Hand Clin. 2010;26(1):85–96. https://doi.org/10.1016/j.hcl.2009.08.005. PMID: 20006247.

Hand and Wrist Injuries in Baseball: Scaphoid Fractures

2

T. Greg Sommerkamp

Definition of Injury/Classification

A scaphoid fracture is defined as a unicortical or bicortical fracture though the body of the scaphoid that can be further classified by anatomical location, orientation, and stability. A stable fracture is typically any scaphoid fracture on dedicated longitudinal oblique CT imaging that lacks displacement of any kind (0 mm), angulation (SL angle <60°, RL angle <15° sagittal ISA <~30°, coronal ISA <~40°, H/L ratio <0.597 +/− 0.042), comminution or arthroscopically visualized interfragmentary motion after nominal stress is applied…the vast majority [1–17]. The stable group consists of all Herbert A1-volar tuber fractures, Herbert A2 incomplete waist fractures, and the majority of Herbert B2 fractures in ~70% (Fig. 2.1). Nonetheless, one must be cognizant of the fact that recent data from arthroscopic inspection studies has revealed that upwards to 30% of stable appearing fractures by CT criteria above are still unstable at the time of arthroscopic examination intraoperatively [15].

The unstable scaphoid fracture is defined as any fracture on dedicated longitudinal oblique CT imaging that is displaced *at all* (>0 mm), angulated (SL angle >60°, RL angle >15°, sagittal ISA >~30°, coronal ISA >~35°, H/L ratio >0.597 +/− 0.042), comminuted, or demonstrates arthroscopically visualized displacement or interfragmentary motion after nominal stress is applied…the relative minority in ~30% [13–15, 17]. The unstable group consists of Herbert B1 and B2 in ~30%, Herbert B3 (proximal pole), Herbert B4, (trans-S-PL), and Herbert B5 (comminuted). Fortunately, with the aid of CT scanning in the oblique or longitudinal axial projection as described by Sanders [6], we have come to realize over the past several decades how displaced and unstable many scaphoid fractures actually are despite innocuous-appearing plain radiographs.

Incidence

The scaphoid is the most commonly fractured carpal bone with a widely varying literature reported incidence of 1.5 to 121/100,000 persons/yr. depending on the study [1, 20]. Even in the new age of information management, there are limited national databases with widely varying inclusion criteria. Wolf et al. in 2010 [20] based on the National Electronic Injury Surveillance System (NEISS) reported a much lower incidence than earlier estimates at 1.47 fractures per 100,00 person-years based on a 5-year review of the database correlating to ~20,000 scaphoid fractures/year in the USA if

T. G. Sommerkamp (✉)
Cincinnati Hand Surgery Specialists, Department of Orthopedics, University of Cincinnati, Cincinnati, OH, USA
e-mail: gsommerkamp@handsurg.com

G. M. Lourie (ed.), *Hand and Wrist Injuries in Baseball*,
https://doi.org/10.1007/978-3-030-81659-9_2

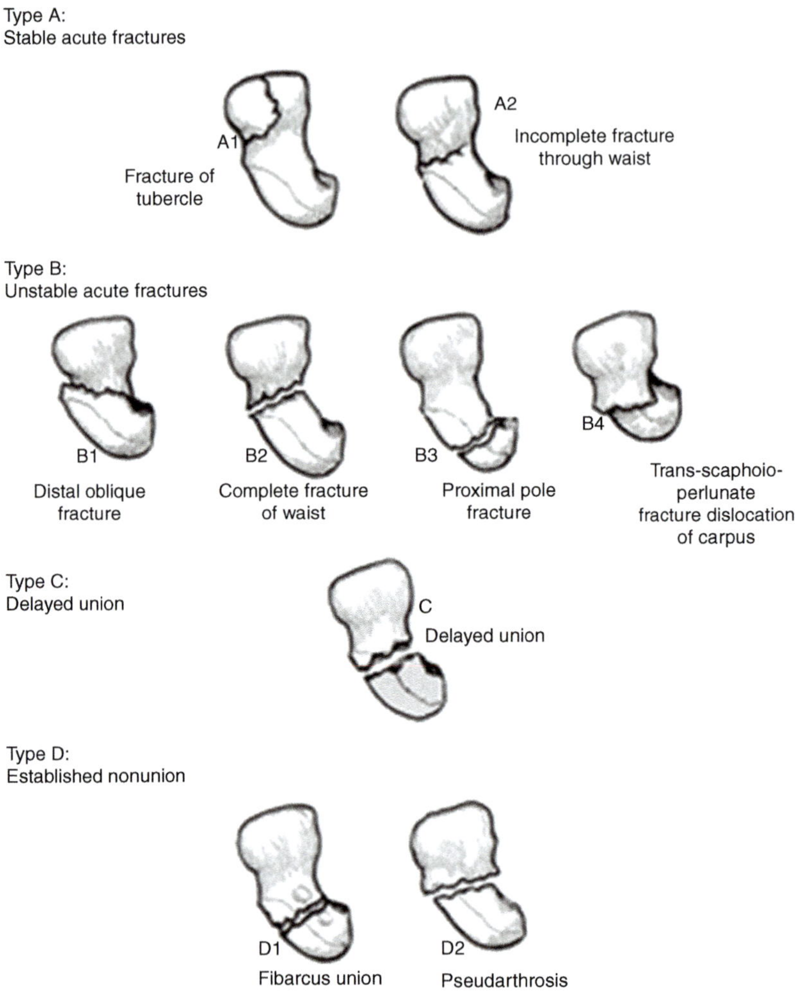

Fig. 2.1 Herbert classification (Reproduced with permission from Elsevier, *Greens Operative Hand Surgery- Fractures of the Carpal Bones*; Fifth Edition. 2005. Ch 17. P 718- Figure 17–11)

suspected fractures were eliminated from the cohort. The highest risk group was young males especially between the ages of 10 and 29 years, and males outnumber females, 2:1. A more recent prospective single center defined, adult capture population reported by Duckworth et al. in 2012 revealed 29 fractures per 100,00 person-years in Edinburgh [21].

Approximately 35% of all scaphoid fractures occurred during sporting activities with the highest incidence sports being basketball followed by biking, football, skateboarding, snowboarding, soccer, and then baseball with baseball only accounting for approximately 2% of all sports-related scaphoid fractures (Fig. 2.2).

Anatomy

This oddly shaped, peanut-sized, carpal bone has nearly 80% of its surface area covered by hyaline cartilage and resides in a unique orientation in the human carpus at an angle of 47° flexion and 20° radial deviation [1]. The tenuous vascular supply enters via the dorsal ridge or spiral groove vessel, originating from the radial or dorsal intercarpal arteries or both, supplying upward to 70–80% of the scaphoid (Fig. 2.3). In 86% of scaphoids, this critical vascular supply enters the dorsal ridge at or distal to the waist, exposing all fractures at or proximal to this point, to the potential complica-

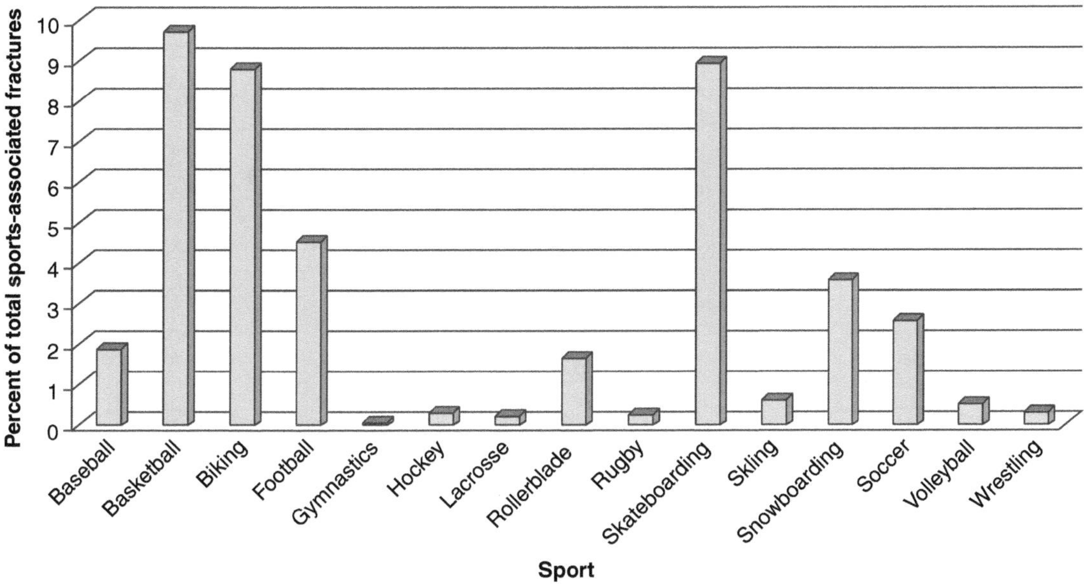

Fig. 2.2 Incidence by sport (Reproduced with permission from Elsevier, Van Tassel et al. [20])

tions of delayed union, nonunion, and/or avascular necrosis [5]. Developmental anatomy must always be kept in mind due to the large number of youngsters in organized youth baseball, and albeit uncommon, scaphoid injuries do still occur. The scaphoid ossification sequence starts in males at age 5–7 and ends by age 15, and in females it starts at 4–6 years and ends by age 13. In a player under 10–12 years, sometimes MRI with or without arthrography is necessary to rule out an occult fracture prior to complete ossification. The intrinsic supporting ligaments of importance are the scapholunate (SL), the radioscapholunate (RSL), and the scaphotrapeziotrapezoidal (STT), in addition to the extrinsic radioscapholunate (RSL) and the long radiolunate (long RL) (Figs. 2.4 and 2.5).

Mechanism of Injury (MOI)

The most common mechanism of injury is a rather violent hyperextension and radial deviation of the wrist from a fall or a protective maneuver against the outstretched arm. Frykman [22] as well as Weber and Chao [4] demonstrated that scaphoid fractures required extreme hyperextension and radial deviation at extreme loads of 209–436 kilograms of force with the wrist hyperextended greater than 95° and radially deviated more than 10°, whereas distal radius fractures were produced at lesser angles of extension and at smaller loads with slower rate of loading. The load appears to be against the radial portion of the palm, with tension loading of the volar tuber/volar cortex consistent with classic beam loading formats. The tensile force volarly then propagates through the body of the scaphoid resulting in compressive loading of the dorsal cortex where the rare bit of comminution typically occurs. The overall force and rate of loading is greater than two times that of a distal radius fracture [4]. Other less common mechanisms include the punchers fracture from direct axial loading of the radial metacarpus through the trapezoid where comminution is a more common finding. In high-energy, displaced fractures, it has been recently demonstrated that contrary to earlier beliefs, the common "humpback collapse" occurs as the proximal pole extends due to the unbridled force of the lunate, while the distal pole remains in relatively neutral alignment due to the stout ligamentous tether and strong confines of the STT joint distally [18].

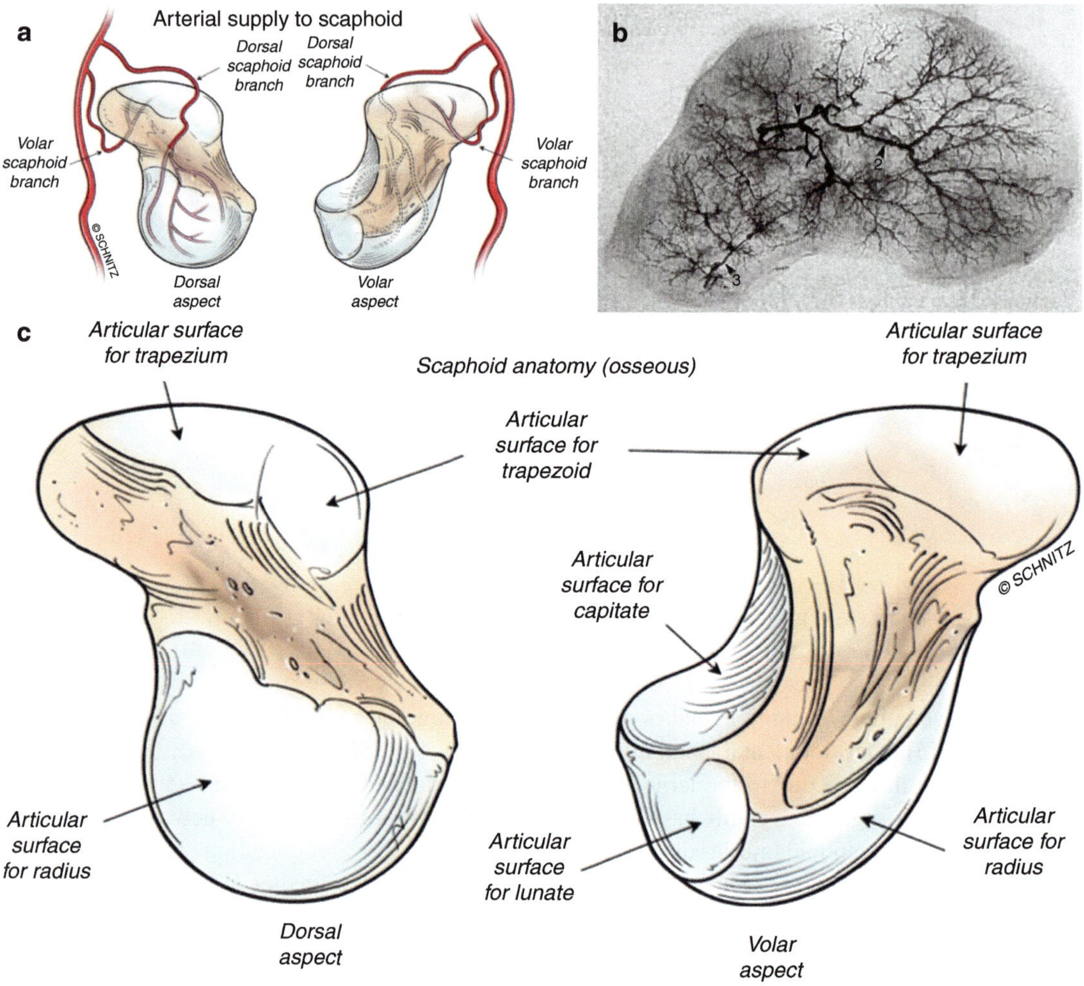

Fig. 2.3 (**a**, **c**) Vascular/osseous anatomy illustration. (**b**) Vascular anatomy (Reproduced with permission from Gelberman and Gross [30])

In baseball, we see these injuries most commonly during outfield fence collisions, foul ball over-railing falls, head first slides into second and third base, and believe it or not, even after tripping down dugout steps after a bench clearing brawl secondary to the visiting pitcher throwing a little inside "high heat." The injury fortunately is fairly infrequent in baseball but does occur at least every 3–5 years in our major league club and approximately once every year or two in our combined five affiliated minor league clubs, and even more frequently in the amateur high school and college ranks.

History/Differential Dx

The player usually presents begrudgingly at the direction of the trainer or position coaches after a sudden drop off in performance metrics with soreness in the radiodorsal aspect of the wrist. The player himself seldom requests evaluation, especially in the minor leagues. Approximately 90% or better do recall some sort of hyperextension/axial load mechanism of injury (MOI), but most dismiss it as a "jammed wrist" and brush themselves off and continue to play. In the MLB

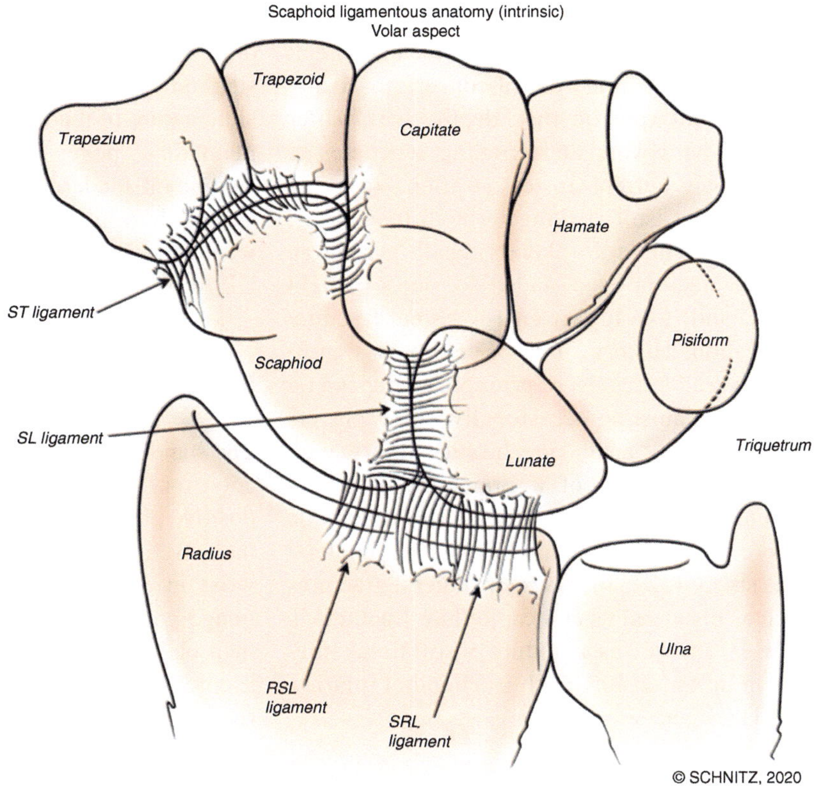

Fig. 2.4 Intrinsic ligamentous anatomy illustration

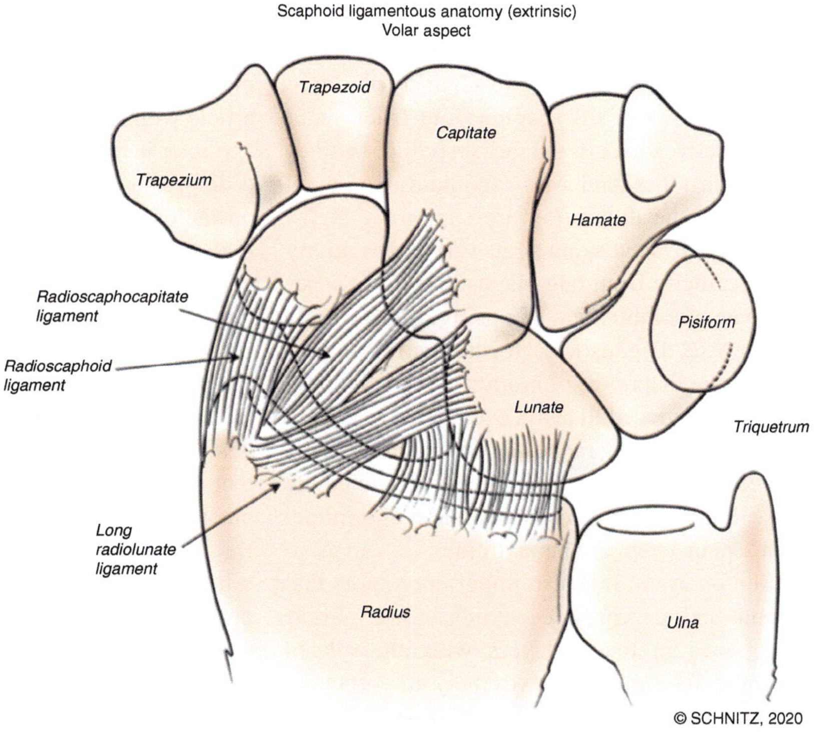

Fig. 2.5 Extrinsic ligamentous anatomy illustration

and the affiliated minor league system, the majority of players are overly reluctant to call attention to any injury out of concern for losing their current spot on the "depth chart," after years of hard work and grueling schedules to attain their current roster position. In other words, "If it isn't sticking through the skin.... play on." Seldom do players recall hearing an audible crack or snap, and if so, one's thought should shift to a higher energy carpal fracture/dislocation. History of prior injury is significant, as well as review of prior pre-trade/sign on physical exams, as occasionally, these players present as an "acute on chronic" injury with acute exacerbation of a premorbid scaphoid nonunion that was relatively asymptomatic before. Associated pathologies include: bilateral injuries in 1–2% of cases, ipsilateral fractures such as distal radius and capitellum fractures in up to 1%, as well as a mixture of soft tissue injuries in up to 30–40% such as chondral injuries, SL, TFCC, etc.

Physical Exam

The most consistent physical exam sign is anatomic snuffbox tenderness in ulnar deviation to bring the waist of the scaphoid out from under the protective cloak of the radial styloid. In addition, volar tuber tenderness and pain upon axial loading of the thumb ray are supportive signs. All of the physical exam signs vary in sensitivity and specificity from one manuscript to the next; however, a combination of positive signs results in improved diagnostic performance. It is important to note that range of motion is typically only minimally reduced, if at all, even in the relatively acute setting. If any range of motion parameter is reduced, it is typically extension that is noted the most. The players typically complain of minimal to no pain even at the extremes of range of motion on exam. It is also important to note that edema and certainly ecchymosis are almost never seen in these players with an isolated scaphoid fracture. It is extremely important to differentiate tenderness over a proximal pole with the wrist in slight flexion from SL ligament tenderness, and one must be very focally discrete during the physical examination. In addition, the surgeon should be keenly appreciative of the stoic nature of these athletes and a propensity to maintain a "poker face" even in the presence of significant tenderness and pain. The last thing any of these highly competitive young athletes want after years of hard work is to head to the DL (disabled list) IR (Injured Reserve).

Imaging

The standard plain radiographic screening evaluation for the player with positive symptoms and positive physical exam signs is a scaphoid series inclusive of a PA, PA in ulnar deviation with the wrist in slight extension, oblique, and lateral image with the wrist in neutral. The fracture is then classified based on its anatomical location according to the Herbert classification schedule (Fig. 2.1). If a true scaphoid fracture is present, approximately 80% of the time plain radiographs will be positive; however, 20% of the time plain radiographs will be negative. An increased RL angle is concerning for not only a scaphoid fracture being present but for the possibility of displacement and instability [4]. Dias's classic article from 1990 [23] revealed a mean percentage error in diagnosis of 43% that showed no sign of improvement at the time of the 3-week follow-up radiographs, and profoundly underscored the high degree of not only inter-observer error but equally as high intra-observer error with poor reproducibility. Tim Herbert further underscored this observation in a personal comment to me at the ASSH meeting in 1989 in Seattle when he said "x-rays tell lies…they tell 'damndable' lies!". Thus, in a professional player with persistent clinical exam findings and negative x-rays, placing him in the suspected or occult scaphoid fracture category, the surgeon has the responsibility to proceed promptly with advanced diagnostic imaging to try and sort out whether a true fracture is present [16]. At the amateur level, one has the option to immobilize in a cast and forego advanced diagnostic imaging and simply repeat plain radiographs at 17–21 days post injury following the long-standing common orthopedic community standard; however, one must realize this option is not without risk. There currently exists no perfect reference standard for the diagnosis of a scaphoid fracture and false negatives, and false positives persist irrespective of which modality is utilized [24, 25]. Repeat radiographs at 17–21 days to rule out an occult fracture are far from accurate, and it has even been shown that x-rays at 6 weeks still have occasional false negatives [26]. Therefore, even at the amateur level, advanced diagnostic imaging should be offered to the player, family, and coaches, sharing with them the current limitations of plain radiography.

With respect to advanced diagnostic imaging, even though far superior to plain radiography, from the outset, it is best to state simply that there is no perfect study for all clinical presentations [25, 27]. MRI and CT scans in the longitudinal oblique axis of the scaphoid are the most applicable and the most well studied with the highest available diagnostic performance characteristics [27]. MRI is typically the best in our hands in the acutely injured athlete where we need to know whether the scaphoid is fractured or not within the first week after the injury. MRI has the highest sensitivity especially early in the course for an occult fracture with an average sensitivity of 0.88 and a specificity of 1.0 [26]; however, false positives do occur in the "bone bruise" category. Microtrabecular fractures without cortical disruption aka "bone bruises" can be interpreted as true fractures and lead to overtreatment; however, it is also well-known that up to 2% of these do pan out to be nondisplaced true fractures by week 8 [24]. CT scans, performed properly in the dedicated longitudinal oblique axis of the scaphoid, have a sensitivity of 0.72 and a specificity of 0.99 and provide not only the diagnosis but graphic osseous detail of displacement, angulation, and/or the presence of comminution [26]. The sensitivity of the CT scan is far better in our hands in the subacute period beyond 7–10 days. The CT scan however must be performed in the dedicated longitudinal oblique axis with the following CT parameters: 0.55 slice thickness, 0.27 slice interval, 0.7 pitch, and ultrahigh resolution.

Quite often these athletes maintain their "game face" early on in the course and don't usually admit to having pain until their performance metrics suffer, and by that time we can usually head straight to a CT scan. In the rare player that presents acutely within the first several days to a week out from the injury, MRI reformatted in the longitudinal oblique axis of the scaphoid is our preferred diagnostic study of choice. If the MRI is negative, we briefly rest the wrist in a splint, and as pain and edema subside, we proceed with a prompt progressive rehabilitation schedule followed by a minor league rehabilitation assignment once AROM and 80% of strength have been restored. If the MRI is positive for a "bone bruise," we immobilize in a short arm thumb spica for 2 weeks, and then perform a CT scan to rule out the presence of an occult fracture. If the CT is negative, we then follow prompt rehabilitation schedule as outlined above. If the CT is positive, and reveals the presence of displacement, angulation, comminution, or presence of a proximal pole fracture, we recommend prompt arthroscopic-assisted reduction and internal fixation (AARIF). If the CT is positive yet demonstrates a truly nondisplaced, non-angulated, non-comminuted waist fracture, the player, the team physician, and the agent are given the option of immobilization in a cast versus prompt AARIF. Unfortunately, there is up to a 30–35% false-negative rate by CT scan with respect to assessment of fracture instability in our studies as well as Rings [14, 15, 17], and therefore even a nondisplaced and non-angulated fracture may still be unstable at the time of arthroscopic inspection/stabilization (Figs. 2.6 and 2.7). The player, team head physician, and agent all must be given strong warnings that even with a completely stable CT appearance if one elects conservative treatment in a cast, there is no guarantee that the fracture is truly stable, and thus might still end up as a delayed union or nonunion [19]. This further underscores the evolving concept of how difficult it is to diagnose scaphoid fracture instability, and how it is best defined so that we may properly advise our patients of the most prudent treatment course going forward. As Ring so eloquently summarized, one "should no longer

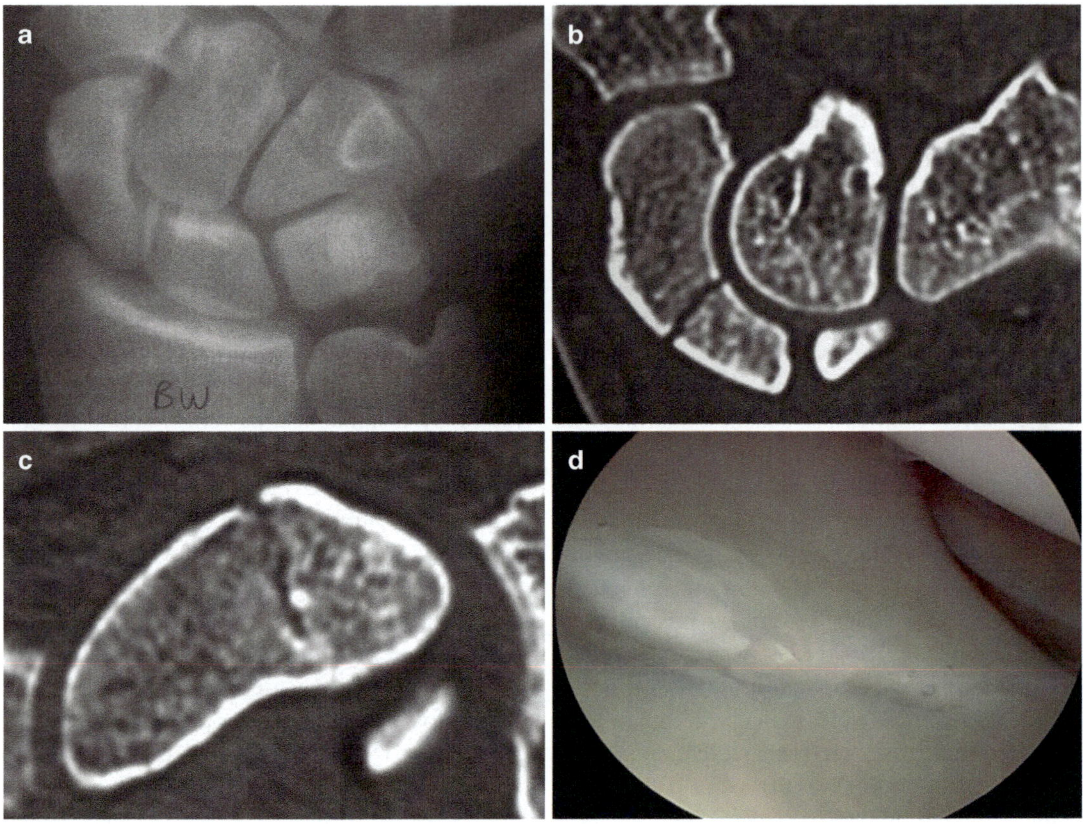

Fig. 2.6 Stable scaphoid fracture by CT + arthroscopy (true negative): (**a**) PA x-ray in UD. (**b**) Coronal CT. (**c**) Sagittal CT. (**d**) RMC arthroscopic view – stable

use the terms nondisplaced and stable interchangeably" as at least 30% of the time or more… one will be wrong. Typically, however, in this select agressive patient population, even in the nondisplaced stable appearing fracture by longitudinal oblique axis CT, the players, agents and team physicians almost universally ask us to proceed with prompt AARIF to shorten overall immobilization times in the hopes of pursuing an earlier rehabilitation schedule.

Treatment: Conservative

It is a basic orthopedic tenet that intracapsular fractures with, by definition, a tenuous vascular supply require stable immobilization and compression of the fragments in order to increase the likelihood of union and hopefully ward off avascular necrosis. Although historically, the orthopedic community's approach to treatment of the fractured scaphoid has not quite reflected it, the scaphoid is not all that dissimilar to its intracapsular counterparts, the femoral neck and the talus, as they unite by primary bone healing, with direct formation of bone across the fracture site without the aid of external callus. With this premise in mind, the only fractures that we recommend cast immobilization for in this active, high demand athletic population are the Herbert A1 and Herbert A2 fractures as documented by CT. Even in the A2 fractures, we recommend follow-up CT scan early in the course at approximately 3–4 weeks to make sure there's rapid progressive trabeculation (STS – scaphoid trabeculation score) [28] consistent with ongoing healing. On rare occasion on serial follow-up CT examination, one will find a Herbert A2 that appears to be more of a complete through and through

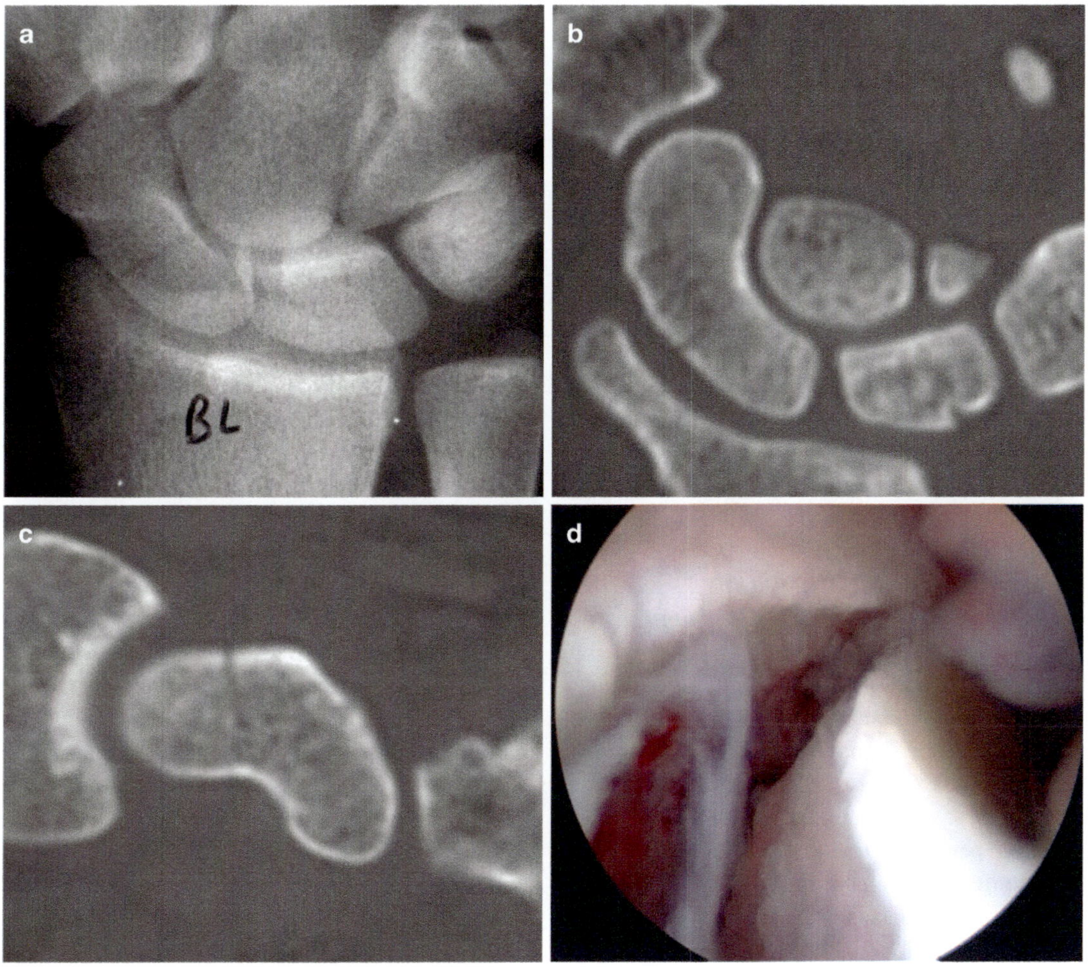

Fig. 2.7 Scaphoid fracture nondisplaced – stable by CT and unstable by arthroscopy (false negative). (**a**) PA x-ray in UD. (**b**) Coronal CT. (**c**) Sagittal CT. (**d**) RMC arthroscopic view – unstable

Herbert B1 or B2 fracture with a higher potential for instability, thus meriting attention for delayed AARIF. We do share with the player, head team physician, and agent that it is certainly fair and ethical to consider conservative management for completely stable appearing Herbert B1, B2 fracture on CT scan; however, a strong warning is given that in our studies as well as Ring's, up to 30–35% of these fractures demonstrate profound instability at the time of arthroscopic inspection which may lead to an increased incidence of nonunion [14, 15, 17]. Obviously, all Herbert B3, B4 fractures are excluded from consideration of conservative treatment and require prompt AARIF.

Treatment: Surgical

Currently, the accepted approach to treatment realizes the need for stable internal fixation in a significant subset of patients with an unstable scaphoid fracture pattern as well as the stable appearing fracture in the high demand athletic population such as the high school, college, and professional baseball player. Herbert [3] even questions the wisdom of considering "nondisplaced" scaphoid fractures as being "stable." In his own classification (Fig. 2.1), Herbert considers all complete fractures (B1 and B2) as unstable whether displaced or not, and considers only incomplete fractures (A1 and A2) as truly stable injury patterns. As shown by Weber and Chao [4], the force and rate of loading required to fracture the scaphoid is almost twice that of the distal radius. After this significant hyperextension-axial load force, it is only by the nature of the very snug capsular constraints surrounding the scaphoid that both fragments end up appearing in a rather benign, "nondisplaced" configuration upon imaging. To consider such an injury as "stable" only because there is no displacement on plain radiographs/CT, is relatively precarious at best.

The unstable scaphoid fracture can be treated by a variety of different methods including open reduction and internal fixation (ORIF), percutaneous fixation with either k-wires or cannulated screws, and arthroscopic-assisted reduction and internal fixation (AARIF) with various cannulated screw systems. The drawbacks of ORIF include extensive soft tissue dissection, disruption of the nondominant volar blood supply, division of the radioscaphocapitate and/or radiolunate ligaments and volar capsule, and prolonged rehabilitation. ORIF should be avoided at all costs, except in the extreme situations of highly unstable, highly comminuted fractures or trans-scaphoid perilunate fracture dislocations, etc. due to the prolonged rehabilitation involved secondary to the resultant scarring, and the obligate persistent alteration in intercarpal angles. Percutaneous fixation avoids the aforementioned drawbacks, yet relies on fluoroscopic guidance alone to assure accurate reduction of the scaphoid fracture fragments and optimal positioning of the implant in the central third axis of the scaphoid. The frank technical limitations of plain radiography as well as fluoroscopy in detailed visualization of the oddly oriented scaphoid finitely limit the accuracy of the percutaneous technique. AARIF avoids all the limitations of ORIF and percutaneous fixation, yet allows direct visualization of the scaphoid fracture site and assures accurate reduction of the fragments prior to, and during, definitive arthroscopically assisted internal fixation. AARIF also assists in accurate targeting of the proximal pole apex or "sweet spot" assuring central third scaphoid axis placement, in addition to allowing detection of concurrent pathology in the radiocarpal or midcarpal joints. Scaphoid AARIF is a convenient therapeutic alternative that avoids many of the inherent pitfalls of ORIF and percutaneous fixation.

Despite their immense popularity and seductively simple surgical techniques, the percutaneous or limited incision techniques have several inherent potential technical pitfalls, including (1) the well-known limitations of plain radiography and fluoroscopy in adequately visualizing scaphoid fracture anatomy and hence their reduction; (2) tendency for problematic freehand screw insertion potentially resulting in further displacement, rotation, or even distraction of the fragments [12]; and (3) the potential in totally freehand systems without jig/barrel guidance for the narrow diameter guide wire to bend resulting in binding of the subsequent instrumentation. In selected cases from our early lab experience, especially with percutaneous or freehand techniques, we have experienced on more than one occasion, the phenomenon where the scaphoid fracture appeared fluoroscopically to be anatomically reduced, only to find a 1–2 mm dorsal gap in the fracture site when directly visualized arthroscopically thru the RMC portal. This is especially true if the axis of the screw is too far volar, resulting in compression of the volar cortex and slight distraction of the dorsal cortex (Fig. 2.8). Just as plain radiographs have given way to CT over the years for accurate definition of precise scaphoid fracture anatomy preoperatively, fluoroscopy has now been supplanted by the additional benefits of arthroscopy in the assessment of fracture reduction intraoperatively. Irrespective of the type of intramedullary implant system used, especially if it is a percutaneously placed screw, it is recommended that one perform at least a brief arthroscopic inspection through the RMC portal to confirm fracture reduction, alignment, and stable compression. The arthroscope is usually much more "critical" of reduction relative to the fluoroscope, as one will frequently find the fracture to be well reduced fluoroscopically yet have residual displacement by arthroscopic inspection. This is key for an oddly shaped carpal bone well-known for sparingly granting surgeons a second chance due to the relatively narrow intramedullary canal central axis with little margin for error.

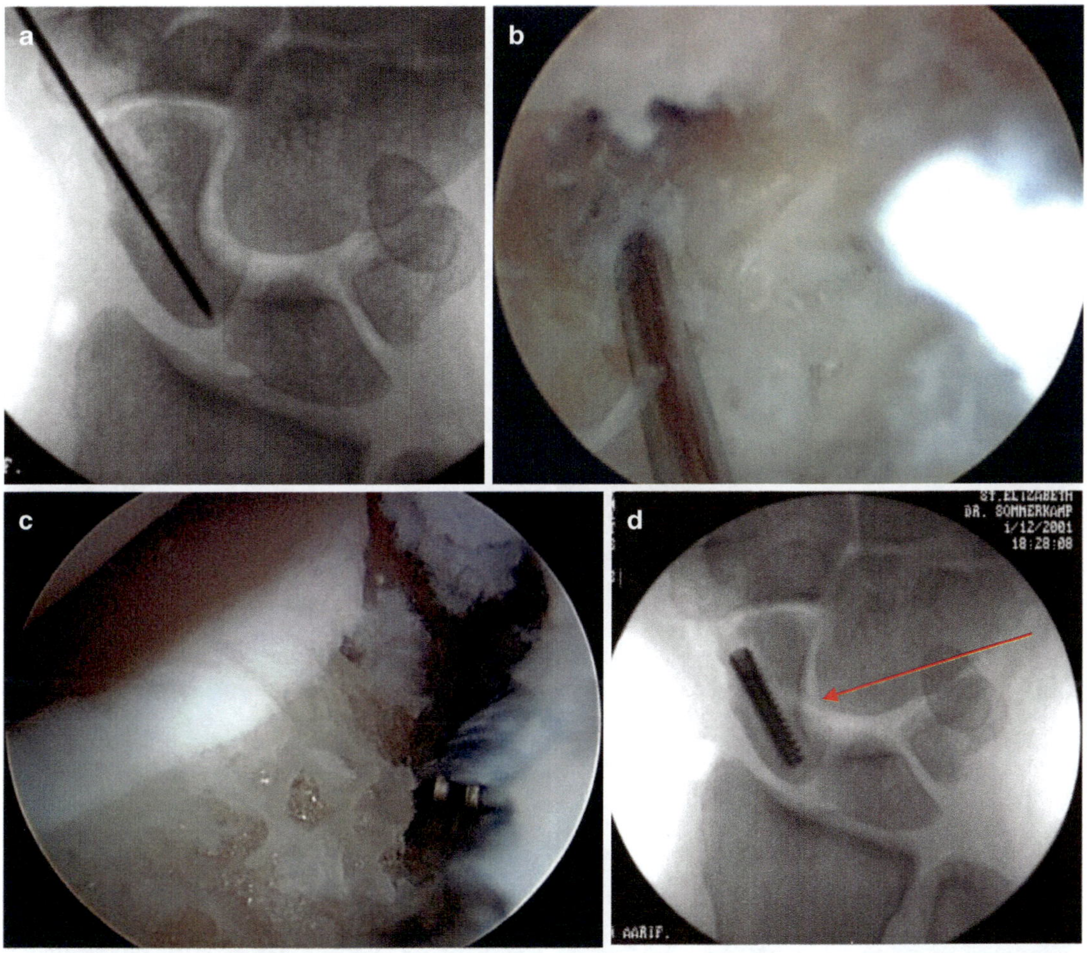

Fig. 2.8 Freehand percutaneous technique (Acutrak). (**a**) X-ray guide wire. (**b**) RMC image gapped. (**c**) After screw still gapped 2 mm. (**d**) Final x-ray – innocuous appearance

To further complement the various "percutaneous" or limited incision techniques which are performed only under fluoroscopic guidance, Whipple [7, 8] introduced the concept of AARIF in 1992 (Fig. 2.9). With the addition of arthroscopy, one can adequately visualize the fracture site and frankly confirm reduction under direct visualization thru the RMC portal. In addition, the proximal pole target site in the apex or "sweet spot" can be directly visualized thru the 3–4 portal aiding in proper central third placement of the screw. Concurrently, one can visualize the remainder of the midcarpal and radiocarpal joints to assess for any coexistent pathology. The Herbert-Whipple screw placed in a retrograde fashion through the distal pole starting hole is used in our hands for the vast majority of scaphoid fractures as long as the proximal pole fragment is greater than 25% in size. For the diminutive proximal pole fracture that is less than 25% in size, we then perform arthroscopically guided freehand placement of the Herbert-Whipple screw from an antegrade dorsal approach with the technical modifications as espoused by Geissler [29] with a guide wire being placed through the 14-gauge needle in the 2–3 portal. If initial fracture displacement is greater than 2 mm and the aforementioned reduction maneuvers are not promptly successful, on rare occasion one must abort AARIF and convert to ORIF. Upon completion of the AARIF, the wrist is placed thru an arc of motion under direct arthroscopic visual-

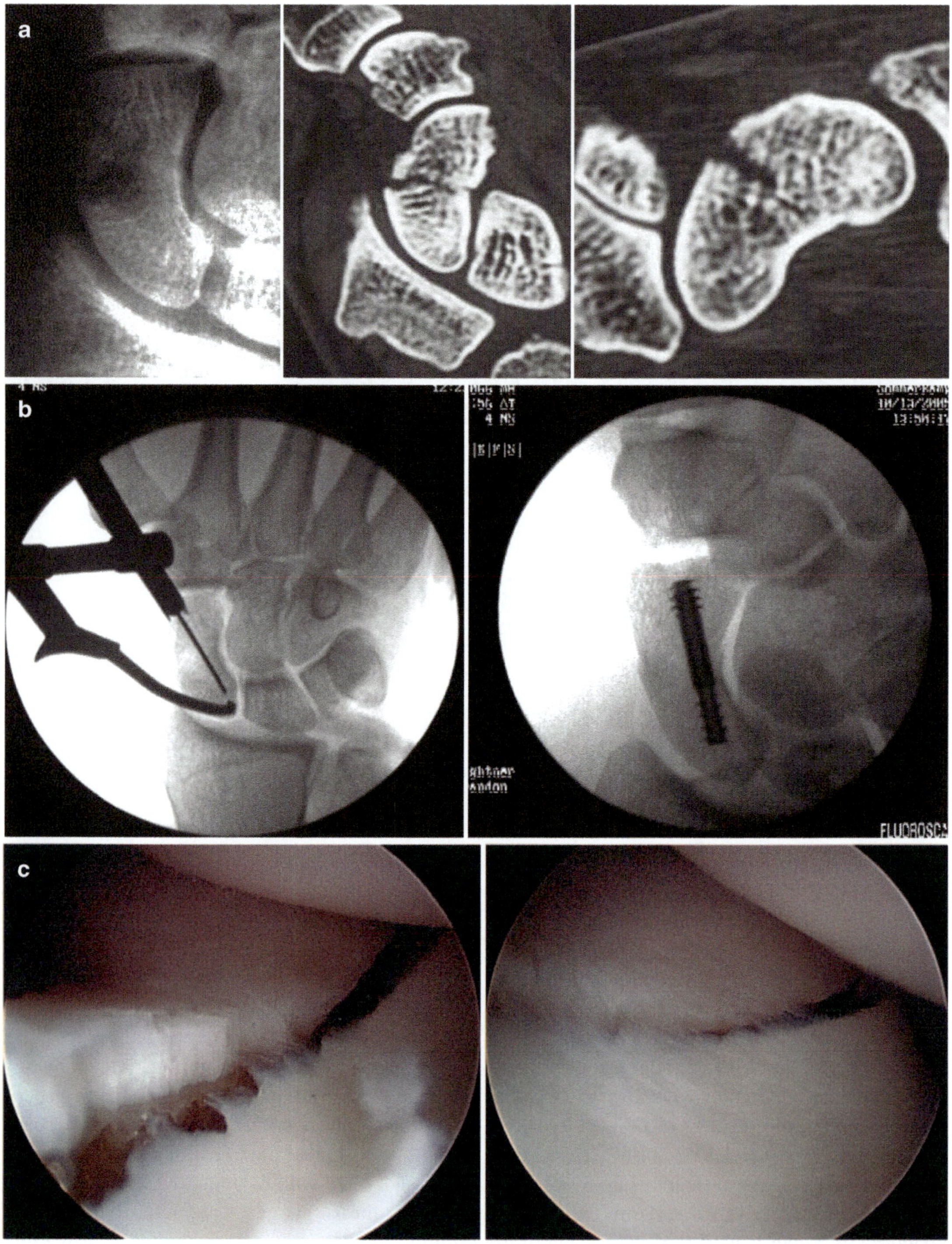

Fig. 2.9 Herbert-Whipple AARIF technique: (**a**) Pre-op XR and CT. (**b**) Intra-op guide wire thru jig + screw placement. (**c**) Arthroscopic RMC portal view pre/post

ization to confirm fracture stability, and thus help guide the surgeon's postoperative rehabilitation planning schedule.

Rehabilitation

Initially, the patient is immobilized in a bulky cotton compression dressing/thumb spica splint for the first week. Sutures are removed at approximately 1 week and AROM is started at approximately 7–10 days, but heavy gripping and power puddy strengthening is avoided until CT-proven cross-sectional fracture trabeculation is present with a scaphoid trabeculation score (STS) of at least 25%, usually at ~3–4 weeks [27]. A follow-up CT scan at approximately 6 weeks usually reveals rapid consolidation with an STS score anywhere between 50% and 100%. The thumb spica splint is discontinued once the STS score is greater than 50%. After AROM is full, grip strengths are greater than 80%, and the STS is greater than 50%, the player is returned to the trainer for initiation of position-specific rehabilitation drills including short toss, long toss, hitting off the T, flip toss hitting, cage hitting, and eventually live batting practice (BP). The rehabilitation schedule can be accelerated for the rare case of the nondominant (glove hand) in the American League pitcher who has a designated hitter.

RTP (Return to Play)

The RTP decision is a multifactorial process lead by the trainer and head team physician with input from the subspecialty surgeon as needed. Usually, by this stage, minimal input is needed from the hand surgeon as long as the player achieves all position-specific rehabilitation drills at a satisfactory level, has no pain and normal grip strength corrected for hand dominance, and is then green lighted for a rehabilitation assignment in the minor leagues. The "rehab assignments" can vary anywhere between 7 to 14 days depending on the players' position and the duration of time on the DL leading up to it.

References

1. Herndon J. Scaphoid fractures and complications. AAOS Monograph Series; 1994. p. 1, 26–27, 69–71.
2. Smith DK, Linscheid RL, Amadio PC, et al. Scaphoid anatomy: evaluation with complex motion tomography. Radiology. 1989;173:177–80.
3. Herbert TJ. The fractured scaphoid. St. Louis: Quality Medical Publishing; 1990. p. 51–67.
4. Weber ER, Chao EY. An experimental approach to the mechanism of scaphoid waist fracture. J Hand Surg [Am]. 1978;3A:142–8.
5. Gelberman RH, Menon J. The vascularity of the scaphoid bone. J Hand Surg Am. 1980;5A:508–13.
6. Sanders WE. Evaluation of the humpback scaphoid by computed tomography in the longitudinal axial plane of the scaphoid. J Hand Surg [Am]. 1988;13A:182–7.
7. Whipple TL. Arthroscopic surgery: the wrist. Fractures of the scaphoid. Philadelphia: Lippincott; 1992. p. 148–56.
8. Whipple TL. The role of arthroscopy in the treatment of intraarticular wrist fractures. Hand Clin. 1995;11(1):13–8.
9. Slade JF, Grauer JN, Mahoney JD. Arthroscopic reduction and percutaneous fixation of scaphoid fractures with a novel dorsal technique. Orthop Clin North Am. 2001;32(2):247–61.
10. Sommerkamp TG. Scaphoid AARIF: arthroscopically assisted reduction and internal fixation of scaphoid fractures. J Am Soc Surg Hand. 2001;1(3):192–210.
11. Sommerkamp TG. Scaphoid AARIF: arthroscopically assisted reduction and internal fixation of scaphoid fractures, delayed unions, and nonunions. Oper Tech Orthop. 2007;17:106–17.
12. Sommerkamp TG. Scaphoid AARIF: arthroscopically assisted reduction and internal fixation of scaphoid fractures. Oper Tech Sports Med. 2010;18:146–54.
13. Swart E, Strauch R. Diagnosis of scaphoid fracture displacement. J Hand Surg Am. 2013;38A:784–7.
14. Buijze GA, Jogsholm P, Ring D, et al. Diagnostic performance of radiographs and computed tomography for displacement and instability of acute scaphoid waist fractures. J Bone Joint Surg. 2012;94:1967–74.
15. Buijze GA, Jorgsholm P, Thomsen N, Ring D, et al. Factors associated with arthroscopically determined scaphoid fracture displacement and instability. J Hand Surg Am. 2012;37A:1405–10.
16. Lozano-Calderon S, Blazar P, Zurakowski D, et al. Diagnosis of scaphoid fracture displacement with radiography and computed tomography. J Bone Joint Surg. 2006;88A:2695–703.
17. Sommerkamp TG. Scaphoid fractures and nonunions: arthroscopic vs. CT assessment of instability. In Submission. J Arthroscopy. 2021.
18. Schwarcz Y, Schwarcz Y, Peleg E, et al. Three-dimensional analysis of acute scaphoid fracture displacement: proximal extension deformity of the scaphoid. J Bone Joint Surg. 2017;99:141–9.
19. Grewal R, Suh N, Mac Dermid J. Use of computed tomography to predict union and time to union in

acute scaphoid fractures treated nonoperatively. J Hand Surg Am. 2013;38A:872–7.
20. Van Tassel DC, Owens BD, Wolf JM. Incidence estimates and demographics of scaphoid fracture in eth US population. J Hand Surg Am. 2010;35A:1242–5.
21. Duckworth AD, Jenkins PJ, McQueen MM, et al. Scaphoid fracture epidemiology. J Trauma. 2012;72:E41–5.
22. Gösta Frykman. Fracture of the Distal Radius Including Sequelae-Shoulder–Handfinger Syndrome, Disturbance in the Distal Radio-Ulnar Joint and Impairment of Nerve Function: A Clinical and Experimental Study. Acta Orthopaedica Scandinavica 2014;38(sup108):1–61.
23. Dias JJ, Thompson J, Barton NJ, Gregg PJ. Suspected scaphoid fractures- the value of radiographs. J Bone Joint Surg Br. 1990;72B:98–101.
24. Buijze G, Jupiter J. Scaphoid fractures- evidenced based management: predictors of Scaphoid fractures. St Louis: Elsevier; 2018. p. 49–60.
25. Ring DR, Lozano-Calderon L. Imaging for suspected scaphoid fractures. J Hand Surg Am. 2008;33A:954–7.
26. Buijze G, Jupiter J. Scaphoid fractures - evidenced based management: diagnostic workup for suspected scaphoid fractures. St Louis: Elsevier; 2018. p. 61–6.
27. Mallee W, Doornberg JN, Ring DR, et al. Comparison of CT and MRI for diagnosis of suspected scaphoid fractures. J Bone Joint Surg. 2011;93A:20–8.
28. Sommerkamp TG. STS- Scaphoid Trabeculation Score - assessment of healing presented at the scaphoid: from stem to stern-the entire spectrum. Boston: ASSH; 2014. p. 18.
29. Geissler WB, Hammit MD. Arthroscopic aided fixation of scaphoid fractures. Hand Clin. 2001;17(4):575–88.
30. Gelberman RH, Gross MS. The vascularity of the wrist: identification of arterial patterns at risk. Clin Orthop (Lippincott Williams Wilkins-Wolters-Kluwer). 1986;202:40–9.

Carpal Fractures Excluding the Scaphoid and Hook of Hamate

3

Matthew C. DeWolf and Randall W. Culp

Introduction

Fractures of the wrist in athletes most commonly involve the scaphoid and hook of the hamate and thus require a full discussion in separate chapter. While other fractures of the carpus are rare, it remains critical for the physician to help determine when a player may return to sport early versus when the athlete must be managed with longer periods of immobilization versus when the athlete requires surgery.

Injuries can be divided into three main groups depending on the mechanism of injury: perilunate injuries, axial injuries, and avulsion injuries [40, 48].

The work-up of carpal fractures typically starts with physical examination. Plain radiographs are enhanced with specific views depending on the type of fracture suspected. If there is concern but no obvious fracture is identified on plain radiographs, CT or MRI scans provide invaluable information.

Many carpal fractures occur with other injuries, including other carpal fractures and carpal dislocations. In any case of carpal dislocation, careful examination of the neurovascular status should be performed with particular attention paid to the median nerve, which can be seen in up to 50% of cases, as median nerve injury can lead to persistent symptoms [11].

Triquetral Fractures

Triquetral fractures are second only to scaphoid fractures and comprise 3–5% of all carpal fractures [4, 6, 8, 21, 38]. Physical examination can be difficult to isolate in these injuries given its proximity to the ulnar side of the wrist, including the TFCC. They are typically identified on radiographs. A 45° pronated oblique XR of the wrist can be helpful in the evaluation [12, 13]. If there is concern for injury that is not identified on plain radiographs, then CT scans are helpful in identifying them.

These fractures can occur within three varieties: dorsal chip fractures, volar avulsion fractures, and body fractures. Dorsal triquetral chip fractures typically occur with extreme palmar flexion and radial deviation and result from the pull of the radiotriquetral and triquetroscaphoid ligaments [6, 20]. They are seen most easily on the lateral view as shown in Fig. 3.1. Alternatively, these fractures can occur with a fall onto an ulnarly deviated wrist that is in dorsiflexion, in which case the ulnar styloid is driven as a chisel into the dorsal cortex of the triquetrum [13–15, 23]. In fact, a large ulnar styloid has been proposed as a predisposition to this type of fracture [14]. Dorsal chip fractures can be an incidental finding on a

M. C. DeWolf (✉)
Philadelphia Hand to Shoulder Center and Thomas Jefferson University, Philadelphia, PA, USA

R. W. Culp
Orthopedic Surgery, Thomas Jefferson University, Philadelphia, PA, USA

G. M. Lourie (ed.), *Hand and Wrist Injuries in Baseball*,
https://doi.org/10.1007/978-3-030-81659-9_3

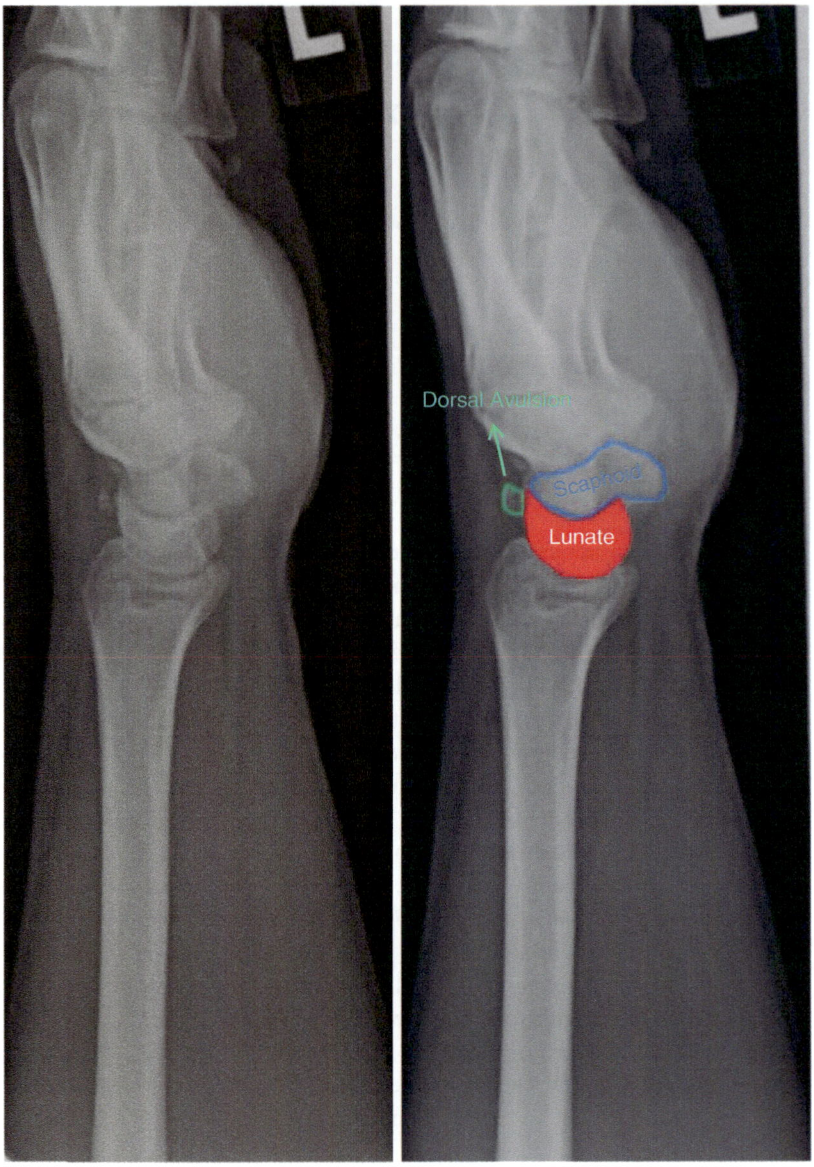

Fig. 3.1 Triquetral fracture. Representation of a dorsal triquetral chip fracture

lateral radiograph. If acute injury is suspected, then short periods of immobilization of 1–2 weeks with interim evaluation can help determine the appropriate time to return to play. However, if there is marked swelling of the wrist, then a MRI should be obtained. If pain persists beyond 8 weeks, MR arthrography is recommended to investigate the possibility of a concurrent intercarpal ligament injury or TFC tear [24].

Volar triquetral avulsion fractures are considered avulsion of the palmar ulnar triquetral ligament or the lunotriquetral ligament. Radiographic evaluation includes radial deviation views. These fractures are indicative of carpal instability, which is the primary focus of treatment. Thus, volar triquetral avulsion fractures do not require specific treatment but should alert the treating provider of possible carpal instability [39, 40].

Triquetral body fractures are typically high-energy injuries that are associated with greater arc perilunate fracture dislocations [25]. It is imperative for the treating physician to be aware and look for these types of fractures in the setting of a perilunate dislocation. Treatment of triquetral body fractures varies depending on the characteristics of the injury. For perilunate injuries, we recommend pinning of the lunotriquetral joint. A displaced triquetral body fracture warrants open reduction internal fixation [11, 36]. For chronic cases that have led to pisotriquetral arthritis, excision of the pisiform has been helpful [1, 41].

Hamate Fractures

Fractures of the hamate are slightly less common than triquetral fractures and occur in 2% of all carpal fractures [16]. The hook of the hamate fractures occurs more frequently and is covered elsewhere. Hamate body fractures typically occur with high-energy axial loads and occur concomitantly with fourth and fifth carpal-metacarpal fracture dislocations. Hamate body fractures can be difficult to detect on plain radiographs, but obtaining CT imaging with the hands in the praying position has been shown to be beneficial for detecting them, as is shown in Fig. 3.2 [3, 22].

Hamate fractures primarily occur during stickhandling sports such as baseball, golf, and tennis [33]. They are frequently misdiagnosed, but the treating physician should be aware when a patient presents with diminished grip strength, ulnar nerve paresthesias, or mild carpal tunnel syndrome [32, 44].

Hamate body fractures can be broken down into four major groups: sagittal oblique fractures, dorsal coronal fracture, proximal pole fractures, and fractures of the medial tuberosity [14, 15, 28]. The most common types of hamate body fractures are coronal body fractures and hamatometacarpal fracture-dislocations [33].

Treatment involved open reduction internal fixation if there is involvement of more than 1/3 of the hamate body or articular involvement, typically performed with compression screws or low profile plates for bone stabilization. K-wires can be used for joint stabilization. Care must be taken when drilling from dorsal to palmar to avoid the motor branch of the ulnar nerve. If there is extensive dorsal comminution, then CMC capsular repair may be indicated.

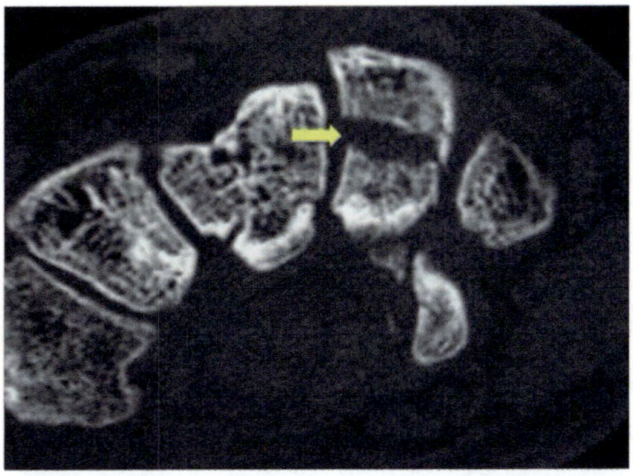

Fig. 3.2 Hamate fractures. The CT shows a comminuted hamate fracture as shown by the arrow. (From Suh Carpal Fractures JHS 2014)

Trapezium Fractures

Fractures of the trapezium comprise 4–5% of carpal fractures [10, 17, 34]. Given the association of trapezium fractures and first metacarpal fractures, care should be taken to look for trapezium fractures in the setting of a first metacarpal fracture and vice versa [10, 27, 35]. These fractures can be described as body fractures, trapezial ridge fractures, or fracture dislocations [40]. These fractures are typically high-energy fractures and occur with a fall onto an outstretched hand in which an axial load on the dorsiflexed wrist drives the metacarpal into the trapezium [18]. Examination will reveal point tenderness at the volar base of the thumb. These fractures are commonly identified on standard views of the hand, but identification can be enhanced with a Bett's view, in which the hand is slightly flexed and the thumb is pronated to give a true lateral of the thumb and to better visualize the trapeziometacarpal articulation [46]. A carpal canal view can be useful to identify trapezial ridge fractures, which are often missed with standard radiographs [26]. CT can be useful for identifying occult cases.

Given the intimate relationship of the trapezium with the first metacarpal at the first CMC joint, treatment varies depending on the morphology of the fracture. Nondisplaced fractures should be treated with thumb spica immobilization for 4–6 weeks. Comminuted fractures with reduced joints can be treated nonoperatively, as seen in Fig. 3.3a–e. Intra-articular fractures,

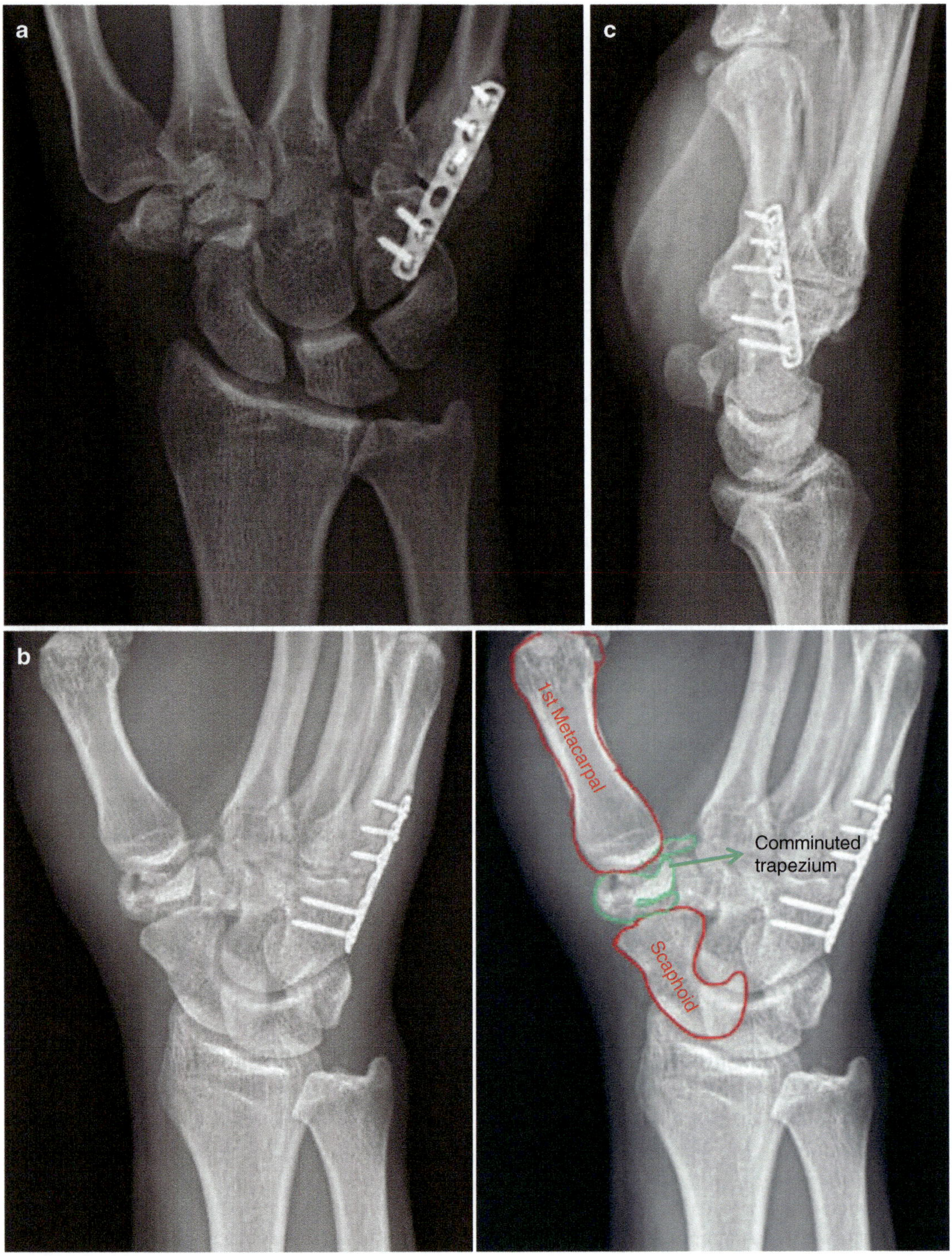

Fig. 3.3 Trapezium fracture. This 30-year-old male "jammed" his right thumb while playing flag football and presented with pain, swelling, and bruising at the base of the thumb. He had a prior CMC arthrodesis for a right small finger fracture. XR showed a comminuted fracture of the trapezium. CT demonstrated comminution of the articular surface and multiple small pieces. Given the amount of comminution, he was treated nonoperatively in a thumb spica splint for 8 weeks. At 16-month follow-up, he was not noted to have any pain in the thumb CMC joint. (**a**) PA of the hand. (**b**) Oblique of the hand. (**c**) Lateral of the hand. (**d**) The coronal CT slice. (**e**) 16-month follow-up XR. At 16-month follow-up, he was not noted to have any pain in the thumb CMC joint

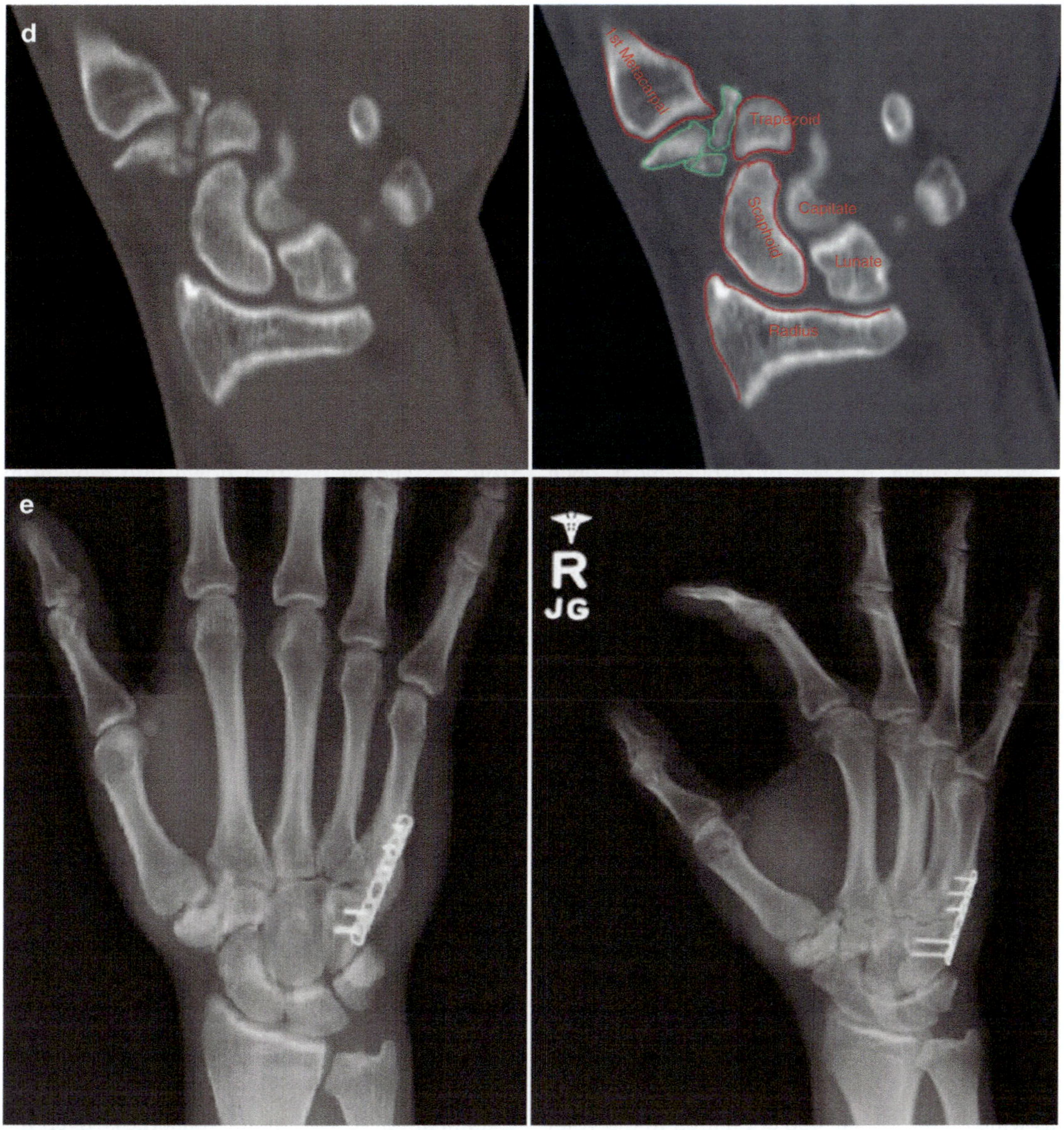

Fig. 3.3 (continued)

including ridge fractures, with >2 mm of displacement or carpometacarpal subluxation should be treated with open reduction internal fixation with pin or minifragment screws. McGuigan and Culp present 11 patients with intra-articular fractures of the trapezium with mean follow-up of 47 months with good results from open reduction internal fixation [27].

Capitate Fractures

Capitate fractures are rare given that it is protected in the center of the hand and comprise 1–2% of all carpal fractures [16]. Given its surrounding protection, isolated fractures are rare. It is more commonly associated with perilunate fracture dislocations.

Isolated fractures result from a direct blow from a baseball pitch or by indirect axial load through the third metacarpal with the wrist flexed. However, these more frequently occur in conjunction with perilunate injury, especially transverse fractures, the so-called scaphocapitate syndrome. Work-up includes a careful physical examination and plain radiographs. However, CT or MRI is frequently required to help identify capitate fractures, as is seen in Fig. 3.4 [2, 9].

Treatment of capitate fractures generally consists of nonoperative treatment for nondisplaced fractures until there are radiographic and clinical signs of healing. In cases of displacement, open reduction internal fixation with a combination of pins and/or screws can be pursued. Cases that go on to nonunion can be treated with open bone grafting and screw fixation, as seen in Fig. 3.5a–c.

It should be noted that the capitate has a retrograde interosseous blood flow, which places the proximal pole at risk for AVN with fractures through the mid-body [19, 45].

Trapezoid Fractures

Trapezoid fractures are exceedingly rare and constitute less than 1% of carpal fractures given that it is protected within the carpus [7]. There are only a few isolated case reports in the literature [29, 31, 37, 47, 49, 50]/[5]. The trapezoid is the keystone of the carpus given that it is twice as wide on the dorsal side compared to the volar side. Given its protection within the carpus, this is most commonly found in conjunction with other carpal fractures or carpometacarpal dislocations. Evaluation starts with physical examination, which would reveal point tenderness at the base of the index metacarpal. Standard radiographs can usually detect fractures of the trapezoid. Special attention should be put on the AP view to evaluate the trapeziometacarpal joint. As with all carpal fractures, CT can augment evaluation if there is concern but no obvious fracture on plain radiograph. Treatment for nondisplaced injuries consists of immobilization, as seen in Fig. 3.6. Nagumo et al. present a case report of an occult fracture in a 21-year-old male baseball player of the trapezoid which was treated with excision of the fragment resulting in improvement in function and pain relief [30]. The individual was able to return to baseball at 8 weeks and was still playing without pain and with full motion of the wrist and fingers at 4-year follow-up [30]. Nammour et al. present a case of a 23-year-old male baseball player who presented with right wrist pain resulting from a dynamic exercise movement in which he moved from a standing position down into a push-up position and was managed nonoperatively in a cast for 6 weeks who went on to have no pain and a return to baseline function at 12-week follow-up [31]. Surgical management consists of a combination of pins and screw fixation to help stabilize both the trapezium and the trapeziometacarpal joint.

Pisiform Fractures

Fractures of the pisiform are also rare, and make up 1% of carpal fractures in the Major League Baseball population. The pisiform has unique anatomy given that it articulates with the triquetrum dorsally, is the origin of the abductor digiti minimi, and serves as the attachment for the flexor carpi ulnaris, and serves as an attachment point for the transverse carpal ligament. Examination reveals point tenderness over the pisiform. The shuck maneuver could raise concern for suspicion for fracture. Given its proximity to the ulnar nerve in Guyon's canal, examination involves evaluation of the ulnar nerve.

Radiographic examination involves standard series including AP and lateral. Additional views include a carpal tunnel view and a reverse oblique view, in which the wrist is placed in 30° of supination to obtain a profile view of the pisiform, as seen in Figs. 3.7 and 3.8.

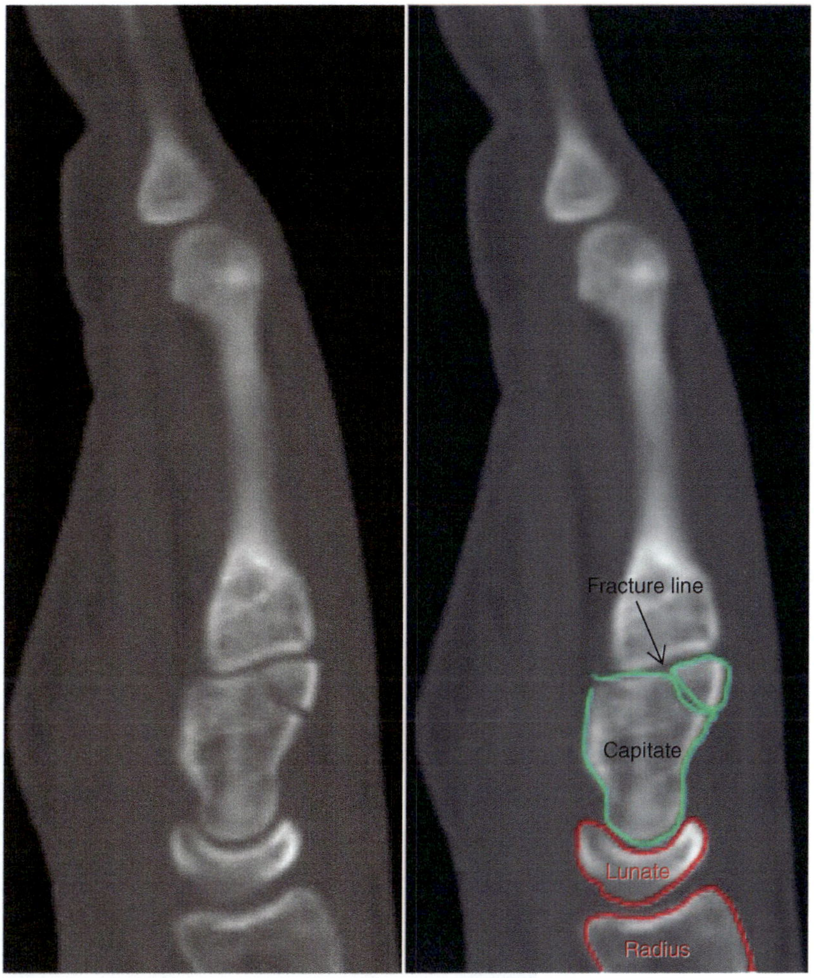

Fig. 3.4 Capitate fracture. 40F who punched a car. Small dorsal fragment. This fracture was treated nonoperatively

Nonoperative management consists of cast immobilization for 4–6 weeks. Treatment can include pisiform excision to provide expedient and safe return to sport, but that is rarely needed.

Lunate Fractures

Lunate fractures are another rare carpal fracture, comprising approximately 1% of all carpal fractures [42]. These fractures occur when the lunate is compressed between the distal radius and capitate with extreme wrist hyperextension and ulnar deviation that occurs when falling on an outstretched hand [24]. Lunate fractures have been described following a blow to the hand by a ball in line with the forearm [43]. Physical examination consists of looking for tenderness on the dorsal aspect of the lunate. Radiographic evaluation consists of AP and lateral with supplemental CT scan as needed. There is no consensus as to causal relationship between acute lunate fractures and avascular necrosis.

Lunate fractures can be managed with short courses of immobilization and re-examination in the setting of small marginal chip fractures, as seen in Figs. 3.9 and 3.10. Displaced fractures and fractures resulting in DISI or VISI deformity demand operative fixation. Therefore, careful examination for DISI and VISI on lateral radiographs is imperative (Table 3.1).

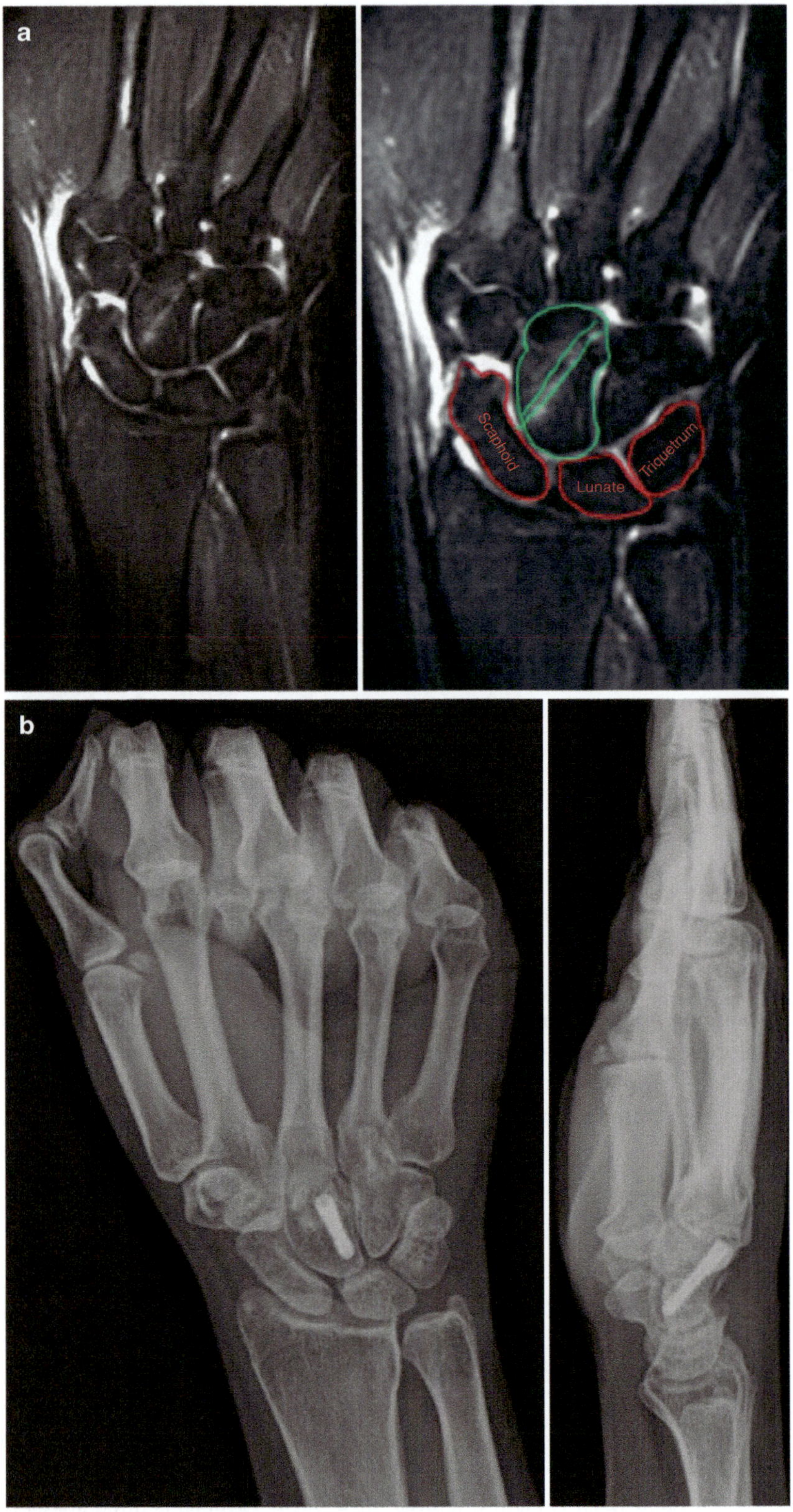

Fig. 3.5 Capitate fracture. 23F RHD with right capitate fracture nonunion after 6 months of nonoperative treatment. Surgery was a dorsal approach through the 3–4 interval, cancellous bone was harvested from the 3rd metacarpal, and fracture was stabilized with Acutrak screw. (**a**) T2 coronal cut of the MRI showing the oblique fracture line. (**b**) PA and Lateral of the right hand postoperatively

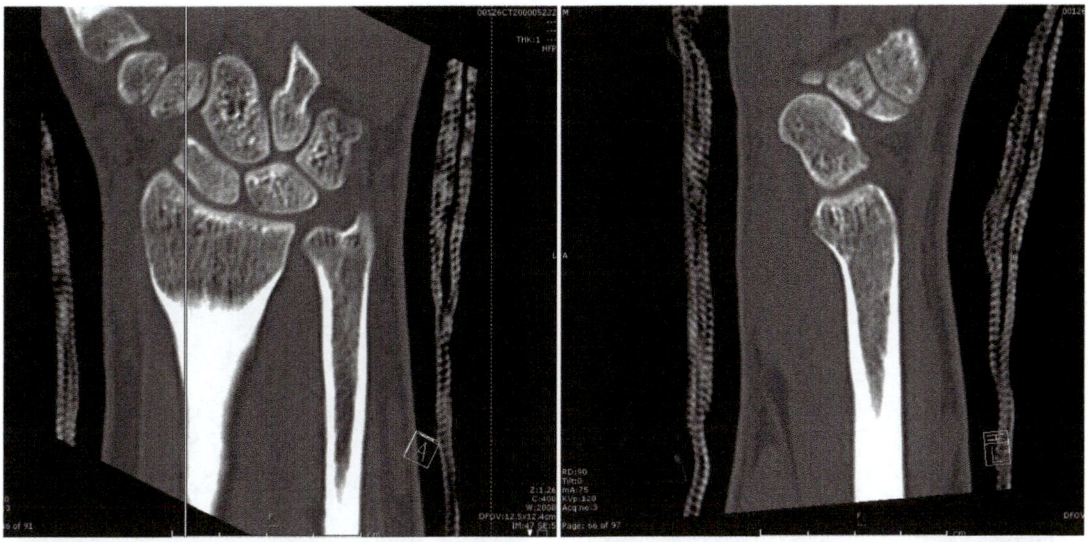

Fig. 3.6 Trapezoid fractures. 27-year-old male with left trapezoid fracture after punching a heavy bag. Initial XR were negative for fracture, but significant pain prompted advanced imaging. CT demonstrated nondisplaced trapezoid fracture. Given the nondisplaced nature, reduction of the trapeziometacarpal joint, and excellent healing potential, this was treated nonoperatively in a short-arm cast. (Case and Imaging Courtesy of Brandon Prioreschi, MD)

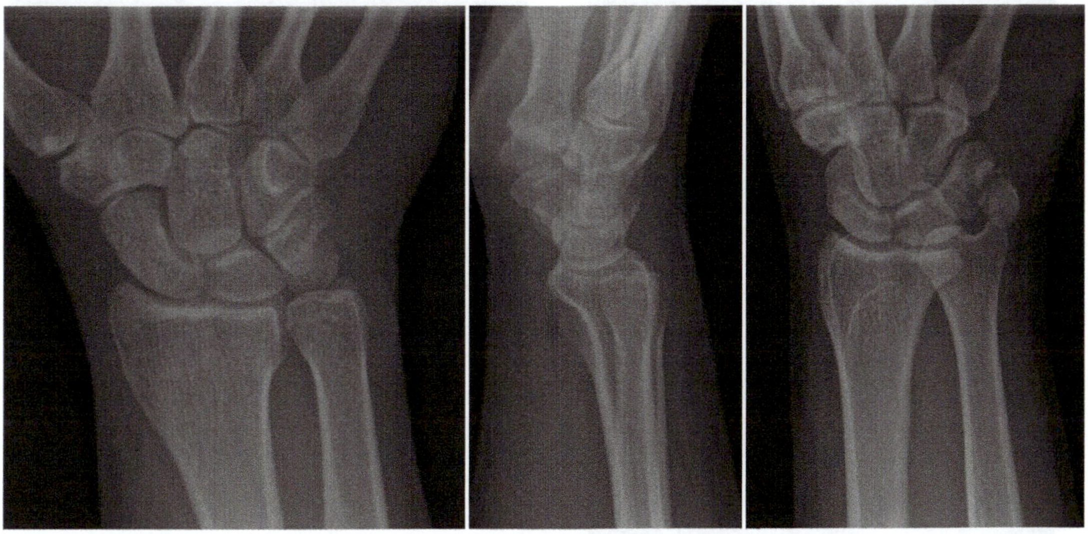

Fig. 3.7 Pisiform fractures. 33M sliding into a base playing softball. Presented with swelling, ecchymosis, and pain over the volar ulnar aspect of the hand. Best visualization of the fracture is on the oblique view

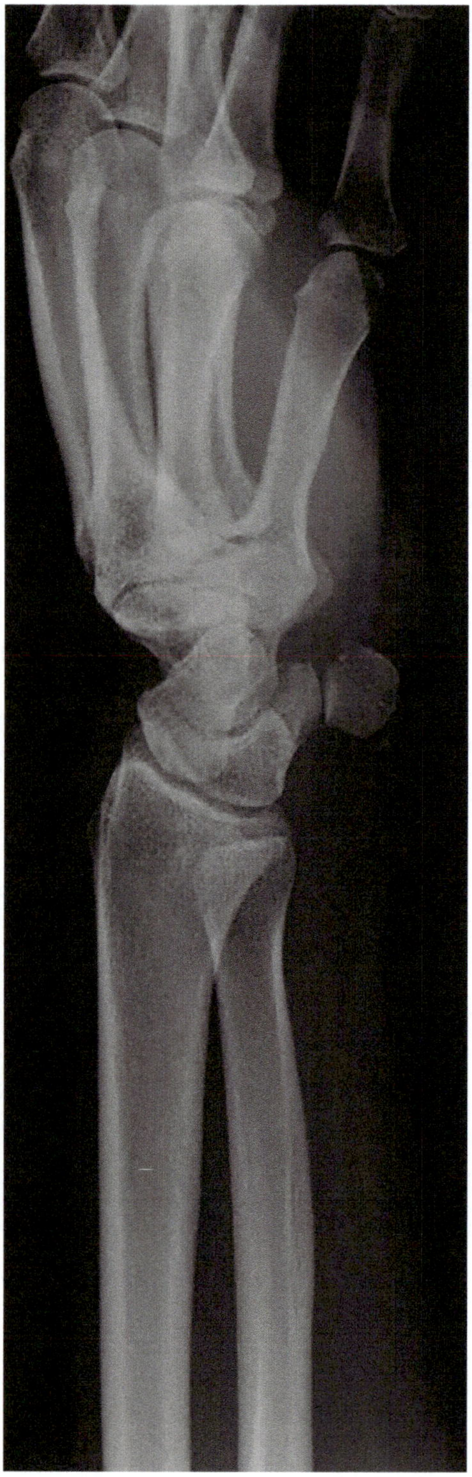

Fig. 3.8 Pisiform fractures. 51F who was evaluated for left-sided volar/ulnar wrist pain. Diagnosed with pisiform avulsion fracture. Treated nonoperatively

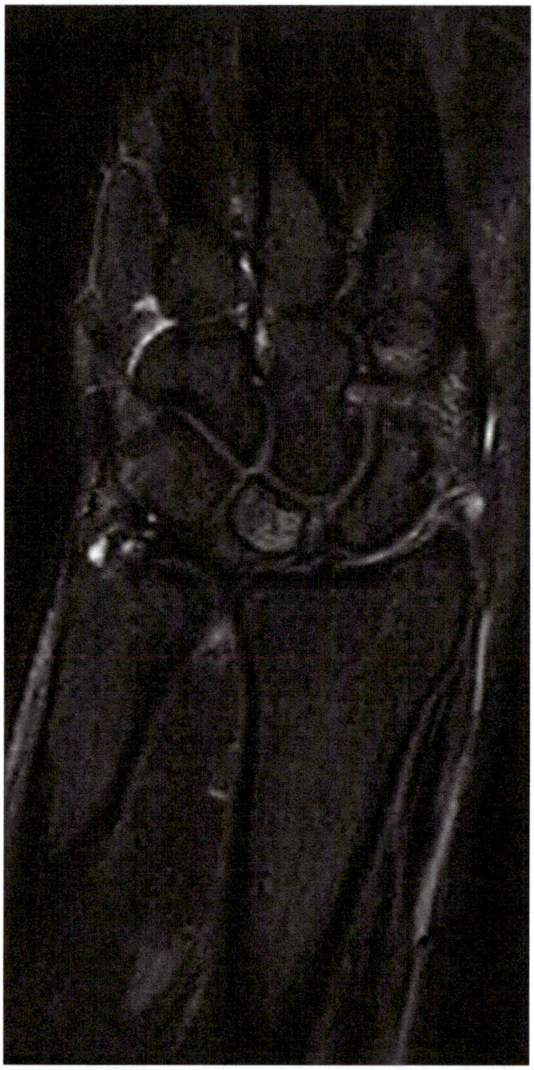

Fig. 3.9 Lunate fracture. 26M professional hockey player presenting with right wrist pain. MRI showed right lunate stress reaction. Treated with splint immobilization and bone stimulator. Pain resolved within 1 month

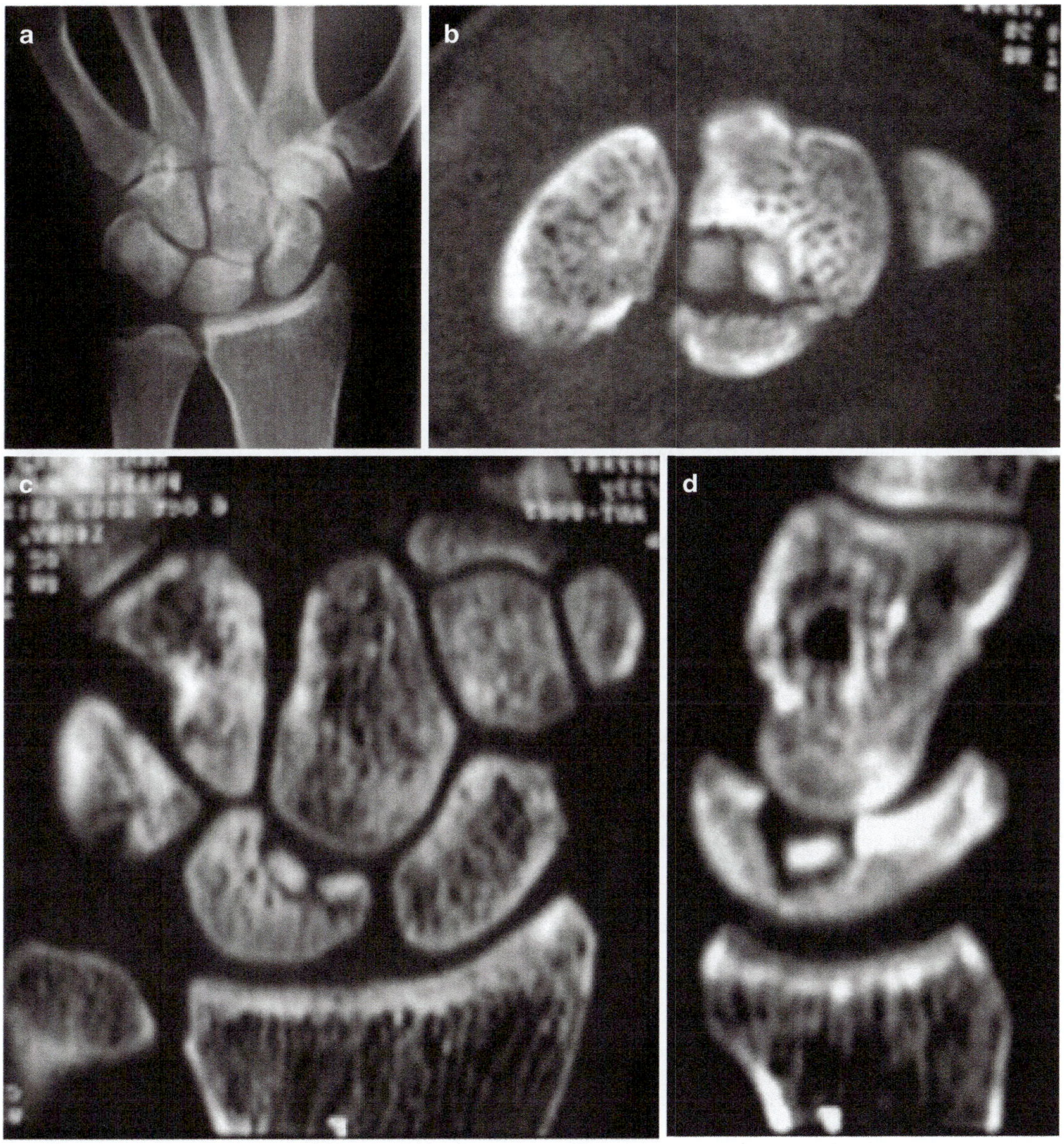

Fig. 3.10 Lunate fracture. The curvature of the lunate surfaces and position of the bone in the proximal row can obscure lunate body fractures on standard radiographs (**a**). CT clearly illustrates a lunate body fracture on axial, coronal, and sagittal views (**b**–**d**). (From Hand Clinics Marchessault 2009)

Table 3.1 Overview and highlights for the management of carpal fractures in the baseball player

Carpal fracture	Additional radiographic views	Treatment	Pitfalls
Triquetrum fractures	45° pronated oblique XR	*Dorsal chip*: short period of immobilization with repeat clinical and radiographic exam at 1–2-week intervals *Body fractures*: operative	Body fractures are associated with perilunate dislocations
Hamate fractures	CT in the "praying position"	Operative treatment	
Trapezium	Bett's view	*Nondisplaced*: cast for 4–6 weeks *Displaced*: operative	Be aware of first CMC dislocation
Capitate fractures	CT scan	*Nondisplaced*: cast for 4–6 weeks *Displaced fractures*: operative	Be aware of perilunate dislocation Retrograde blood supply – be aware of AVN
Trapezoid	Evaluate trapeziometacarpal joint	Operative	Be aware of high energy
Pisiform	Carpal tunnel review and reverse oblique view	*Nonoperative:* immobilization for 4–6 weeks Excision allows expedient return to play	
Lunate	Frequently need CT scan	*Marginal chip fractures*: short course of immobilization *Body fractures or associated DISI/VISI*: operative fixation	

Acknowledgment The authors would like to thank Jeffrey Marchessault, MD; Matt Conti, BS; and Mark E. Baratz, MD, for their prior article titled Carpal Fractures in Athletes Excluding the Scaphoid, which served as a useful guide and outline for the writing of this chapter.

References

1. Aiki H, Wada T, Yamashita T. Pisotriquetral arthrosis after triquetral malunion: a case report. J Hand Surg Am. 2006;31:1157–9.
2. Albertsen J, Mencke S, Christensen L, et al. Isolated capitate fracture diagnosed by computed tomography. Case report. Handchir Mikrochir Plast Chir. 1999;31:79–81.
3. Andresen R, Radmer S, Sparmann M, et al. Imaging of hamate bone fractures in conventional X-rays and high-resolution computed tomography: an in vitro study. Investig Radiol. 1999;34:46–50.
4. Bartone NF, Greico RV. Fractures of the triquetrum. J Bone Joint Surg. 1956;38:353–6.
5. Blomquist GA, Hunt TR III, Lopez-Ben RR. Isolated fractures of the trapezoid as a sports injury. Skelet Radiol. 2013;42(5):735–9. https://doi.org/10.1007/s00256-013-1581-z.
6. Bonnin JG, Greening WP. Fractures of the triquetrum. Br J Surg. 1944;31:278–83.
7. Boulas HJ, Milek MA. Hook of the hamate fractures. Orthop Rev. 1990;19(6):518–22.
8. Bryan RS, Dobyns JH. Fractures of the carpal bones other than the lunate and navicular. Clin Orthop Relat Res. 1980;14:107–11.
9. Calandruccio JH, Duncan SF. Isolated non- displaced capitate waist fracture diagnosed by magnetic resonance imaging. J Hand Surg Am. 1999;24:856–9.
10. Cordrey LJ, Ferror-Torrells M. Management of fractures of the greater multangular. J Bone Joint Surg Am. 1960;42:1111–8.
11. Culp RW, Lemel M, Taras JS. Complications of common carpal injuries. Hand Clin. 1994;10(1):139–55.
12. DeBeer JD, Hudson DA. Fractures of the triquetrum. J Hand Surg Br. 1987;12:52–3.
13. Fairbank TJ. Chip fractures of the os triquetrum. Br Med J. 1942;2:310–1.
14. Garcia-Elias M. Dorsal fractures of the triquetrum—avulsion or compression fractures? J Hand Surg Am. 1987;12:266–8.
15. Garcia-Elias M. Chapter 36. Fractures of the carpal bones with exception of scaphoid. In: Injuries of elbow, forearm, wrist, and hand, vol. 27. Madrid (Spain): Editor Mapfre; 1987. p. 459–76.
16. Garcia-Elias M. Carpal bone fractures (excluding scaphoid fractures). In: Watson HK, Weinberg J, editors. The wrist. Philadelphia: Lippincott Williams & Wilkins; 2001. p. 174–81.
17. Garcia-Elias M, Henriquez-Lluch A, Rossignani P, et al. Bennett's fracture combined with fracture of the

trapezium. A report of three cases. J Hand Surg Br. 1993;18:523–6.
18. Geissler WB. Carpal fractures in athletes. Clin Sports Med. 2001;20(1):167–88.
19. Gelberman RH, Panagis JS, Taleisnik J, et al. The arterial anatomy of the human carpus. Part I: the extraosseous vascularity. J Hand Surg Am. 1983;8:367–75.
20. Greening WP. Isolated fracture of the carpal cuneiform. Br Med J. 1942;1:221–2.
21. Hocker K, Menschik A. Chip fractures of the triquetrum. J Hand Surg Br. 1994;19:584–8.
22. Kato H, Nakamura R, Horii E, et al. Diagnostic imaging for fracture of the hook of the hamate. Hand Surg. 2000;5(1):19–24.
23. Levy M, Fischel RE, Stern GM, et al. Chip fractures of the os triquetrum. The mechanism of injury. J Bone Joint Surg Br. 1979;61:355–7.
24. Marchessault J, Baratz C. Carpal fractures in athletes excluding the scaphoid. Hand Clin. 2009;25:371–88.
25. Mayfield JK, Johnson RB, Kilcoyne RK. Carpal dislocations: pathomechanics and progressive perilunar instability. J Hand Surg Am. 1980;5:226–41.
26. McClain EJ, Boyes JH. Missed fractures of the greater multangular. J Bone Joint Surg Am. 1966;48:1525–8.
27. McGuigan FX, Culp RW. Surgical treatment of intraarticular fractures of the trapezium. J Hand Surg Am. 2002;27:697–703.
28. Milch H. Fracture of the hamate bone. J Bone Joint Surg. 1934;16:459.
29. Miyawaki T, Kobayashi M, Matsuura S, Yanagawa H, Imai T, Kurihana K. Trapezoid bone fracture. Ann Plast Surg. 2000;44:444–6.
30. Nagumo A, Toh S, Tsubo K, Ishibashi Y, Sasaki T. An occult fracture of the trapezoid bone. J Bone Joint Surg. 2002;84-A(6):1025–7.
31. Nammour M, Desai B, Warren M, Godshaw B. Approach to isolated trapezoid fractures. Ochsner J. 2019;19:271–5.
32. Nisenfield FG, Neviaser RJ. Fracture of the hook of hamate: a diagnosis easily missed. J Trauma. 1974;14(7):612–6.
33. O'Shea K, Weiland AJ. Fractures of the hamate and pisiform bone. Hand Clin. 2012;28:287–300.
34. Palmer AK. Trapezial ridge fractures. J Hand Surg Am. 1981;6:561–4.
35. Pointu J, Schwenck JP, Destree G, et al. Fractures of the trapezium. Mechanism, pathology and indications for treatment. French J Orthop Surg. 1988;2:380–91.
36. Porter ML, Seehra K. Fracture-dislocation of the triquetrum treated with a Herbert screw. J Bone Joint Surg Br. 1991;73:347–8.
37. Pruzansky M, Arnold L. Delayed union fractures of the trapezoid and body of the hamate. Orthop Rev. 1987;16:624–8.
38. Rhee PC, Camp CL, D'Angelo J, Desai VS, Shin SS, Sheridan D, Conte S. Epidemiology and impact of hand and wrist injuries in major and minor league baseball. Hand (N Y). 2019:1–7. https://doi.org/10.1177/1558944719864450.
39. Smith DK, Murray PM. Avulsion fractures of the volar aspect of triquetral bone of the wrist: a subtle sign of carpal ligament injury. AJR Am J Roentgenol. 1996;166(3):609e614.
40. Suh N, Ek ET, Wolfe SW. Carpal fractures. J Hand Surg. 2014;39:785–91.
41. Suzuki T, Nakatsuchi Y, Tatweiwa Y, et al. Osteochondral fracture of the triquetrum: a case report. J Hand Surg Am. 2002;27:98–100.
42. Teisen H, Hjarbaek J. Classification of fresh fractures of the lunate. J Hand Surg Br. 1988;13:458–62.
43. Teisen H, Hjarbaek J, Jensen EK. Follow-up investigation of fresh lunate bone fracture. Handchir Mikrochir Plast Chir. 1990;22:20–2.
44. Terrono A, Ferenz CC, Nalebuff EA. Delayed diagnosis in non-union of the body of the hamate: a case report. J Hand Surg Br. 1989;14(3):329–31.
45. Vander Grend R, Dell PC, Glowczewskie F, et al. Intraosseous blood supply of the capitate and its correlation with aseptic necrosis. J Hand Surg Am. 1984;9:677–80.
46. Vigler M, Aviles A, Lee SK. Carpal fractures excluding the scaphoid. Hand Clin. 2006;22:501–16.
47. Watanabe H, Hamada Y, Yamamoto Y. A case of old trapezoid fracture. Arch Orthop Trauma Surg. 1999;119:356–7.
48. Wolfe SW, Hotchkiss RN, Pederson WC, Kozin SH. Green's operative hand surgery. 6th ed. Philadelphia: Elsevier/Churchill Livingstone; 2011. p. 680–704.
49. Wulff RN, Schmidt TL. Carpal fractures in children. J Pediatr Orthop. 1998;18:462–5.
50. Yasuwaki Y, Nagata Y, Yamamoto T, Nakano A, Kikuchi H, Tanaka S. Fracture of the trapezoid bone: a case report. J Hand Surg [Am]. 1994;19:457–9.

Hook of the Hamate Fractures

4

Timothy B. Griffith and Gary M. Lourie

Introduction

Fractures involving the hook of the hamate represent only 2–4% of carpal fractures, following the scaphoid, triquetrum, and trapezium in order of frequency [1]. However, delay in diagnosis and ultimate treatment can lead to significant morbidity. This is apparent in baseball where its concentrated higher incidence and deleterious impact on return to play can pose serious consequences. Recent studies support this finding. Camp, in a report on the top 50 injuries seen in professional baseball presented at the 2018 MLB Winter Meetings, found that fractures of the hook of the hamate were found in the top ten and encompassed a significant stay on the Injured List (IL) [2]. Rhee et al. similarly found in their epidemiological study that hook fractures represented 72% of wrist fractures and significant time on the Injured List [3]. Clearly, a finer comprehension of the fracture of the hook of the hamate emphasizing earlier diagnosis and more expedient treatment, along with optimum rehabilitation and possible better prevention, may affect the overall morbidity of this injury [4]. The purpose of this chapter is to describe the incidence of the fracture of the hook of hamate in baseball, the pertinent clinical anatomy, the mechanism of injury, history and differential diagnosis, the exam, imaging including advanced studies when applicable, treatment, post-injury rehabilitation, complications, and/or adverse results, along with a protocol for early return to play with minimal risk.

T. B. Griffith
Peachtree Orthopedic Clinic, Atlanta, GA, USA
e-mail: tgriffith@pocatlanta.com

G. M. Lourie (✉)
The Hand and Upper Extremity Center of Georgia, Atlanta, GA, USA

G. M. Lourie (ed.), *Hand and Wrist Injuries in Baseball*,
https://doi.org/10.1007/978-3-030-81659-9_4

Incidence of Fractures of the Hook of the Hamate

The reported incidence of the hamate fracture in the general population ranges between 2% and 4%, ranking far behind the scaphoid. It is difficult to determine the exact incidence in baseball, though believed to be higher, due to reporting inadequacies, missed diagnoses, and as a recent publication cited a higher incidence in certain cultural batting grips; however, recent reports have helped delineate its heightened occurrence and potential morbidity [5]. The hook versus body fracture of the hamate remains the more common presentation in racquet sports such as tennis and even more so in two-handed sports such as baseball where the nondominant hand that approximates the knob or end of the bat is subjected to significant force. Camp et al. reported on the top 50 injuries in professional baseball, citing hook fractures of the hamate in the top ten injuries localized to the wrist and hand and emphasizing its prolonged time on the IL

(53 days) [2]. Rhee et al. reported a 72% incidence of the hook fracture in professional baseball players when compared to other carpal fractures, far more common than the scaphoid fracture seen in the general population. Mean days missed averaged over 50 days [3]. This number carries even more significance when one acknowledges the 50-day Injured List is seen in professional baseball where our athletic trainers are keenly aware of this injury and the need for expedient diagnosis and treatment. In the senior author's (GML) experience with the Atlanta Braves, the 40–50-day return to play with the hook of hamate fracture compares favorably to the average 126 days seen in community referrals due to delay in diagnosis and even further delay in referral to the hand surgeon for definitive treatment [6].

In summary, the incidence of the hook fracture in the baseball player may be more than the 2–4% incidence seen in the general population; however, what is certain is that it carries a higher occupational morbidity in this specific cohort and this chapter will highlight those important aspects.

Clinical Anatomy

The casual observer would believe the hook of the hamate to be a small insignificant fragment; textbooks described it as a long sliver of bone that arises from the body of the hamate, measures 1 by 3 cm, and projects into the palm 1–2 cm distal and lateral to the pisiform. It can be found topographically in two ways described in the literature. Wright credited Kaplan, using his cardinal line (Kaplan's cardinal line), drawn from the pisiform to the proximal aspect of the thumb web space. Where this line bisects a line dropped from the ulnar aspect of the ring finger corresponds to the tip of the hook [7]. Carter, in a more simplified manner, described where the examiner places his or her interphalangeal joint of the thumb over the pisiform and flexes the thumb in a line directed to the index finger metacarpal head. Where the tip of the examiner's thumb strikes the patients palm corresponds to the tip of the hook [8].

General texts describe the hook submerged beneath the skin, subcutaneous fat, and the palmaris brevis muscle [8]. That description is inaccurate, as the hook is connected to strategic structures very close to vital neurovascular structures that if iatrogenically damaged can have catastrophic consequences (Fig. 4.1). Further, this area is often the location of many anatomic variants involving the hypothenar muscles, the ulnar nerve, and the ulnar artery. Stark likened the hook to the mast of a ship being anchored by the attachment of the pisohamate ligament, the flexor, and the opponens digiti quinti, along with the transverse carpal ligament [9]. These four structures act like stays for the mast, stabilizing the hook, but when fractured can theoretically distract the fractured hook impairing osseous healing. When the hook is intact, it serves as a pulley or trochlea for the small and ring flexors which pass around its radial border, exiting the carpal tunnel and traveling obliquely across the palm to their respective attachments (Fig. 4.2). Three clinical findings emphasize this anatomic landmark and its potential advantage. First, the hook of the hamate pull test described by Wright utilizes this close proximity of the two structures

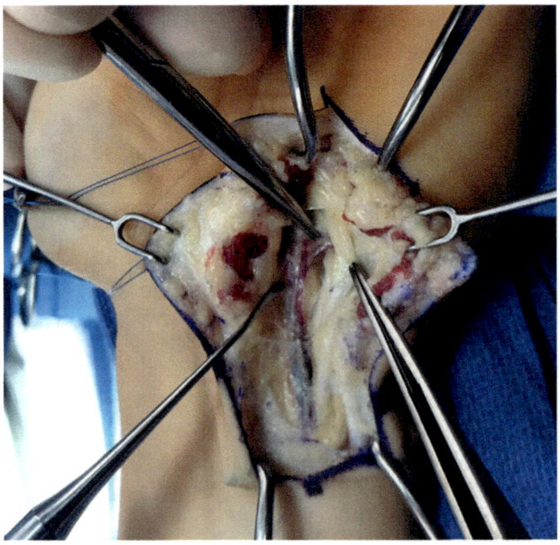

Fig. 4.1 Intraoperative photograph Guyon's canal (ulnar tunnel) revealing rich anatomical region

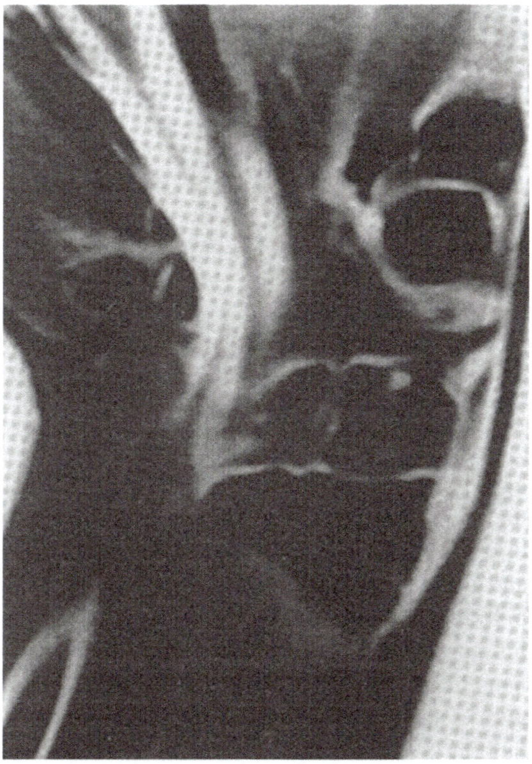

Fig. 4.2 MRI demonstrating flexor tendons arching around the hamate which serves a pulley

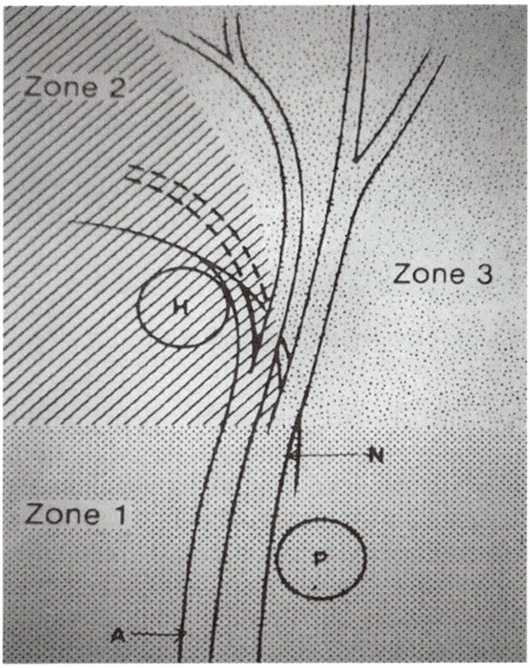

Fig. 4.3 Illustration of Guyon's canal

to confirm a fractured hook [10]. Second, the documented incidence of attritional flexor tendon ruptures seen in untreated hook nonunion serves to accentuate this intimate anatomic relationship. Milek reported on a 17% flexor tendon rupture in untreated nonunion of the hook due to the close proximity of these structures [11]. Lastly, Calandruccio in a cadaveric study created a model to simulate flexor tendon forces with and without the hook present and found theoretic advantage in preserving the hook to optimize its pulley function and increase flexor efficiency [12]. Though this was an in vitro study and most surgeons advocate excision of the hook with fracture, it does reinforce the intimate relationship between the hook and the ulnar flexors.

The flexors traverse the radial aspect of the hook being housed in the carpal tunnel. The ulnar border of the hook is attached to the pisohamate ligament, representing the distal aspect and the floor of Guyon's canal also referred to as the ulnar tunnel and is the location of the ulnar neurovascular structures. The floor of Guyon's canal is formed by the pisohamate ligament along with the transverse carpal ligament, while the roof is formed by the palmaris brevis and more proximal the volar carpal ligament. The proximal and distal boundaries are the pisiform and hook of the hamate, respectively (Fig. 4.3). The ulnar neurovascular structures; the ulnar artery and nerve traverse the canal in the acronym relationship "ANT," from lateral to medial, the artery, the nerve, and the tendon of the flexor carpi ulnaris in that order. It is important for the surgeon to be well versed with the classic anatomy along with common variants that if not recognized can result in iatrogenic damage. Classic description usually has the ulnar nerve bifurcating in the canal with the deep motor branch traversing around the hook to dive deep into a muscle hiatus formed by the flexor and opponens digit quinti. The superficial branch, still close to the tip, continues into the palm to give sensation to the ulnar digits. The ulnar artery also bifurcates in the canal with the superficial branch contributing to the superficial arch, the main supply to the hand through its digi-

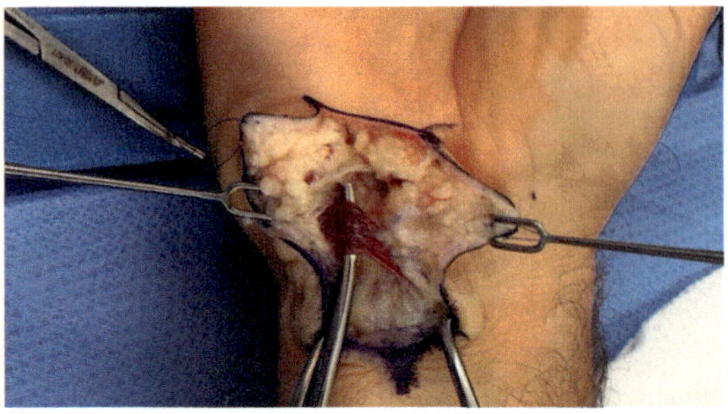

Fig. 4.4 Accessory abductor digiti minimi

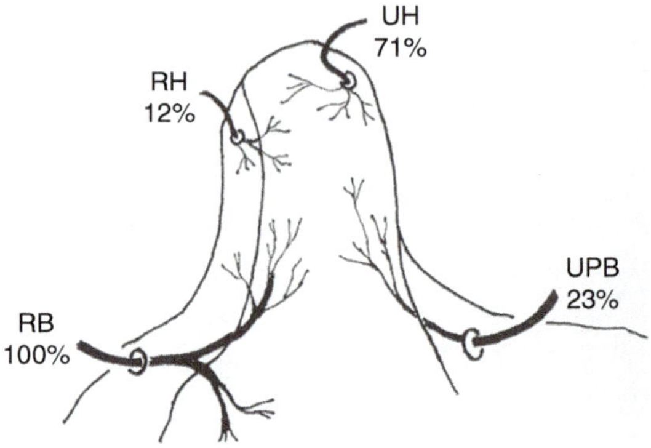

Fig. 4.5 Vascular foramina hamate hook (Failla, MD)

tal arterial branches. The deep branch accompanies the deep motor branch and usually keeps to its radial (lateral) position, though Levina described a case where the deep arterial branch coursed volar and ulnar to the nerve creating a "noose" that with exercise and effort related dilatation of the artery compressing and creating an exertional ulnar nerve dysfunction that resolved at rest [13]. Other important anatomic variations of the canal have been described. The motor branch, usually located deep and ulnar to the hook, can rarely give off a radial branch creating a neural loop as described by Rogers et al. [14]. Further variation in Guyon's canal involving muscular structures can occur up to 22.4% of the time most commonly being represented by an accessory abductor digit quinti that can course through the canal volar to the neurovascular structures [15] (Fig. 4.4). The surgeon operating in this area should familiarize him or herself with these anatomic variations. Finally, the intraosseous blood supply to the hook has been described by Failla and holds clinical implications [16]. In a cadaver study, he found that the radial base foramina are large and consistent, whereas the ulnar tip foramina were absent nearly 30% of the time creating a watershed area leaving the fracture fragment prone to avascular changes and probable nonunion (Fig. 4.5).

Mechanism of Injury

The mechanism of injury of the hook fracture in the baseball player is similar to other racquet sports and involves the direct traumatic contact of the knob of the bat to the volar ulnar base of the palm, the location of the hook. In baseball, this is typically the nondominant or bottom hand and usually occurs with a checked swing on a high inside pitch, though some give a history of lunging for a low outside pitch [17]. The dominant hand may rarely be involved and occurs with a fall on the outstretched hand, seen in fielding a hit ball or in an errant slide into the base. This mechanism is different than the direct impact of the bat on a misdirected swing and is due to an indirect mechanism with the fracture due to an avulsion imparted by the transverse carpal ligament onto the bone. The senior author (GML), noting in the Atlanta Braves organization a higher incidence of hook fractures in Latin players, observed the characteristic grip displayed more often in these players, that being the knob of the bat held in the hand (palm) rather than the more conventional grip which places the knob on the ulnar border of the hand (Figs. 4.6 and 4.7). We hypothesized that this grip termed the "palmar hamate grip" has the potential to place significant forces on the hook predisposing it to fracture. This theory was tested in our recent study comparing forces on the hook with pressure-sensitive monitors between the palmar hamate grip and the conventional grip. Striking results were found with the palmar hamate group demonstrating a 335% increase in force on the sensor overlying the hook of the hamate when compared to the conventional grip [5]. These findings deserve notice and will be discussed in later sections.

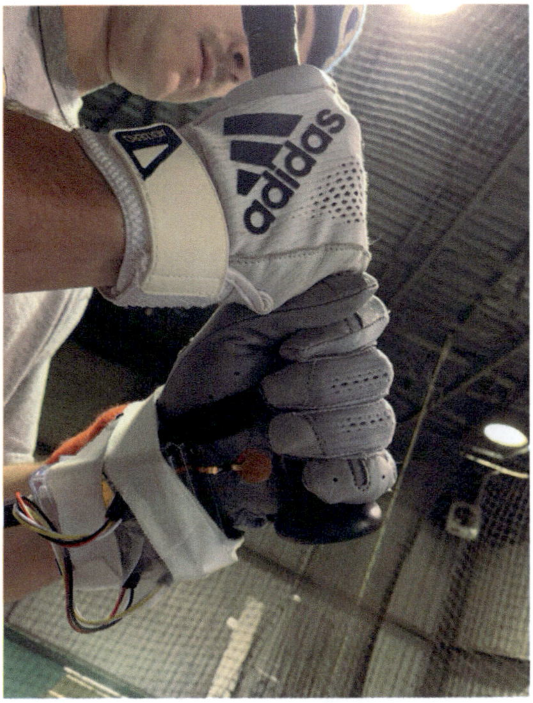

Fig. 4.6 Conventional batting grip, the knob on the ulnar border of the palm

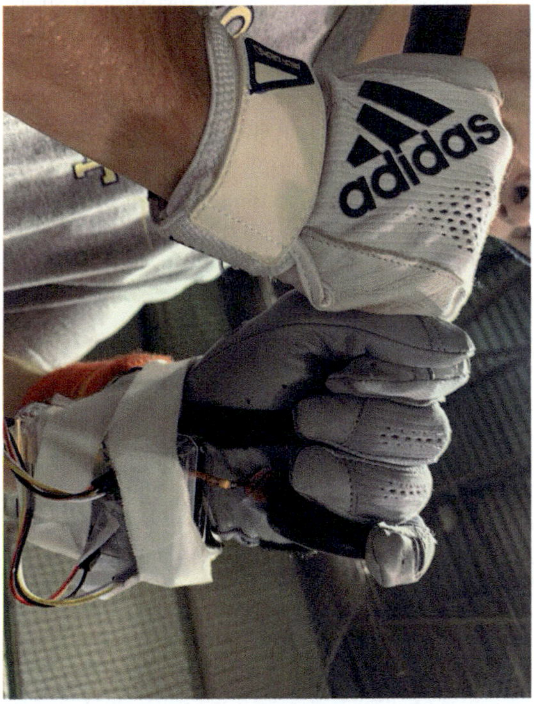

Fig. 4.7 Palmar hamate grip, the knob is situated in the palm directly over the hook of the hamate

History

Players presenting with the hook fracture may present in an acute or less often a more chronic, insidious presentation. The majority of the time, the player will recall an awkward swing involving the nondominant or bottom hand. In the acute setting with displacement of the fracture, the player may experience numbness in the ring and small finger due to the close proximity of the hook to the ulnar nerve. Similarly, the close location of the ring and small flexors to the fracture may cause the player to present with weakness in flexion and in some cases actual rupture of the tendon.

The player will describe a vague, deep aching pain in the volar ulnar palm. In many players, especially players who use the palmar hamate grip, the pain will be located to an often large calloused area where the knob of the bat is held. The discomfort is very often not present at rest or even low-impact activities, but grasping the bat or maximal flexing of the ring and small finger will exacerbate the symptoms. In players in which the fracture is located at the base of the hook where it attaches to the body of the hamate, the described pain may be located to the dorsal ulnar aspect of the hand very close to the base of the small finger metacarpal which can confuse the trainer and clinician. Many of these symptoms form the basis for the specialized parts of the exam that are important to understand and help to solidify the diagnosis.

Physical Exam

The exam for the player suspected of a hook of the hamate fracture follows similar orthopedic principles for any bony injury. Inspection and palpation, along with neurovascular assessment and special testing, make up the basic assessment. In viewing the palm, often a callous can be seen in the player using the palmar hamate grip especially if the player describes this area as the site of maximal tenderness. If the fracture is acute, swelling and ecchymosis can be seen in the palmar ulnar aspect of the hand over the hook. If the injury is chronic, injuries to neighboring structures due to progressive attrition or compression may be apparent on inspection. Loss of the normal cascade of the digits at rest may signal flexor tendon injury or even rupture [11]. Pallor or cyanosis of the digits may denote vascular injury due to the unstable hook compressing the artery and/or vein. Dryness or loss of sweating in the ulnar two digits could signify sensory nerve injury, and atrophy of the hypothenar muscles can occur with injury to the motor branch of the ulnar nerve.

Palpation is the next part of the exam. Tenderness to palpation of the hook in the palm is suggestive of its fracture. Topographic location of the hook is confirmed by placing the examiner's thumb interphalangeal joint on the pisiform in the palm in a line pointed toward the index finger metacarpal head [8] (Fig. 4.8). The pulp of the examiner's thumb will now be on the tip of the hook of the hamate. The hook is usually 1.5–3 centimeters distal to the pisiform. Carter and others have also recommended assessing for pain to palpation over the dorsal and medial border of the hamate as a fracture of the base of the hook can be far tenderer in this location rather than the palm [8]. This finding can also confuse the clinician and miss the diagnosis of hook fracture thinking the injury to be a ring or small metacarpal injury.

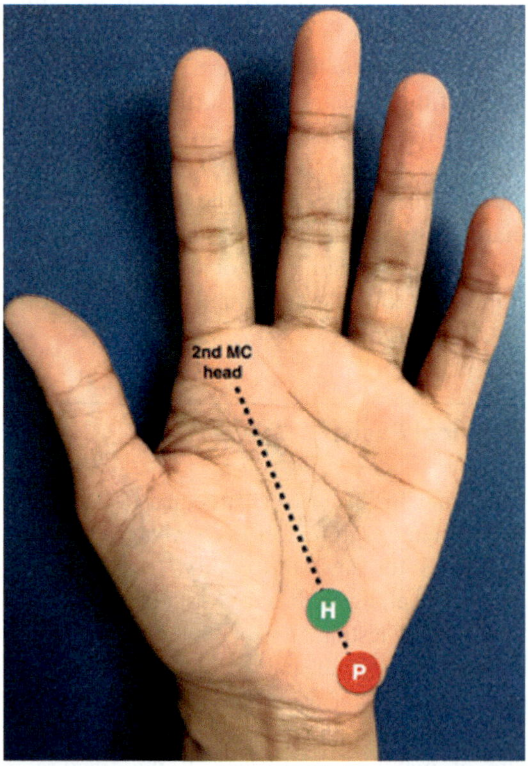

Fig. 4.8 Palpation of the hook topographic location

The hook of the hamate pull test, a specialized test described by Wright, is very accurate in confirming fracture of the hook [10]. The examiner places the injured hand in ulnar deviation and resists the flexion of the ring and small finger. Pain in this maneuver is both highly sensitive and specific for fracture (Fig. 4.9). The ulnar deviation of the wrist places the flexors close to the fractured hook causing pain with resistance. It is why the clinician should assess flexion of the two ulnar digits as part of the exam as there is a 17% flexor rupture rate due to the displaced hook fracture causing attritional injury [11]. The exam is completed with vascular assessment of the digits utilizing Allen's test, which assesses the patency of the arterial structures perfusing the hand. This is due to the close proximity of the fractured hook to the ulnar artery and the rare, but possible, thrombosis of the vessel. Assessment of ulnar nerve function assessing intrinsic muscle strength along with sensation to the two ulnar digits is recommended, again due to potential nerve compression from the hook fracture.

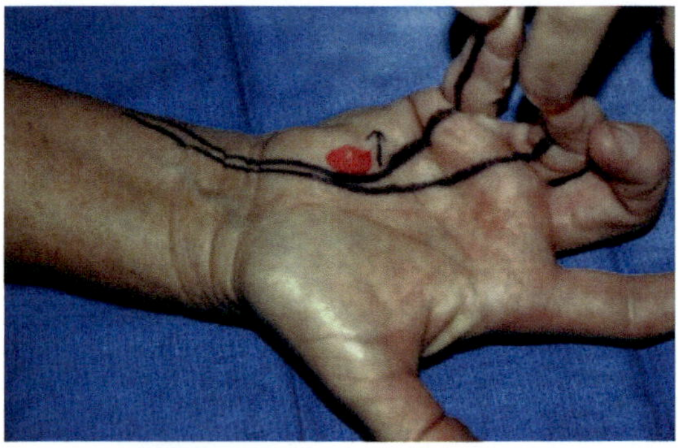

Fig. 4.9 Hook of the hamate pull test

Radiographs/Advanced Imaging

With a tentative diagnosis of hook fracture, standard x-rays are first ordered. A posteroanterior (PA), lateral, and oblique view will usually not show the hook fracture but are useful to rule out any other bony injury. A carpal tunnel view (picture) may show the hook of the hamate, but the injured player with pain and swelling often is unable to position the wrist in adequate extension to profile the hook (Fig. 4.10). Papilion described a useful radiographic view, termed the semi-supine oblique view that can reliably show the fracture [18]. The hand is positioned in radial deviation, thumb palmar abduction, and slight supination and if done properly will show the hook fracture reliably (Fig. 4.11). The gold standard, however, remains the CT scan, and the best projection is an axial cut with both hands positioned together in the "prayer position" [19] (Fig. 4.12). This allows the uninjured hand to be used as a comparison. Finally, an MRI scan may show the fractured hook, and though the CT scan is more specific, the MRI may be beneficial in ruling out other soft-tissue injuries.

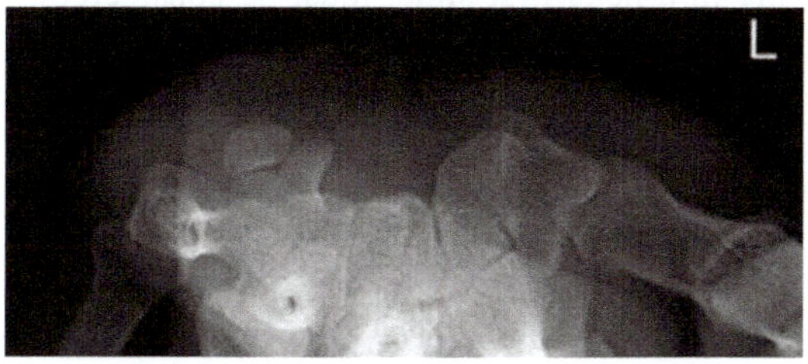

Fig. 4.10 Radiograph carpal tunnel view

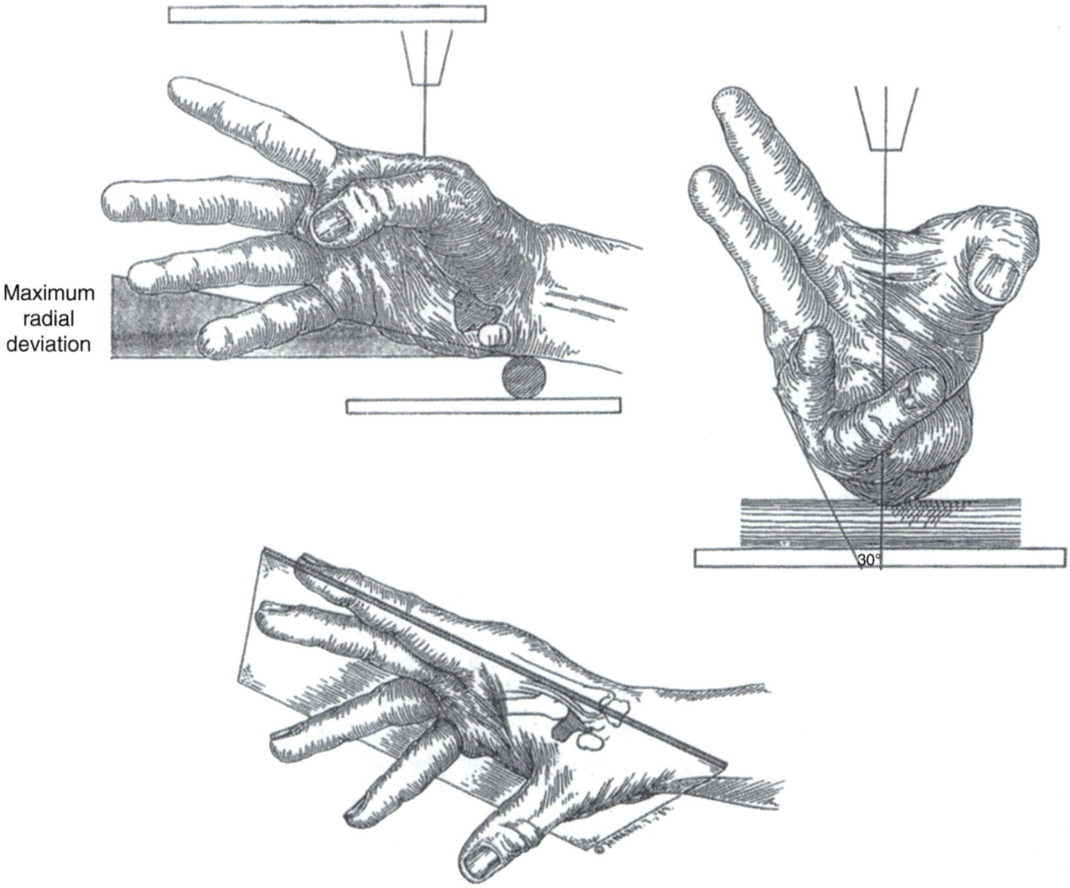

Fig. 4.11 Papilion semi-supine oblique view

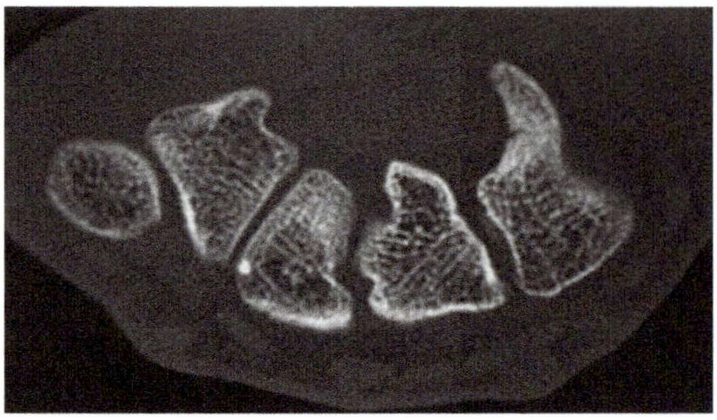

Fig. 4.12 Gold standard CT axial prayer position

Differential Diagnosis

The differential diagnosis of the hook fracture involves consideration of the other causes of ulnar-sided wrist pain. Most of these diagnoses are covered in this book; however, ulnar-sided wrist pain can be a challenge, so a brief mention of other causes is warranted. Injuries to the triangular fibrocartilage complex (TFCC) often involve the nondominant hand in the baseball player and need to be ruled out. Though the mechanism of injury may be similar, the TFCC injury usually presents with pain on wrist rotation and the tenderness is over the medial ulnar aspect of the wrist. Injuries to the lunotriquetral ligament can mimic the hook fracture, but the tenderness usually is dorsal-ulnar over the ligament. Triquetral hamate impaction syndrome, also described in the bottom nondominant hand, usually presents with tenderness over this joint and is exacerbated with passive dorsiflexion and ulnar deviation on exam [20]. Tendinitis involving the flexor carpi ulnaris (FCU) can be a source of injury but usually is repetitive in its onset, with tenderness evoked over the tendon in the volar-ulnar aspect of the forearm. The pisiform bone, because of its sesamoid nature, sits within the FCU and articulates with the triquetrum (pisotriquetral joint), and injuries to this complex can result in chondral injury. A recent report described an MLB player with locking of this joint due to a loose body, and its close proximity to the hook of the hamate makes its existence important in the differential diagnosis [21]. These injuries are usually situated on the volar and medial aspect of the wrist. However, as a fracture of the base of the hook may simulate a dorsal wrist injury as described by Carter, it is imperative that the surgeon or the trainer rule out injury to the extensor carpi ulnaris (ECU), which can present as tendinitis, or if injury to the subsheath occurs, subluxation may be present [8, 22]. Finally, fractures of the fifth metacarpal, because of their close proximity to the hook, need to be ruled out. Similarly, dorsal triquetral avulsion fractures, often occurring in a head first slide, must be considered in the ballplayer presenting with injury in this region.

Treatment (Conservative Versus Surgical)

With a diagnosis of a hook fracture, confirmed treatment commences. Most hand surgeons associated with baseball opt for the time-proven surgical procedure of removal of the fractured hook as the definitive treatment, but this procedure is not without adverse results, so limited support for other options exist. Bishop reported on eight patients seen with hook fractures of which greater than 90% healed with immobilization for 6 weeks in a short arm cast incorporating the ring and small fingers [23]. They advocated this treatment for acute nondisplaced fractures; however, none of the reported patients were baseball players where significant forces are imparted on the hook pre and post injury [23]. Other authors have not been able to replicate these results, but Triplet felt that higher success could be achieved in cast treatment by incorporating the thumb in the cast [24]. They showed in a cadaveric study that immobilizing the thumb in a simulated hook fracture could increase stability by negating the deforming forces of the transverse carpal ligament on the base of the hook where it attaches. Fujioka suggested that the use of low invasive pulsed ultrasound stimulation could possibly accelerate the rate of healing of the hook, though this was a case report only [25]. Most hand surgeons feel that in the high demand patient, specifically the baseball player, that surgical excision is the treatment of choice to return the player to pre-injury levels of success. There are, however, a few reports that advocate fixation of the fracture hook rather than excision, citing the potential retention of the hook to serve as a pulley for the flexors. Open reduction and internal fixation was proposed by Watson and Cecarelli in separate publications [26, 27]. Calandruccio confirmed this theoretical advantage in a cadaveric study which showed the biomechanical increased flexor strength advantage in retention of the hook compared to the unretained hook [12]. Despite these small studies and biomechanical support, internal fixation has not gained support in the treatment of the ballplayer with a fractured hook of the hamate. The gold standard remains excision of the hook. Many studies support this recommendation [4, 7–9, 28–31].

Successful surgical excision of the hook demands a thorough knowledge of the clinical anatomy found in this area. One would think excision is a simple procedure, but the close proximity of the ulnar nerve, specifically the deep motor branch and the ulnar artery, make this procedure complex. In addition, being aware of the significant variation in neurovascular and muscular structures can help avoid iatrogenic damage and adverse results. We have used an incision that adequately identifies and protects the ulnar nerve and artery found in Guyon's canal [32, 33] (Fig. 4.13). The procedure is done under a tourniquet to allow for hemostasis and better visualization. Next, we identify the piso-hamate ligament and trace its insertion to the hook. Intraoperative radiographic confirmation of the hook allows the surgeon to now carefully remove the hook in a subperiosteal fashion [29]. Others have recommended an extraperiosteal removal [7]. Gentle retraction of the deep motor branch is necessary, and with removal of the hook, the remaining bone is smoothened to avoid tendon fraying. The flexor tendons are visualized in the carpal canal and assessed for fraying or rupture. Intraoperative radiographic confirmation of hook removal is advocated by the senior surgeon for official records. The Papilion view described earlier in this chapter will show the pre- and postoperative removal accurately [18] (Figs. 4.14 and 4.15). The hook is photographed as part of the permanent record (Fig. 4.16). This recommended technique used by the senior surgeon has helped to avoid adverse results and complications in over 75 surgeries. Jones has

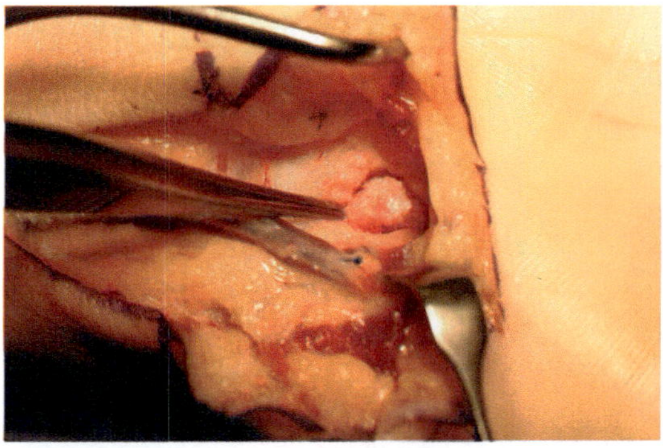

Fig. 4.13 Intraoperative view demonstrating the close proximity of the hook to the neurovascular structures

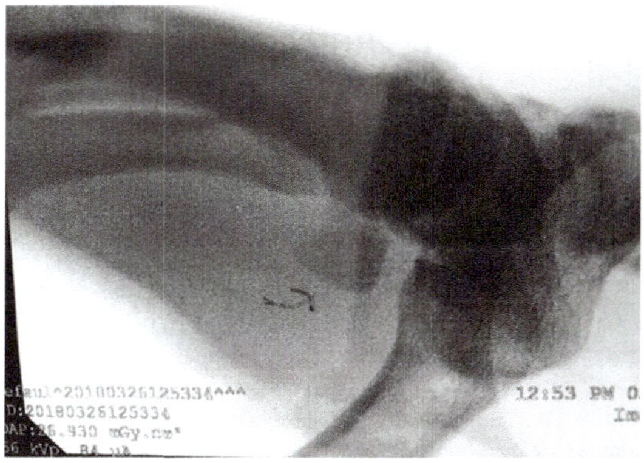

Fig. 4.14 Papilion view preoperatively showing the fractured hook

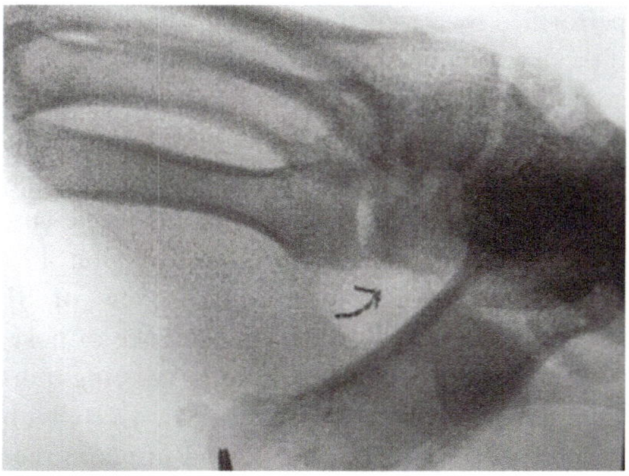

Fig. 4.15 Papilion view postoperatively confirming adequate excision of the hook

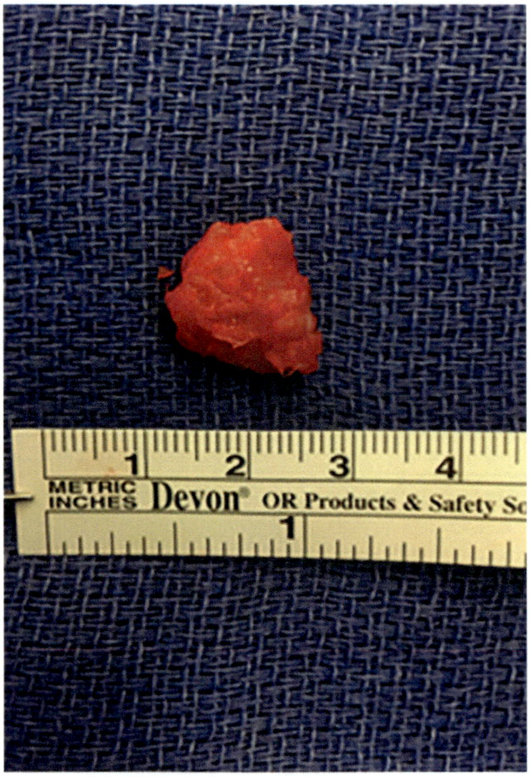

Fig. 4.16 The hook after its excision

described this method in his publication and is a useful resource for the hand surgeon [32]. The excision of the hook of the hamate should be performed by a well-trained hand surgeon. Even if these recommendations are followed carefully, complications and adverse results can occur. Wright in a survey of hand surgeons reported a 3% rate of complications, all due to nerve or vascular injury and all thought to be due to the surgical exposure rather than the excision [7]. Goldfarb in another exhaustive review of 81 patients reported up to a 25% incidence of postoperative complications, the majority being transient ulnar nerve neuropraxia [34]. Even with these reported findings, most hand surgeons recommend excision of the hook once the diagnosis is made. This applies for both acute, subacute, and established nonunion. The senior author has reported on a rare hook fracture presentation, in which the fracture is incomplete, usually the fracture line based radially with sclerosis seen ulnarly at the base suggesting attempted healing or even a stress injury [35]. Though many have advocated a wait and see approach, our series along with one by Zemel recommends early excision in the high demand athlete to allow for earlier return to play due to the high rate of failure with conservative treatment [36].

Our postoperative protocol involves a short arm cast for 3 weeks followed by a removable splint and initiation of scar massage as the tender scar in this regions seems to be the biggest impediment to sport-specific rehabilitation. This important protocol is covered in the last chapter of this book written by our Atlanta Brave's trainer. Their input and skill is crucial to the success of returning the player to the field. Range of motion is commenced at 3 weeks followed by strengthening. When 85% of contralateral grip strength is achieved, a gradual hitting sequence is initiated with most, but not all, studies reporting return to play at 6–8 weeks.

Results

Earlier studies reported a high level of satisfaction and equally high return to level of play equal or better than pre-injury status. In the 1970s through the 1980s, Stark et al. along with Carter et al. reported on a mixed cohort of patients not exclusive to baseball, but with successful return to pre-injury activity in the majority of patients [8, 9]. The data in these studies was very limited and scant follow-up given. Bishop et al. published on a more thorough series in the 1980s and again showed with limited follow-up greater than 90% return to pre-injury athletic status [31]. Little mention of adverse results or residual symptoms was reported in these earlier reports. More recent studies by Wiekert, Shin, and Osterman reported on 60 athletes, the majority baseball players [28–30]. This combined cohort showed high satisfaction rate and successful return at 6–8 weeks to a level similar to pre-injury status with improved DASH scores. Of the 60 players, there were only three reported adverse results, two patients with scar sensitivity and one with transient ulnar nerve sensory findings, all which resolved at final follow-up. The excellent results of these earlier studies have been tempered by three recent publications. Wright et al., in their review, reported a 3% complication rate including injury to the ulnar nerve, the superficial arch, and the median nerve [7]. The authors felt these findings were due more to the exposure than the actual excision, but regardless of cause, this only highlights the complexity of this surgery and the need for experienced knowledge of this region. Bansal et al. echoed these findings in a more recent exhaustive review of 81 patients, of which more than half were baseball players [34]. Though the median return to play was 6 weeks, 11 patients (14%) did not return until 12 weeks or later. Twelve patients (15%) with documented full recovery continued to describe continued intermittent discomfort in the affected hand. The authors further described a 25% incidence of postoperative complications with the majority being ulnar nerve dysfunction. Erickson et al., in the most complete study to date, further supported the more sobering findings reported by Bansal [17, 34]. In a study dedicated to only baseball players and more specifically professional players, 261 players undergoing hook excision between 2010 and 2017 were analyzed using the MLB Health and Injury Tracking System (HITS) database [17]. This study is the first to provide data on player performance after excision of the hook of the hamate. The median return to play was 7 weeks, which is similar to smaller studies, though 81% returned to sport at the previous level, 3% returned to a lower level, and 16% did not return. In evaluating player performance, player utilization significantly increased after surgery, but player efficiency, including batting average (BA), on-base percentage (OBP), and on-base plus slugging percentage (OPS), all significantly decreased. These findings must be tempered when compared to earlier studies which paint a much more optimistic picture. The authors still recommend the excision of the hook in the high-level baseball player, but moving forward perhaps hand surgeons and trainers can affect both the prevalence and the consequences of this injury.

Prevention/Management Optimization

Though in the general population, the hook of the hamate fracture is rare, we have shown its higher occurrence in baseball players and with that a higher morbidity rate. To reduce this morbidity, working on better ways to prevent this fracture outright and lessen time to diagnosis and treatment may better affect this experience. The mechanism of injury in the hook fracture involves the knob of the bat in the nondominant or bottom hand being driven into the palm, usually in an awkward swing, causing the injury. In our Atlanta Braves experience, we have documented in the palmar hamate grip, in which the knob of the bat is actually in the palm rather than outside the palm on the ulnar border of the hand, that the rate of hook fracture is much higher. Further in our studies in measuring this force of the knob with pressure-sensitive sensors in the two different grips, we found a dramatic 4–5× greater PSI (pounds/square inch) with the palmar hamate than the conventional grip [5]. We have sought to counsel our players with this grip in hopes of changing to the conventional one. Most of our players who enjoy this grip remain resistant to a change, but perhaps imparting this knowledge to coaches managing younger players may make an impact. In players who will not make the change, possibly adding a pad to this area in the batting glove may help lessen the chance of fracture. A recent new bat, the Axe Bat™ (AXEBAT US, Kent, Washington), has a redesigned handle similar to an axe that theoretically reduces the force imparted to the hook of the hamate and may, with more widespread use, lessen the incidence of this fracture in the high-level baseball player (Fig. 4.17).

Prevention may be the best way to lessen the morbidity of the hook fracture, though realistically asking a high-level player to change his grip or bat may be difficult. A more accurate way to decrease its deleterious impact remains earlier diagnosis with expedient referral to the hand surgeon to proceed with treatment. In the senior author's experience, this delay is multi-

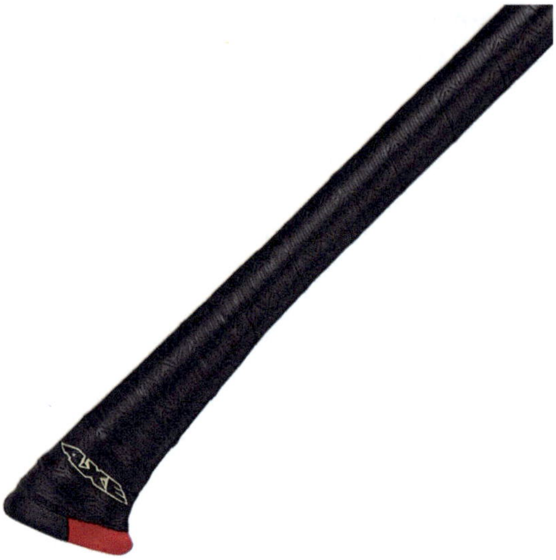

Fig. 4.17 Axe Bat, tapered handle

faceted and starts with failure to recognize the injury, failure to confirm the injury on exam, delay in radiographic confirmation, and finally inordinate delay in referral to the hand surgeon for recommended treatment that still remains excision. The continued use of attempted unsuccessful conservative treatment, usually prolonged casting, plays large into the delay in returning the high-level player to pre-injury status. This adverse delay is highlighted in the senior author's (GML) comparative experience between the Braves and routine community hook fracture referrals. Our Braves' trainers, being skilled in the history of this fracture and its mechanism of injury, are quick to assess the player, order the proper radiograph (Papilion modified supinated oblique or CT), confirm the diagnosis, and refer for surgery. This results in approximately a span of 50 days from injury to return to play. This is compared to our community experience in which there is an inordinate delay in diagnosis coupled with an even further delay in referral resulting on average 126 days from injury to return to play. It is our continued goal to educate primary care doctors and providers to this injury and the need for expedient referral [6].

Conclusion

The hook fracture in the baseball player has a higher prevalence in incidence than the normal population. This seemingly innocuous injury, if missed or undertreated, can result in increased morbidity. The goal of this chapter has been to document its pertinent clinical anatomy, mechanism of injury, important details of the exam, radiographic and advanced imaging, and treatment. The relationship with the hand surgeon and his or her trainer is crucial to make the diagnosis and begin expedient treatment. Return to play is usually successful, though recent publications do describe a more sobering experience. Pearls in prevention and more efficient management may affect this finding. Education of our first-line health providers hopefully will also help in this overall experience.

References

1. Suh N, Ek ET, Wolfe SW. Carpal fractures. J Hand Surg Am. 2014;39(4):785–91. https://doi.org/10.1016/j.jhsa.2013.10.030.
2. Camp CL, Dines JS, van der List JP, Conte S, Conway J, Altchek DW, Coleman SH, Pearle AD. Summative report on time out of play for Major and Minor League Baseball: an analysis of 49,955 injuries from 2011 through 2016. Am J Sports Med. 2018;46(7):1727–32. https://doi.org/10.1177/0363546518765158.
3. Rhee PC, Camp CL, D'Angelo J, Desai VS, Shin SS, Sheridan D, Conte S. Epidemiology and impact of hand and wrist injuries in major and minor league baseball. Hand. 2019;23:1558944719864450. https://doi.org/10.1177/1558944719864450.
4. Klausmeyer MA, Mudgal CS. Hook of hamate fractures. J Hand Surg Am. 2013;38(12):2457–60. https://doi.org/10.1016/j.jhsa.2013.06.004.
5. Alexeev M, Kane SM, Lourie GM. Force exerted on the hook of the hamate in competitive baseball players. King/Hancock Orthop J. 2020;23:21.
6. Metz J, Lourie GM. Hand injuries in baseball. In: Ahmad CS, Romeo AA, editors. Baseball sports medicine. Philadelphia: Lippincott Williams & Wilkins; 2018.
7. Smith IIIP, Wright TW, Wallace PF, Dell PC. Excision of the hook of the hamate: a retrospective survey and review of the literature. J Hand Surg Am. 1998;13(4):612–5. https://doi.org/10.1016/S0363-5023(88)80107-2.

8. Carter PR, Eaton RG, Littler JW. Ununited fracture of the hook of the hamate. JBJS. 1977;59(5):583–8. https://doi.org/10.2106/00004623-197759050-00002.
9. Stark HH, Jobe FW, Boyes JH, Ashworth CR. Fracture of the hook of the hamate in athletes. JBJS. 1977;59(5):575–82. https://doi.org/10.2106/00004623-197759050-00001.
10. Wright TW, Moser MW, Sahajpal DT. Hook of hamate pull test. J Hand Surg Am. 2010;35(11):1887–9. https://doi.org/10.1016/j.jhsa.2010.08.024.
11. Milek MA, Boulas HJ. Flexor tendon ruptures secondary to hamate hook fractures. J Hand Surg Am. 1990;15(5):740–4. https://doi.org/10.1016/0363-5023(90)90147-J.
12. Demirkan F, Calandruccio JH, DiAngelo D. Biomechanical evaluation of flexor tendon function after hamate hook excision. J Hand Surg Am. 2003;28(1):138–43. https://doi.org/10.1053/jhsu.2003.50005.
13. Levina Y, Lourie GM, Matthias RC Jr. Dynamic nerve compression of guyon canal secondary to variation of the deep branch of the ulnar artery: etiology, diagnosis, treatment, and outcome. J Hand Surg Glob. 2020;2(4):256–9. https://doi.org/10.1016/j.jhsg.2020.04.010.
14. Rogers MR, Bergfield TG. Aulicino PL. a neural loop of the deep motor branch of the ulnar nerve: an anatomic study. J Hand Surg Am. 1991;16(2):269–71. https://doi.org/10.1016/S0363-5023(10)80108-X.
15. Dodds GA III, Hale D, Jackson WT. Incidence of anatomic variants in Guyon's canal. J Hand Surg Am. 1990;15(2):352–5. https://doi.org/10.1016/0363-5023(90)90122-8.
16. Failla JM. Hook of hamate vascularity: vulnerability to osteonecrosis and nonunion. J Hand Surg Am. 1993;18(6):1075–9. https://doi.org/10.1016/0363-5023(93)90405-R.
17. Erickson BJ, Mcelheny K, Chalmers PN, Carr JB, D'Angelo J, Rowe D, Poulis G, Lourie GM, Carlson M. Performance and return to sport after excision of the fractured hook of the hamate in professional baseball players. Am J Sports Med. 2020;48(12):3066–71. https://doi.org/10.1177/0363546520949204.
18. Papilion JD, DuPuy TE, Aulicino PL, Bergfield TG, Gwathmey FW. Radiographic evaluation of the hook of the hamate: a new technique. J Hand Surg Am. 1988;13(3):437–9. https://doi.org/10.1016/S0363-5023(88)80026-1.
19. Egawa M, Asai T. Fracture of the hook of the hamate: report of six cases and the suitability of computerized tomography. J Hand Surg Am. 1983;8(4):393–8. https://doi.org/10.1016/S0363-5023(83)80197-X.
20. Lourie GM, Booth C, Nathan R. Triquetrohamate impaction syndrome: an unrecognized cause of ulnar-sided wrist pain; its presentation further defined. Hand. 2017;12(4):382–8. https://doi.org/10.1177/1558944716670138.
21. Thompson RG, Poulis GC, Lourie GM. Locked wrist: a case report and literature review on pisotriquetral loose bodies. J Wrist Surg. 2020;9(06):518–22. https://doi.org/10.1055/s-0040-1710394.
22. Lourie GM. Tendinopathy and tendon instability in the athlete's wrist: the ECU and ECRB. In: Carlson M, Goldfarb C, editors. The Athlete's hand and wrist. Chicago: American Society for Surgery of the Hand; 2014.
23. Whalen JL, Bishop AT, Linscheid RL. Nonoperative treatment of acute hamate hook fractures. J Hand Surg Am. 1992;117(3):507–11. https://doi.org/10.1016/0363-5023(92)90363-T.
24. Triplet JJ, Gellman H, Clause D, Halikis NM. The effect of thumb immobilization on fractures of the hook of the hamate: a cadaver study. Hand. 2020;15(3):365–70. https://doi.org/10.1177/1558944718795307.
25. Fujioka H, Tsunoda M, Noda M, Matsui N, Mizuno K. Treatment of ununited fracture of the hook of hamate by low-intensity pulsed ultrasound: a case report. J Hand Surg Am. 2000;25(1):77–9. https://doi.org/10.1053/jhsu.2000.jhsu025a0077.
26. Watson HK, Rogers WD. Nonunion of the hook of the hamate: an argument for bone grafting the nonunion. J Hand Surg Am. 1989;14(3):486–90. https://doi.org/10.1016/S0363-5023(89)80008-5.
27. Ceccarelli R, Dumontier C, Camuzard O. Minimally invasive fixation with a volar approach using a cannulated compression screw for acute hook of hamate fractures. J Hand Surg Am. 2019;44(11):993–e1. https://doi.org/10.1016/j.jhsa.2019.01.014.
28. Bachoura A, Wroblewski A, Jacoby SM, Osterman AL, Culp RW. Hook of hamate fractures in competitive baseball players. Hand. 2013;8(3):302–7. https://doi.org/10.1007/s11552-013-9527-4.
29. Devers BN, Douglas KC, Naik RD, Lee DH, Watson JT, Weikert DR. Outcomes of hook of hamate fracture excision in high-level amateur athletes. J Hand Surg Am. 2013;38(1):72–6. https://doi.org/10.1016/j.jhsa.2012.10.011.
30. Burleson A, Shin S. Return to play after hook of hamate excision in baseball players. Orthop J Sports Med. 2018;6(10):2325967118803090. https://doi.org/10.1177/2325967118803090.
31. Bishop AT, Beckenbaugh RD. Fracture of the hamate hook. J Hand Surg Am. 1988;13(1):135–9. https://doi.org/10.1016/0363-5023(88)90217-1.
32. Fredericson M, Kim BJ, McAdams TR, Date ES. Injury to the deep motor branch of the ulnar nerve during hook of hamate excision. Orthopedics. 2006;29(5):456–8. https://doi.org/10.3928/01477447-20060501-08.
33. Dashe J, Jones NF. A modified surgical approach through Guyon's canal and the proximal ulnar border of the carpal tunnel allows for safe excision of the hook of the hamate. J Hand Surg Am. 2019;44(12):1101–e1. https://doi.org/10.1016/j.jhsa.2019.07.015.

34. Bansal A, Carlan D, Moley J, Goodson H, Goldfarb CA. Return to play and complications after hook of the hamate fracture surgery. J Hand Surg Am. 2017; 42(10):803–9. https://doi.org/10.1016/j.jhsa.2017.06.108.
35. Barber JA, Loeffler B, Gaston RG, Lourie GM. Excision of incomplete hook of the hamate fractures. Orthopedics. 2019;42(2):e232–5. https://doi.org/10.3928/01477447-20190125-05.
36. David TS, Zemel NP, Mathews PV. Symptomatic, partial union of the hook of the hamate fracture in athletes. Am J Sports Med. 2003;31(1):106–11. https://doi.org/10.1177/03635465030310010201.

Carpometacarpal (CMC) Injuries Digits 2–5

5

George A. Cibulas II and Melvin P. Rosenwasser

Introduction

Over the last 10 years, many epidemiologic reports and studies have been published on the increasing rates of injury in Major League Baseball (MLB). These injuries lead to more time on the disabled list and affect the economics and competitiveness of the organization [1]. In one study, looking at both major and minor league baseball (MLB/MiLB), about 50,000 injuries were reported over 7 seasons (8000 injuries in the MLB) resulting in weeks to a whole season loss of playing time. Injury to the wrist, hand, finger, or thumb accounted for 14% of injuries. This is the second highest locus of injury behind the shoulder/clavicle (15%) [2]. While injury to the carpometacarpal joints of digits 2–5 are relatively uncommon in the MLB (<5%), they are challenging to treat and return to play while preventing short and longterm complications [3].

Carpometacarpal Bossing

Carpal bossing is a bony protrusion on the dorsal surface of the wrist involving the radial carpometacarpal (CMC) joints (CMC joints of the index and long finger) that is classically associated with CMC arthritis. Patients often present with an asymptomatic mass on the dorsum of the wrist over the CMC joint made more prominent by wrist flexion [4]. Typically, symptoms include snapping of the extensor tendons over the carpal boss, ganglion cyst at the CMC joint, or inflammation of the extensor tenosynovium [5, 6].

In an elite MLB athlete, however, the player may present with radial CMC symptoms without a notable carpal boss, or an associated ganglion cyst. Localized pain is seen in hitters who must go through a full arc of radial and ulnar deviation during the batting swing. The index and long finger CMC joints are stable but do have micromotion in the coronal plane during battings (Fig. 5.1). The ability to finish the batting swing with authority is compromised if there is pain associated with the carpal boss.

In athletes presenting with symptoms over a carpal boss an associated sessile ganglion cyst or an intraosseous lesion should be ruled out. Standard anteroposterior x-ray views of the hand and wrist should be supplemented with a modified lateral view of the wrist in which the hand is supinated 30–40° with ulnar deviation of 20–30°, which highlights the profile of the carpal boss (Fig. 5.2) [5]. Computed tomography (CT) and magnetic resonance imaging (MRI) may be useful for confirmation and to rule out other pathology (Fig. 5.3) [8].

A symptomatic carpal boss is treated with rest and often an intra-articular corticosteroid injection.

G. A. Cibulas II · M. P. Rosenwasser (✉)
Department of Orthopedic Surgery, New York Presbyterian/Columbia University Irving Medical Center, New York, NY, USA
e-mail: mpr2@cumc.columbia.edu; mpr2@columbia.edu

G. M. Lourie (ed.), *Hand and Wrist Injuries in Baseball*,
https://doi.org/10.1007/978-3-030-81659-9_5

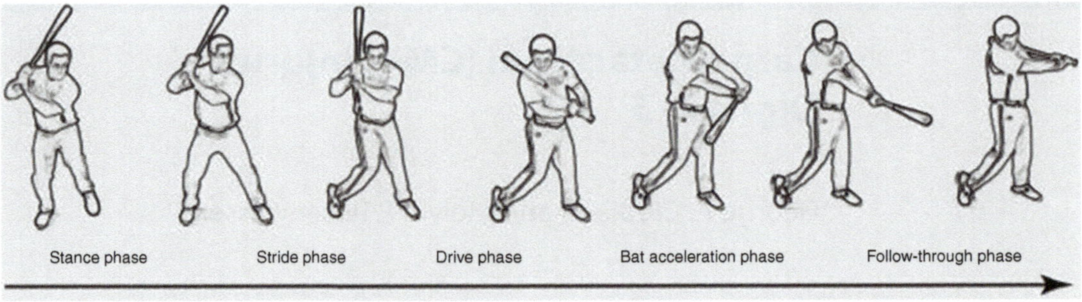

Fig. 5.1 Batter's swing progression with high forces in radial and deviation focused on the second CMC joint. Note the position of the wrist (radial and ulnar deviation) in the coronal plane during phase progression (With permissions from Am J Orthop [7])

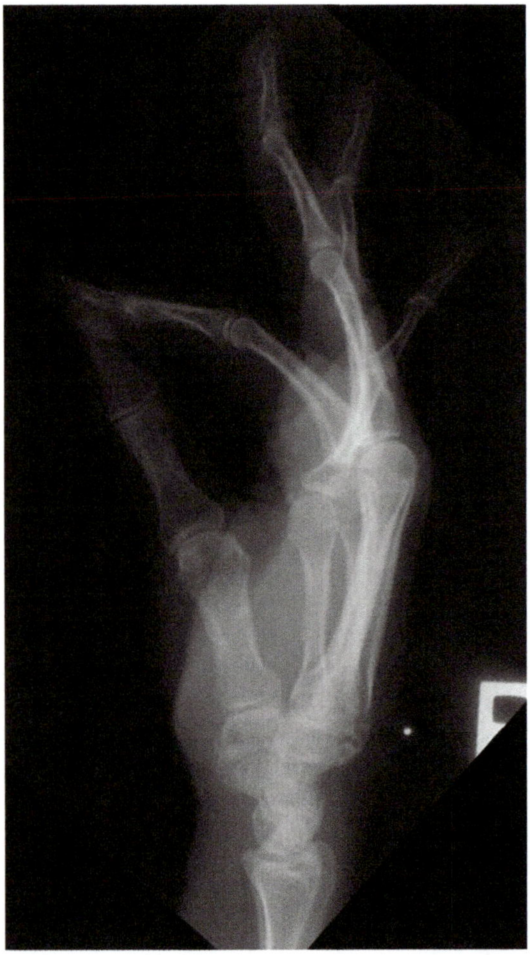

Fig. 5.2 Lateral x-ray of the right wrist. Note the prominent metacarpal boss adjacent to the radiographic marker (located over the second CMC joint)

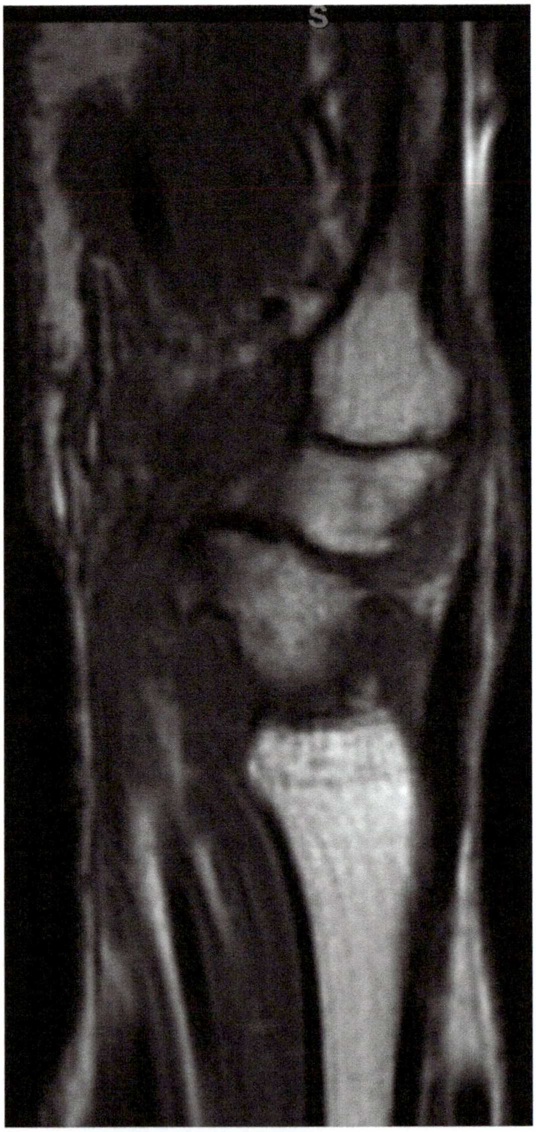

Fig. 5.3 Sagittal MRI imaging of a second CMC metacarpal boss

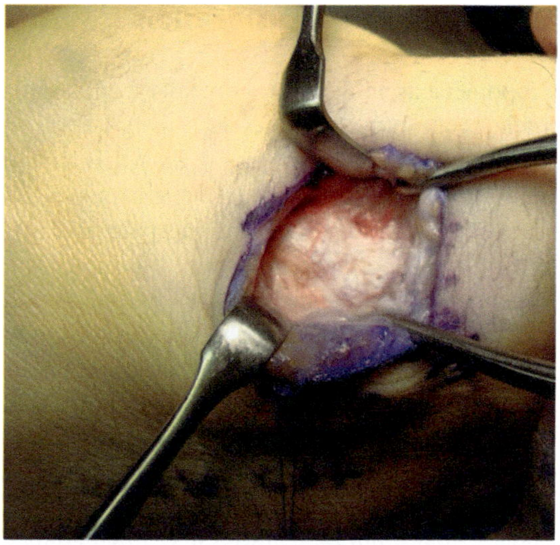

Fig. 5.4 5-cm incision made in line with base of the second CMC joint overlying the symptomatic boss

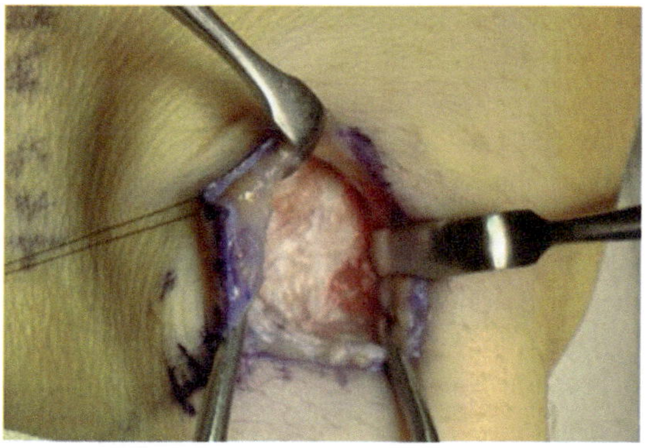

Fig. 5.5 Intraoperative photo demonstrating arthritic changes at the second CMC joint

Persistent symptoms limiting play will indicate surgery. Historically, this has consisted of surgical wedge resection [9]. While studies have shown positive results with this procedure. The nature of the operation can destabilize the CMC further which may delay or prevent return to play as a MLB player [6, 9, 10]. Thus, for the symptomatic ballplayer with a painful carpal boss, a CMC arthrodesis with or without adjunctive bone grafting is the preferred treatment option [11]. Outcomes have demonstrated pain relief and return to the previous level of performance in baseball and other sports.

CMC arthrodesis begins with a longitudinal incision over the base of the second CMC joint extending proximally and distally about 5 cm

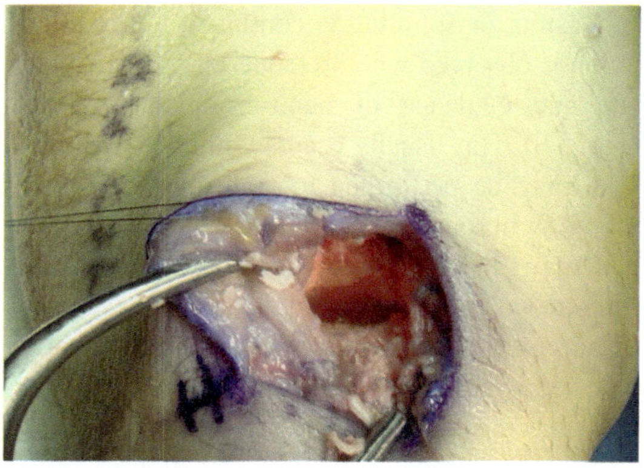

Fig. 5.6 Prepared second CMC joint after removal of articular cartilage

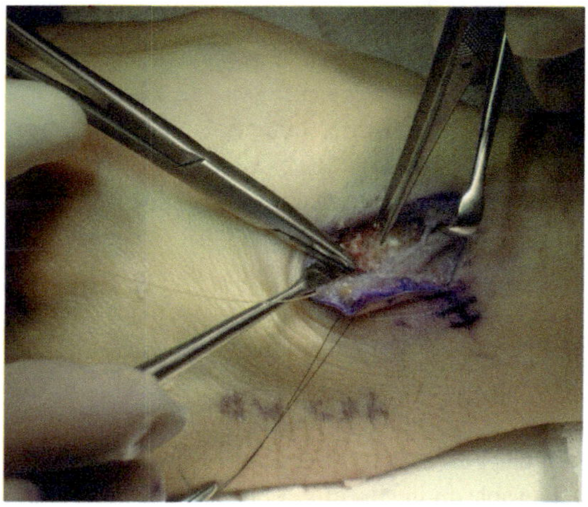

Fig. 5.7 Impacted crushed cancellous bone graft within the second CMC joint

(Fig. 5.4). The dorsal ridge of the base of the second metacarpal hides the articulation and needs to be unroofed via osteotomy. The articulation can then be visualized (Fig. 5.5). Next, removal of the remaining articular cartilage is performed carefully with curettes and a high-speed bur (Fig. 5.6). The joint is then packed with allograft cancellous croutons utilizing an impaction grafting technique in order to fill the prepared joint cavity (Fig. 5.7). It is not necessary to add adjunctive fixation as there is minimal motion at this joint once splinted. If additional fixation is preferred, percutaneous or buried K-wires would be sufficient. More obtrusive hardware such as dorsal plates have not been necessary to facilitate fusion at this site.

Casting or splinting is continued until clinical union is observed with no tenderness at the fusion site and evidence of bone bridging on x-ray (Fig. 5.8). This usually occurs within 8 weeks. CT scan may be performed to confirm adequacy of union. A fibrous union, as may occasionally happen, may still be sufficient to relieve all local symptoms and allow return to play. The case presented is of an elite college golfer who had incapacitating pain for 3 years at his left second CMC with bossing and now 1.5 years after successful CMC arthrodesis. He has painless wrist motion and is back playing high-level tournament golf and has near symmetric radial and ulnar deviation (Fig. 5.9).

Conclusion: Injuries in baseball players at the second and third CMC joint are infrequent among MLB athletes but persistent pain does affect performance in batting. Unfortunately these symptoms do not always respond to conservative treatments and rest. These injuries are often acute on chronic in etiology and ultimately demonstrate carpal bossing. Earlier presentations may have normal imaging. MLB batters must repetitively load the second CMC joint (in the coronal plane) which can generate articular cartilage damage. Chronic focal pain at that joint which is temporarily relieved by a lidocaine/coticosteroid injection may be treated successfully by a CMC arthrodesis allowing return to play at same level within 4 months making it achievable during the offseason.

Carpometacarpal Dislocation

Carpometacarpal dislocation results from a traumatic event and constitutes less than 1% of all hand injuries [12]. This injury in the MLB athlete is even more infrequent. However, given its severity and potential for chronic pain and disability, it is important to recognize this injury and understand the treatment options. Clinical and anatomic reports have described the anatomy and kinematics of the CMC joints of the hand. A forceful blow to the closed fist is the most commonly described mechanism leading to fracture and/or dislocation of the ring and small finger CMC joints [13]. This may be seen in baseball players after a fall on a closed fist, direct contact with a ball, base, or collision with another player.

The CMC joints of the index and long finger are stable joints and allow only 1–3 degrees of motion in the anterior-posterior plane [14]. Thus, the second and third CMC joints along with the distal carpal row form the stable keystone of the transverse and longitudinal arches of the hand. The CMC joints of the ring and small fingers have a saddle configuration and looser ligamentous attachments, which permit greater mobility and an increased risk of being injured [15].

Ulnar-sided CMC joint dislocations or fracture-dislocations can be missed because of the diffuse

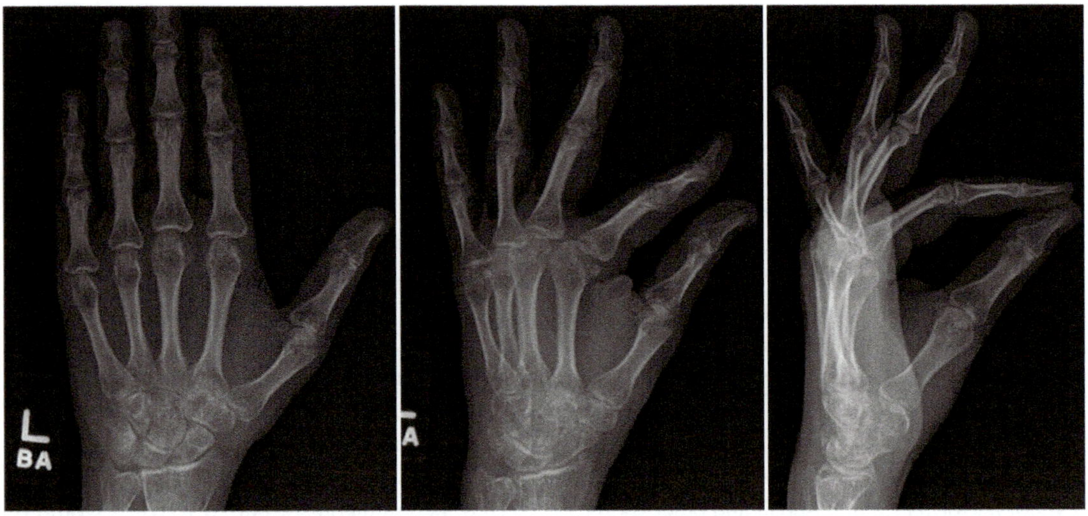

Fig. 5.8 AP, oblique, and lateral radiographs of a successful second CMC fusion with bone bridging at 3 months post-procedure

swelling that can occur in the hand and the misinterpretation of initial radiographs. A careful examination with ballottement of the base of the fourth and fifth metacarpals is required to assess stability of the reduction. Hand radiographs are obtained in the anteroposterior (AP), true lateral, and oblique planes (Fig. 5.10). If initial imaging does not confirm a CMC injury, but clinical exam suggests injury, additional oblique views or computed tomography (CT) scan should be obtained [16, 17].

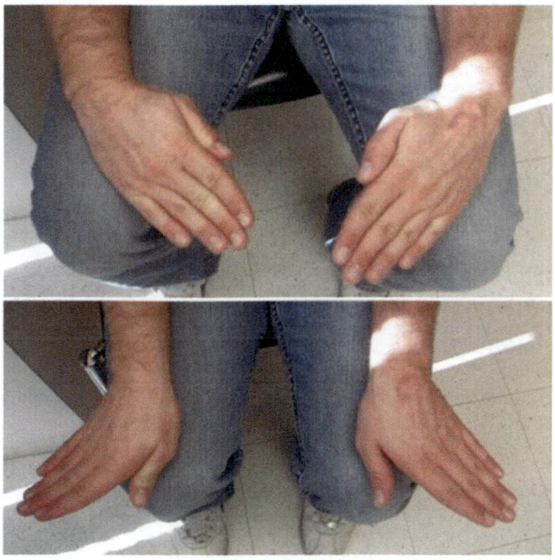

Fig. 5.9 1.5 years after left second CMC arthrodesis with preserved radial and ulnar deviation

Injury pattern (dislocation vs fracture-dislocation), open vs. closed injury, time to diagnosis, and ability to perform early closed stable reduction must be considered when deciding to proceed with conservative or surgical management of these injuries. Traditionally, most CMC dislocations are treated surgically with either open or closed reduction and percutaneous pinning [18]. If the injury pattern is diagnosed early (within 7–10 days of injury), is closed, and is a pure dislocation without associated fracture, then successful outcomes are reported after closed reduction and casting for a period of 6–8 weeks [19, 20]. There are no reports of treating these injuries in MLB players.

If this injury is irreducible or redisplaces after closed reduction, operative repair is indicated.

Closed reduction and percutaneous pinning is effective in maintaining alignment and stability of the fourth and fifth CMC base. It is not necessary to directly transfix the small intra-articular fragments. If the articular fracture remains malaligned after closed reduction, then an open reduction can be performed with a longitudinal incision over the base of the fifth carpometacarpal joint. Be careful to identify and protect dorsal ulnar sensory branches of the ulnar nerve. After fracture and/or joint reduction divergent K wires are placed percutaneously (Fig. 5.11).

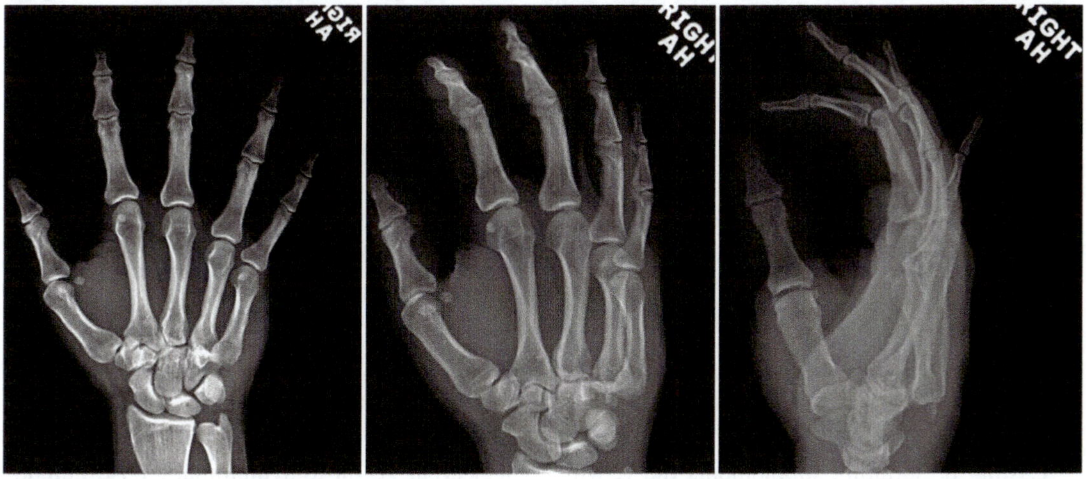

Fig. 5.10 AP, oblique, and lateral imaging of the right hand demonstrating dorsal dislocation of the fourth and fifth metacarpals with associated metacarpal base fracture

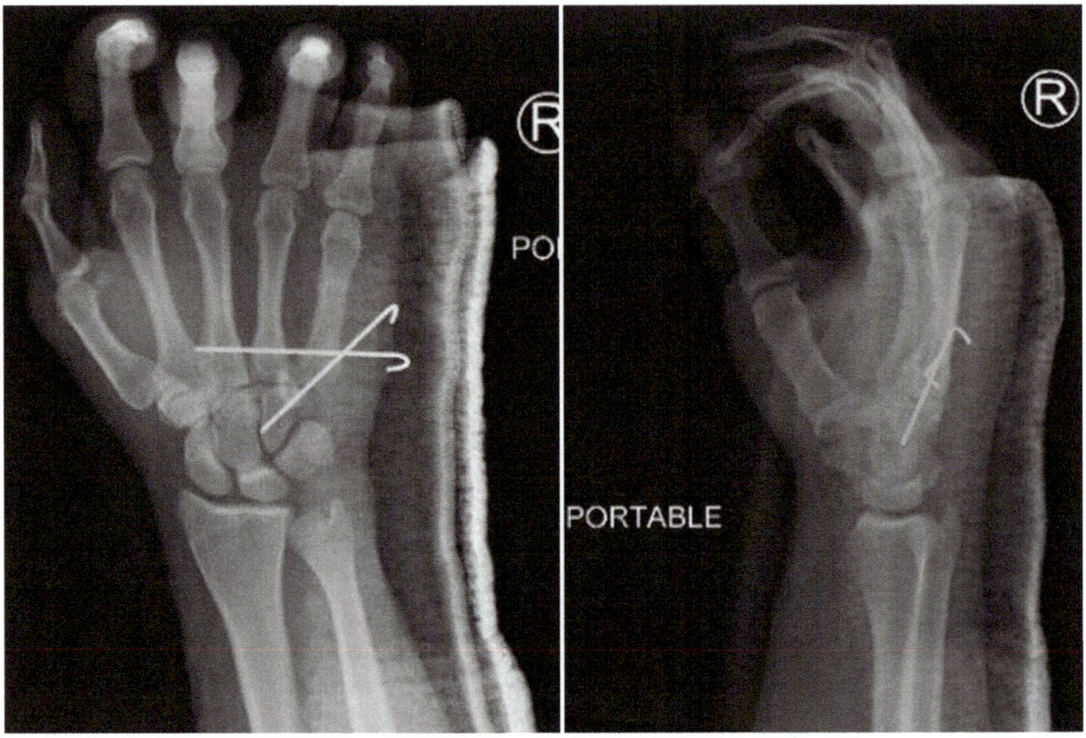

Fig. 5.11 AP and lateral right-hand radiographs post closed reduction and pinning of the fourth and fifth metacarpals with divergent K-wires

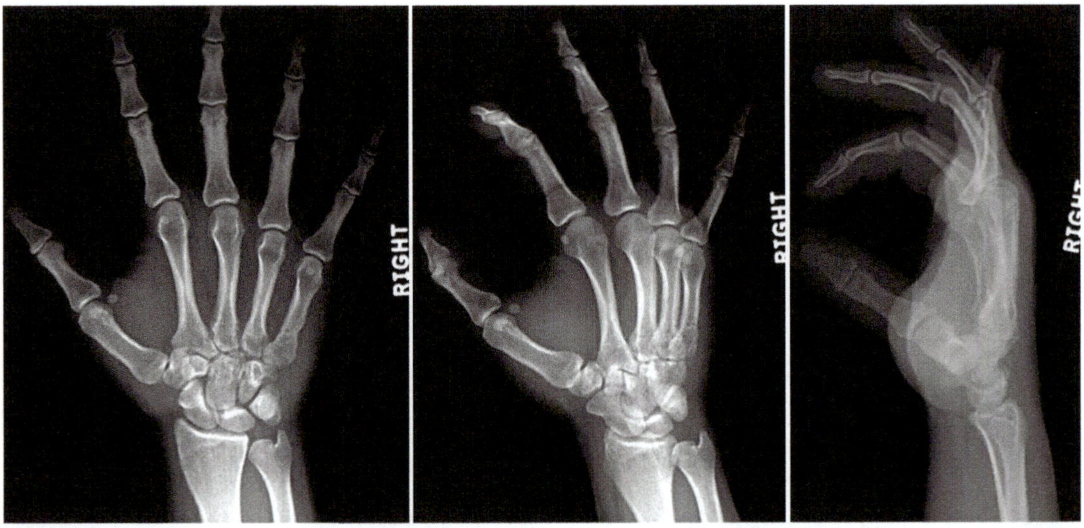

Fig. 5.12 AP, oblique, and lateral imaging of the right hand 3 months after closed reduction and percutaneous pinning of the fourth and fifth metacarpals

Casting or splinting supplements the K-wire fixation until capsular and/or bony healing is complete in 4 weeks. Rarely will a reduced intra-articular fracture at the base of the fifth metacarpal go on to symptomatic posttraumatic osteoarthritis requiring a late arthrodesis.

Athletes may return to play at 2 months post injury (Fig. 5.12).

When treating these injuries in the baseball athlete, surgery or closed reduction and casting are equivalent with regard to return to play. Both methods require 6–8 weeks of immobilization. These injuries when recognized and treated appropriately will allow the athlete to resume competition in a predictable fashion.

References

1. Conte S, Camp CL, Dines JS. Injury trends in Major League Baseball over 18 seasons: 1998–2015. Am J Orthop. 2016;45(3):116–23.
2. Camp CL, Dines JS, van der List JP, et al. Summative report on time out of play for major and minor league baseball: an analysis of 49,955 injuries from 2011 through 2016. Am J Sports Med. 2018;46(7):1727–32.
3. Rhee PC, Camp CL, D'Angelo J, et al. Epidemiology and impact of hand and wrist injuries in major and minor league baseball. Hand (N Y). 2019:1–7.
4. Roulet S, Bacle G, Marteau E, Laulan J. Surgical treatment of carpal boss by simple resection: results in 25 cases at a mean of 8 years' follow-up. Hand Surg Rehabil. 2017;36(2):109–12. https://doi.org/10.1016/j.hansur.2016.12.004.
5. Park MJ, Namdari S, Weiss AP. The carpal boss: review of diagnosis and treatment. J Hand Surg Am. 2008;33(3):446–9. https://doi.org/10.1016/j.jhsa.2007.11.029.
6. Vermeulen GM, de With MC, Bleys RL, Schuurman AH. Carpal boss: effect of wedge excision depth on third carpometacarpal joint stability. J Hand Surg Am. 2009;34(1):7–13. https://doi.org/10.1016/j.jhsa.2008.09.010.
7. Chang ES, Bishop ME, Baker D, West RV. Interval throwing and hitting programs in baseball: biomechanics and rehabilitation. Am J Orthop. 2016;45(3):157–62.
8. Zanetti M, Saupe N, Nagy L. Role of MR imaging in chronic wrist pain. Eur Radiol. 2007;17(4):927–38. https://doi.org/10.1007/s00330-006-0365-4.
9. Cuono CB, Watson HK. The carpal boss: surgical treatment and etiological considerations. Plast Reconstr Surg. 1979;63(1):88–93.
10. Citteur JM, Ritt MJ, Bos KE. Carpal boss: destabilization of the third carpometacarpal joint after a wedge excision. J Hand Surg Br. 1998;23(1):76–8. https://doi.org/10.1016/s0266-7681(98)80225-8.
11. Loréa P, Schmitz S, Aschilian M, Chirila-Dobrea A, Petrea AD. The preliminary results of treatment of symptomatic carpal boss by wedge joint resection, radial bone grafting and arthrodesis with a shape memory staple. J Hand Surg Eur Vol. 2008;33(2):174–8. https://doi.org/10.1177/1753193408087068.
12. Siddiqui YS, Zahid M, Sabir AB, Kumar GM. Multiple carpometacarpal fracture dislocation of the hand – an uncommon pattern of injury which is often missed: a case report with review of literature. J Clin Diagn Res. 2011;5:618–20.
13. Jebson PJL, Engber WD, Lange RH. Dislocation and fracture-dislocation of the carpometacarpal joints. Orthop Rev. 1994:19–28.
14. Gunther SF. The carpometacarpal joints. Orthop Clin North Am. 1984;15:259–77.
15. El-Bacha A. The carpometacarpal joints (excluding the Trapeziometacarpal). In: Tubiana R, editor. The Hand, vol. 1. Philadelphia: W. B. Saunders; 1981. p. 158–68.
16. Storken G, Bogie R, Jansen EJP. Acute ulnar carpometacarpal dislocations. Can it be treated conservatively? A review of four cases. Hand (N Y). 2011;6(04):420–3.
17. Fisher MR, Rogers LF, Hendrix RW. Systematic approach to identifying fourth and fifth carpometacarpal joint dislocations. AJR Am J Roentgenol. 1983;140(02):319–24.
18. Horneff JG III, Park MJ, Steinberg DR. Acute closed dislocation of the second through fourth carpometacarpal joints: satisfactory treatment with closed reduction and immobilization. Hand. 2013;8(2):227–31.
19. Jumeau H, Lechien P, Dupriez F. Conservative treatment of carpometacarpal dislocation of the three last fingers. Case Rep Emerg Med. 2016:1–3.
20. Jimenez I, Sanchez-Hernandez J, Kiimetoglou D. Nonoperative treatment of ulnar carpometacarpal fracture-dislocations. J Wrist Surg. 2020;9:160–3.

6 Phalangeal and Metacarpal Fractures of the Digits

R. Glenn Gaston and A. Jordan Grier

Introduction

The metacarpals and phalanges are among the most commonly observed sites of fracture of the upper extremity in adults in the United States with an incidence of 20.9 fractures per 10,000 annually [1]. Together, metacarpal and phalangeal fractures comprise an estimated 41% of fractures below the elbow in the general population [1, 2]. Injuries of the hand and wrist account for 3–9% of all traumatic athletic injuries, with rates as high as 25% observed in adolescent athletes [3, 4]. Fractures of the metacarpals and phalanges account for over 40% of fractures among professional athletics injuries observed both in the United States and abroad [5, 6]. Male athletes have a particular predilection toward sustaining fractures of metacarpals (87:13, male/female athletes) and phalanges (80:20, male/female athletes) [5].

Fractures of the hand pose a particular challenge in baseball players due to the unique demands of fielding, throwing, and batting coupled with the limited ability to play wearing splints or casts. Fractures of the metacarpals and phalanges are observed at all levels of baseball; therefore, the treating surgeon must possess a sound understanding of the unique demands of their patient's tier of competition. The hand and fingers account for 8.5% of all baseball-related injuries, and over 30% of all fractures observed at the high school level [7]. Comparable rates of injury have been observed at the professional level with hand and finger injuries representing 10% of all baseball-related injuries, and 32.5% of all fractures [8, 9]. Of the observed hand and finger injuries, metacarpal fractures account for 2.6–4.7% of injuries, while phalangeal fractures account for 1.3–3.7% [8, 9]. Injuries of the upper extremity are of particular concern to players, coaches, trainers, and treating physicians as they account for significantly longer time lost to the Injured List relative to that observed in lower extremity and axial skeleton injuries, with average time out of competition in some series ranging from 51 to 59 days for metacarpal fractures and 31 to 61 days for phalangeal fractures [8, 9].

Optimal treatment of metacarpal and phalangeal fractures in baseball athletes is multifactorial in nature. Prompt diagnosis provides for appropriate early care and counseling of the athlete. The treating surgeon must acknowledge the unique needs and circumstances of athletes at different levels of competition from amateur to elite while remaining continually grounded in sound evidence-based medical practices. Strickland has cited the vocal, and occasionally unreasonable, external pressure often encountered by treating physicians from multiple stakeholders including

R. G. Gaston (✉) · A. J. Grier
OrthoCarolina Hand Center, Charlotte, NC, USA
e-mail: Glenn.gaston@orthocarolina.com; Jordan.grier@orthocarolina.com

G. M. Lourie (ed.), *Hand and Wrist Injuries in Baseball*,
https://doi.org/10.1007/978-3-030-81659-9_6

parents, coaches, fans, and sometimes even the athletes themselves [10]. His commentary provides an invaluable perspective and serves as a reminder that the treatment of athletes must remain grounded in solid orthopedic principles to provide for the best short- and long-term treatment outcomes for the patient.

Anatomy

The architecture of the palm and digits lends itself well to the unique motions required for fielding, throwing, and batting. The carpometacarpal (CMC) joints serve as a stout transition from the distal row of the carpus to the metacarpals [11]. This is particularly true on the radial side of the hand where the index and long finger CMC joints exhibit particularly rigid ligamentous complexes. On the ulnar side of the hand, the ring and small finger CMC joints display increased mobility, allowing for 15–20° of flexion and supination which results in deepening of the palm [12]. This unique motion about the ulnar CMC joints, coupled with reciprocal flexion and pronation of the thumb CMC joint, allows for the palm deepening required for accommodation of objects such as grasping a baseball or bat handle.

The coronal and sagittal plane alignment of the metacarpals compliments the anatomy and function of the CMC joints. When viewed in the coronal plane, the long axes of the metacarpals are slightly divergent in nature, with the most radial portions of the index and most ulnar portion of the small finger metacarpal heads lying further from midline than their associated CMC joints. This orientation serves to increase the overall surface area of the palm relative to the width of the carpus. When viewed in the sagittal plane, the metacarpals appear in near parallel alignment. However, when viewed in the axial plane, the metacarpals appear to align in a concave arch configuration [13]. The depth provided by the carpal arch compliments the supination of the fourth and fifth CMC joints to allow for more effective object acceptance into the palm.

The diaphysis of the metacarpal is quite stable, and frequently displays relatively little displacement with low-energy injuries as a result of the attachments of the adjacent dorsal and palmar interossei [14]. Distally, the finger metacarpals are attached via the deep transverse intermetacarpal ligaments, which further stabilizes the metacarpal arch and allows for relative preservation of the bony architecture of the palm even in the setting of fractures. While the interossei origins can serve as partial stabilizers of the metacarpal diaphysis, their distal tendinous expansions impart a deforming force in the sagittal plane as a result of their course volar to the axis of rotation of the metacarpal head. The characteristic apex dorsal angulation of metacarpal fractures is in part attributed to this deforming force imparted by the interossei, along with a similar force from the lumbrical as it passes volar to the deep transverse intermetacarpal ligament. Varus and valgus stability of the metacarpophalangeal joints is conferred by a robust collateral ligament complex consisting of proper and accessory fibers which run in 30° and 90° angles, respectively, from the collateral recess of the metacarpal to the base of the proximal phalanx and volar plate.

The general bony morphology of the phalanges consists of a base, narrow diaphysis, and head [15]. The specific architecture of the proximal and middle phalanges is relatively similar and distinct from that observed in the distal phalanx. Radiographically, the proximal and middle phalanges exhibit a 2:1 size ratio [13]. The proximal phalanx is unique in that it does not have any direct extrinsic tendinous insertions, resulting in a predictable apex volar deformity secondary to the deforming forces of the central slip distally and interossei proximally when extraarticular fractures of the diaphysis occur. The insertions of the central slip of the extensor apparatus dorsally and flexor digitorum superficialis (FDS) palmarly contribute to unique fracture morphology in extraarticular fractures of the middle phalanx. Middle phalangeal fractures occurring proximal to the FDS insertion generally result in apex dorsal angulation as a result of the vector of pull of the FDS slips. Conversely, apex volar angulation is observed in middle phalangeal fractures occurring distal to the FDS insertion. The anatomy of the distal phalanx is distinct from that of the proximal and middle phalanges, consisting of a wide base which narrows through the diaphysis

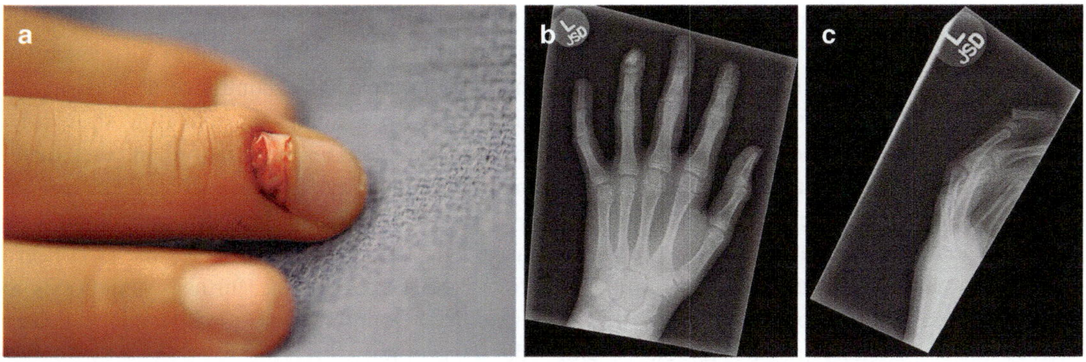

Fig. 6.1 Clinical image of the ring finger demonstrating a visible nail plate deformity concerning for injury to the underlying nail bed and distal phalanx (**a**) PA and lateral radiographs of the ring finger distal phalanx demonstrate a displaced physeal fracture in the same patient who was observed to have interposed nail bed at the time of fracture fixation consistent with a Seymour fracture (**b** and **c**)

and distal tip (often referred to as the "tuft"). Tendinous insertions on the distal phalanx include the terminal tendon of the dorsal apparatus and the flexor digitorum profundus tendon more volarly and distal, both of which may act as deforming forces in fractures of the distal phalanx. The nail plate and underlying nail matrix must also be taken into consideration when treating fractures of the distal phalanx as this tissue may become interposed in fracture sites in both children and adults. In skeletally immature patients, the classic "Seymour" fracture has been described as a physeal fracture associated with entrapment of the nail matrix between the epiphyseal and metaphyseal fracture fragments resulting in non-anatomic alginment (Fig. 6.1a–c). Lacerations of the nail matrix require prompt attention and repair in order to avoid future nail deformity which may impair function of the finger and result in an unacceptable cosmetic deformity in some patients.

Mechanism of Injury

Metacarpal fractures have been observed to occur more frequently than phalangeal fractures in baseball at the minor and major league levels [9, 16]. Fractures of the metacarpal commonly occur as a result of a direct blow from the baseball to the dorsum of the band in batters [17]. This typically affects the lead hand (bottom hand) as the dorsum of the hand faces toward the pitcher and is in line with the trajectory of the incoming pitch. Metacarpal fractures may also occur as a result of direct impact with another player (e.g., collisions at home plate, tagging an opposing player, unintended collision between outfielders, etc.), impact of the hand on a solid object such as a base or with the outfield wall, or a fall onto an outstretched hand.

Phalangeal fractures have a lower incidence than metacarpal fractures but are at risk during similar activities to those which place the metacarpals at risk. Proximal and middle phalangeal fractures occur less frequently than do fractures of the distal phalanx. Due to the relatively unprotected position of the distal phalanx at the tip of the finger, it is at particular risk from events such as fielding a ground ball, sliding into a base, or collisions with players or objects [18].

Differential Diagnosis

Athletes reporting pain about the hand or digits warrant evaluation with a thorough history and physical examination. Particular attention should be paid to the mechanism of injury, reported areas of pain, and associated symptoms. In addition to fractures of the metacarpals and phalanges, care should be taken to rule out alternate or associated diagnoses of the affected extremity. Pain and swelling about the dorsum of the hand may be indicative of a metacarpal fracture, or fractures, but may also be suggestive of injury to the extensor tendons over the dorsum of the hand. Carpal fractures may also present with pain referred distally to the hand and fingers, and care should be taken to rule out any associated carpal pathology such as a fracture of the scaphoid. More distally, pain about the metacarpal head and neck should prompt careful evaluation of the MCP collateral ligament complex as well as the sagittal bands. Distally in the finger, careful attention should be turned to exclusion of associated injuries of the flexor tendons, flexor pulley system, and injuries to the dorsal apparatus (i.e., central slip, lateral bands, terminal tendon).

Physical Examination

When fractures of either the metacarpals or phalanges are suspected, physical examination should begin at the carpus and proceed distally. The hand and fingers should be carefully inspected and compared to the contralateral extremity to note any areas of asymmetry. Particular attention should be paid to areas of swelling, skin changes (erythema, induration, ecchymosis, pallor), skin turgor, open wounds (lacerations, abrasions), loss of normal metacarpal arch contour, altered MCP joint contour, malrotation of the digits, and temperature change. Open metacarpal and phalangeal fractures are relatively uncommon in baseball but should be formally ruled out as this may indicate the athlete for urgent operative intervention for irrigation and debridement of the fracture site. The carpus should be palpated for any focal areas of tenderness suggesting underlying bony or soft tissue injury. Formal examination of the distal radioulnar joint (DRUJ) should be conducted including assessment of the ulnar styloid, triangular fibrocartilage (TFC), extensor carpi ulnar (ECU), and integrity dorsal and volar radioulnar ligaments.

Examination of the hand and fingers should include formal assessment of the digital extensor tendons, sagittal bands, dorsal apparatus of the digit, and flexor tendon system. Range of motion of the MCP, PIP, and DIP joints should be assessed for pain with motion or differences in mobility relative to the contralateral extremity. A detailed neurovascular examination should be performed including sensation in the distal median, ulnar, and radial nerve distributions. Peripheral pulses and capillary refill should be assessed, especially in catchers, and if concern for vascular injury exists, further evaluation with handheld Doppler ultrasound should be conducted promptly.

Imaging

If sufficient concern exists for fracture of either the metacarpals or phalanges, imaging with plain radiographs should be conducted. Posteroanterior (PA), lateral, and oblique radiograph of the hand should be obtained for evaluation of metacarpal fractures. Obtaining oblique radiographs in both pronation and supination is occasionally indicated to provide added detail with respect to the metacarpal anatomy. Oblique radiographs also provide added detail regarding the integrity of the CMC joints, and may detect subtle injuries not readily apparent on standard PA and lateral radiographs [19]. A 30° pronated view is especially helpful for evaluating the fourth and fifth CMC joints. The Brewerton PA view may also be indicated when concern for metacarpophalangeal joint injury exists. This view is obtained by capturing a PA image of the hand with the MCP joints flexed to 60°, and the X-ray beam directed 75° relative to the plate [14]. PA, lateral, and oblique radiographs of the finger should be obtained for suspected phalangeal fractures. Advanced imaging with computed tomography (CT) scans of the hand and/or digit may be obtained if concern for intraarticular fracture exists and radiographic examination alone is deemed insufficient in fully characterizing the injury pattern. CT may be particularly helpful for injuries about the CMC and MCP joints where significant overlap of adjacent structures may obscure visualization on plain radiographs.

Conservative Treatment

Nondisplaced and minimally displaced metacarpal fractures with preserved length, rotation, and alignment are often amenable to nonsurgical treatment though many non-biologic factors such as level of the athlete, time remaining in season, and hand dominance may influence the decision. Angulation of 30–40° of the ring and small finger metacarpals, and 15–20° of index and long finger metacarpals, is generally well-tolerated. While these parameters are often acceptable for the general population, this may not be acceptable for optimum hand function for hitting, fielding, and throwing due to the discomfort associated with a prominent metacarpal head in the palm [17]. Principles of conservative treatment including edema control and maintenance of active and passive range of motion (ROM) of the MCP, PIP, and DIP joints are strictly adhered to in the early post-injury period to allow for timely return to sport. A removable radial gutter orthosis for index and long finger metacarpal fractures, and ulnar gutter orthosis for ring and small finger metacarpal fractures generally, provides adequate support for the player to continue with other daily activities in the early post-injury period. The addition of buddy taping may be considered to discourage malrotation, particularly in more unstable fracture patterns such as long oblique or spiral fractures. Initiation of active ROM with the MCP joints immobilized and IP joints free is initiated on the first 2–3 days following injury to prevent joint stiffness and facilitate return to a baseball-specific rehabilitation program. Follow-up radiographs should be obtained at 2 and 4 weeks post-injury to assess for evidence of radiographic healing. The player is usually converted to a removable orthosis with the MCP joint free at 3 weeks post-injury. Return to play is generally allowed at 6 weeks post-injury provided the player demonstrates at least 75% MCP, PIP, and DIP range of motion (or has returned to their baseline if preexisting deficits were present) and radiographs demonstrate callous formation at the fracture site. Protective dorsal hand splints can be fabricated for players who desire extra protection of the dorsal hand while batting, but formal orthosis wear is otherwise not strictly recommended or tolerated for pitching and fielding.

Similar guidelines are followed for conservative treatment of phalangeal fractures. Nondisplaced or minimally displaced, extraarticular, length-stable fractures are generally considered amenable to nonoperative treatment. Initial treatment for stable fracture patterns generally consists of buddy taping for a period of 2–3 weeks, with an active ROM program beginning no later than 3 weeks after injury. Return to baseball-specific activities is generally allowed between 4 and 6 weeks after injury once painless active ROM of the MCP, PIP, and DIP joints has been achieved. Return to gameplay is allowed between 4 and 6 weeks as well as pending the player's progress with a baseball-specific rehabilitation program under the direction of their trainer.

Surgical Treatment

Surgical treatment of metacarpal fractures is indicated for injuries resulting in malrotation of the digits, open fractures, fractures with shortening >4–5 mm, intraarticular fractures of the metacarpal head, CMC fracture dislocations, and fractures with associated neurovascular or tendon injuries requiring repair. Relative indications for treatment of metacarpal fractures include angulation greater than 20–30° of index and long finger metacarpal shaft fractures, or 30–40° of angulation of ring and small finger metacarpal fractures, prominent metacarpal head in the palm, and multiple metacarpal fractures. Furthermore, elite athletes (we consider professional, college players with aspirations of professional play, and occasionally high school athletes with opportunities for scholarships) may elect surgical management for nondisplaced and minimally displaced fractures in an effort to return to sport sooner. Athletes should be carefully examined for prominence of the metacarpal head in the palm at the level they would grip a bat or the baseball. If athletes are sufficiently bothered by the position of the metacarpal head in the palm, then consideration may be given to operative fixation following a thorough discussion of risks and benefits with the player and the team. Multiple fixation constructs are available for treatment of metacarpal fractures, and the optimal treatment strategy is the one which will allow for stable fixation and early range of motion. Achievement of stable fixation allows for early range of motion, and expeditious progression toward return to play.

Metacarpal Head Fractures

Most metacarpal head fractures are approached via either a longitudinal split of the extensor tendon or a parasagittal approach through the sagittal bands. The authors' preference is to approach the long and ring finger metacarpal head by dividing the ulnar sagittal band and retracting the extensor tendon to expose the fracture site and the metacarpophalangeal joint. The sagittal band is repaired at the time of closure with 3-0 or 4-0 nonabsorbable suture to prevent postoperative extensor tendon subluxation. The index and small finger metacarpal heads are preferentially approached via a longitudinal split in the interval between the common extensor tendon and accessory digital extensor (extensor indicis proprius for the index finger, extensor digiti quinti for the small finger). At the time of closure, the longitudinal split is repaired with 3-0 or 4-0 absorbable suture in a figure-of-eight fashion. Intraarticular fractures of the metacarpal head are treated with anatomic reduction and fixation with either headless interfragmentary compression screws, plate and screw constructs, or smooth Kirschner wires. Plate and screw constructs may be left in place permanently if they do not result in any discomfort in the hand upon return to play. If removal is ultimately desired by the athlete, this is generally performed at least 6 months from the time of fixation and only if the fracture has gone on to clinical and radiographic union. Kirschner wires used for fracture fixation are generally removed between 3 and 4 weeks after surgery; however, these may be left in place for up to 6 weeks if required for achievement of fracture union prior to removal. Rarely, volar shear fractures of the metacarpal head can be encountered. These are best approached with a palmar approach, releasing the A1 pulley, and releasing the volar plate distally. The fracture is then fixed with headless compression screws when possible and the volar plate repaired at the time of closure.

Metacarpal Shaft Fractures

Fractures of the metacarpal shaft are approached via a longitudinal dorsal approach due to the relatively subcutaneous nature of the metacarpal shaft. The common digital extensor tendon is mobilized in line with the incision and retracted radially or ulnarly at the discretion of the treating surgeon. Fixation can be achieved with either interfragmentary screws, plate and screw constructs, or intramedullary fixation using smooth Kirschner wires or a cannulated screw. The fixation construct utilized should be tailored to the fracture pattern present. Provisional reduction is achieved using a combination of longitudinal traction and rotation of the digit. Reduction is maintained with either smooth wires or a small, pointed reduction clamp. Care should be taken to ensure provisional fixation allows for placement of the desired fixation construct and does not result in fracture comminution or displacement.

Interfragmentary lag screw fixation of spiral and long oblique fractures is preferred when the fracture length is at least twice that of the diameter of the bone at the length of the fracture. Fixation generally requires two to four interfragmentary screws depending on the fracture pattern (Fig. 6.2a, b). Screws are placed in a lag-by-technique fashion by over-drilling the near cortex such that the screw glides through the near cortex to engage and compress via the distal cortical hole. The first screw placed should allow for compression perpendicular to the fracture site, with subsequent screws placed proximally and/or distally for added torsional stability.

Metacarpal plating is suitable for treatment of short oblique, transverse, and comminuted fractures of the metacarpal shaft. Plate and screw constructs can be applied to either the dorsal or lateral aspects of the metacarpal depending on the fracture morphology. The plate selected

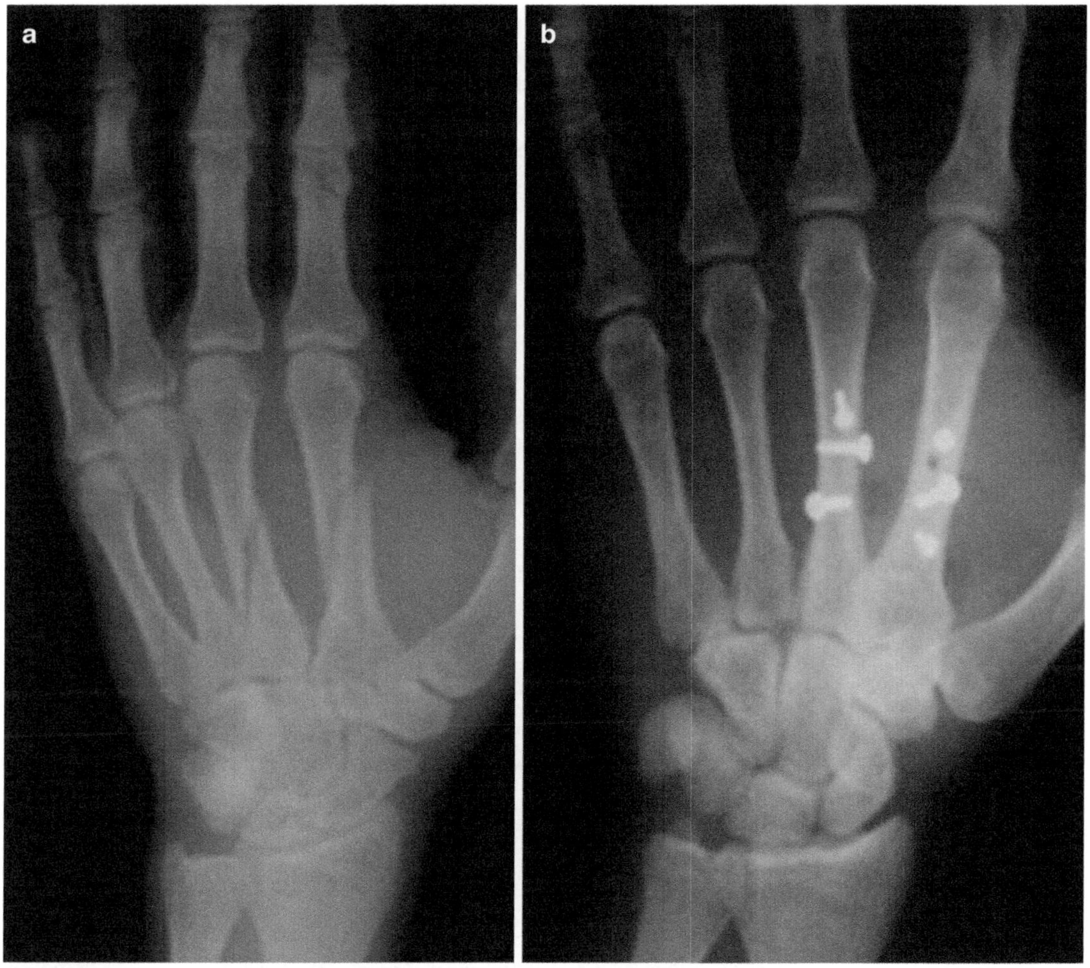

Fig. 6.2 Oblique fractures of the index and long finger metacarpal shaft (**a**) treated with interfragmentary lag screw fixation (**b**)

should allow for fixation of six to eight cortices on both sides of the fracture to ensure adequate stability will be present to allow for early active motion (Fig. 6.3a–d). Plate contouring may be required to accommodate the dorsal bow of the metacarpal shaft to ensure that fixation does not result in fracture malreduction. Care must also be taken to ensure that screw heads are sufficiently recessed within the plate, and no prominent plate edges are present in order to avoid mechanical abrasion of the extensor tendons which may result in pain or tendon rupture. Following completion of fixation, closure of the interosseous fascia over the plate construct should be undertaken when possible to minimize hardware prominence which may be bothersome while wearing either a fielding glove or batting glove.

Intramedullary pinning may be selected for the treatment of transverse, short oblique, and comminuted fractures of the metacarpal shaft. Intramedullary fixation provides sufficient stability to allow for mobilization of the athlete while minimizing trauma to the surrounding soft tissues. Pinning can be performed in an antegrade, retrograde, or transverse fashion depending on the fracture morphology present. Antegrade pinning is best suited for proximal and mid-diaphyseal metacarpal shaft fractures (Fig. 6.4a–i). A longitudinal incision is made centered over the base of the metacarpal. The extensor tendon and travers-

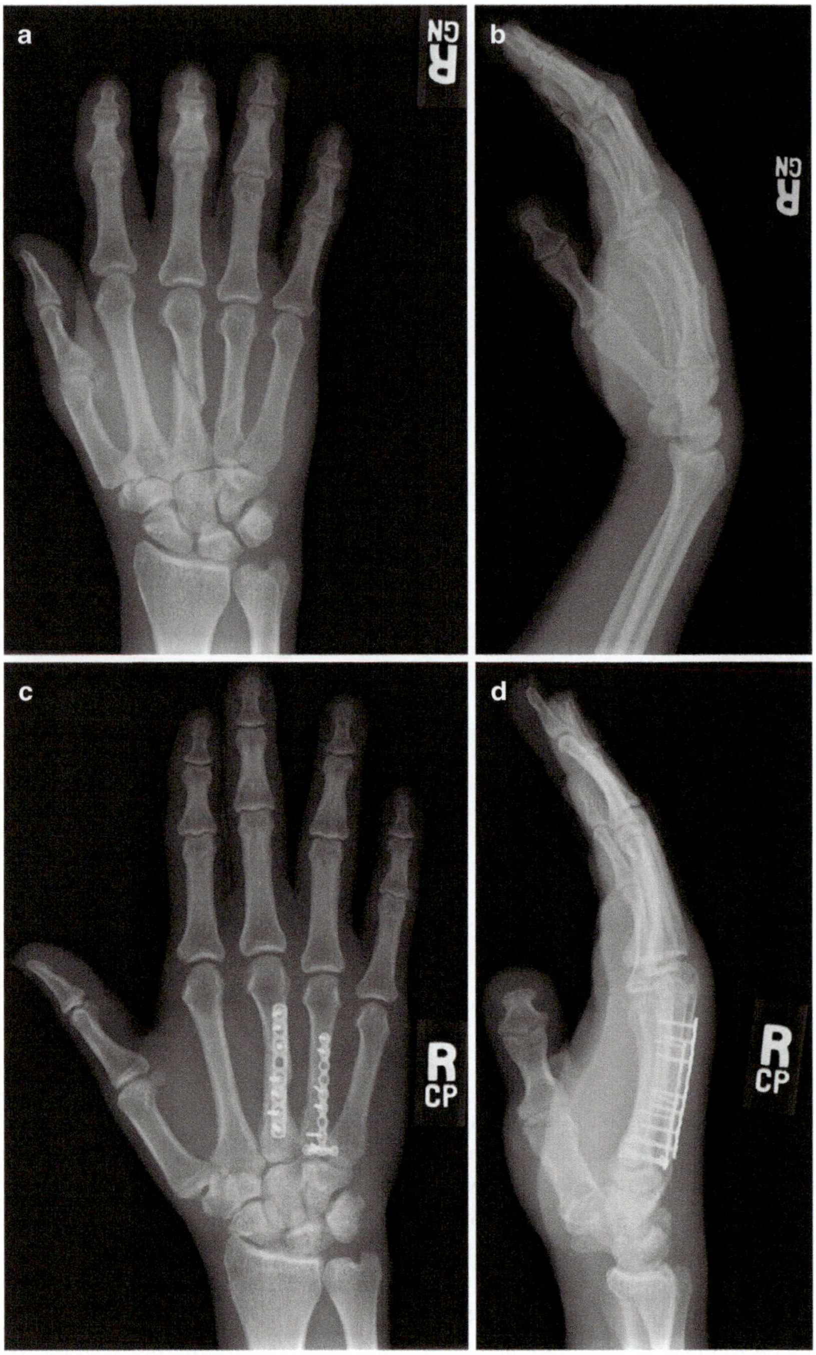

Fig. 6.3 (**a**–**d**) Oblique fractures of the long and ring finger metacarpal shafts (**a** and **b**) treated with open reduction and internal fixation with a plate and screw construct (**c** and **d**)

ing dorsal sensory nerve branches are identified and carefully protected. A starting awl or small diameter drill (1.2–1.8 mm) is used to create a small window in the dorsal metacarpal base. Depending on the size of the patient and fracture morphology, either 0.035″ or 0.045″ smooth wires may be selected for fixation. Wires are prebent to match the native bow of the metacarpal for which they are to be used and then advanced in an antegrade fashion into the medullary canal using the previously created pilot hole. Generally, either two 0.045″ wires or three 0.035″ wires are

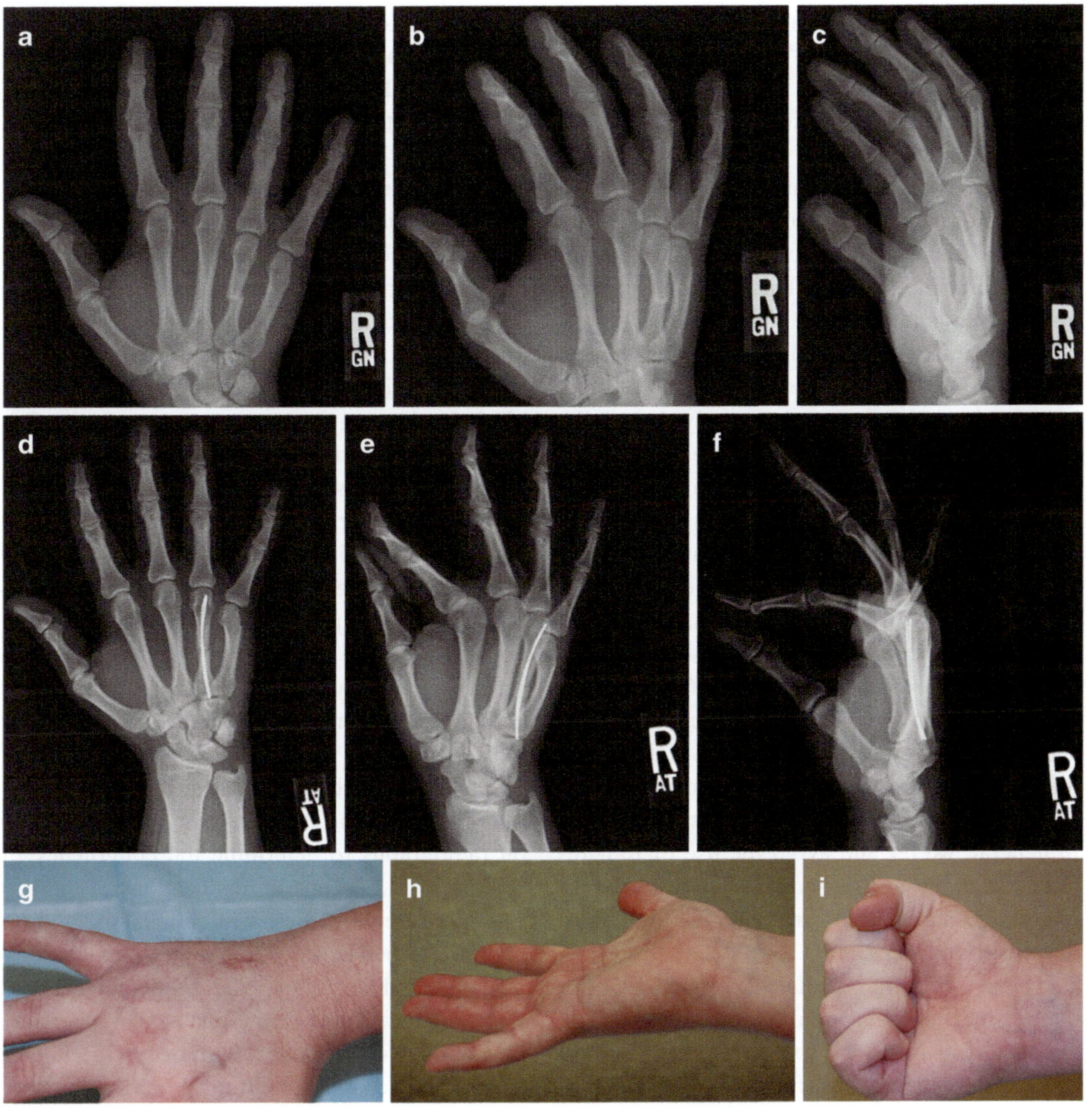

Fig. 6.4 (**a–i**) Transverse fracture of the ring finger metacarpal shaft (**a–c**) treated with antegrade intramedullary wire fixation (**d–f**). At 6-week postoperative follow-up, the patient demonstrated a well-healed wound and full active digital motion (**h–i**)

inserted to achieve stable fixation. Wires may be cut flush with the dorsal cortex of the metacarpal and left in place permanently or left slightly proud for later retrieval following fracture union. Retrograde pinning of the metacarpal is performed percutaneously by passing two 0.035″ or 0.045″ smooth wires from the radial and ulnar collateral recesses into the medullary canal of the metacarpal. Care must be taken to avoid inadvertent penetration of the articular surface of the metacarpal head when obtaining the starting point of the wire as hardware placed in this position may be a source of pain, limited motion, and chondral loss which could be deleterious to the athlete's future return to sport in both the short and long term. The authors' preference is to cut the wires below the skin to decrease the risk of pin tract infection and allow for early range of motion without irritation from wire prominence when this fixation is used. Wires are generally retrieved between 3 and 6 weeks following fixation provided evidence of clinical and radiographic healing is present. Retrieval may be performed with the athlete wide-awake under local anesthetic block to avoid the need for formal return to the operating room. Transverse pinning is useful for maintenance of length, rotation, and alignment of comminuted or significantly length-unstable fracture patterns. This fixation construct is most frequently utilized for the border digits, where the intact long and ring finger metacarpals are used to maintain the desired reduction of the index and small fingers, respectively. Generally, one to two 0.045″ smooth wires are placed both proximal and distal to the fracture site in a transverse, quadricortical fashion across the diaphysis of adjacent metacarpals. Wires are cut below the skin to avoid irritation and decrease the risk of superficial soft tissue infection. Similar to retrograde wire fixation, transverse wires are generally retrieved between 3 and 6 weeks following fixation provided evidence of clinical and radiographic healing is present. Retrieval of transverse wires may also be performed with the athlete wide-awake under local anesthetic block. In general, we try and avoid the use of K-wires for athletes during the season given the risk of refracture once the pins are removed and return to sport commences.

The use of intramedullary screw fixation for the treatment of metacarpal fractures has become our treatment of choice for transverse and short oblique metacarpal shaft fractures (Fig. 6.5a–f). Similar to intramedullary nail fixation of other long bones, the ability to provide rigid, length-stable, diaphyseal fit fixation of the metacarpal with minimal soft tissue trauma allows for earlier mobilization and return to weightbearing activities compared to smooth wire or plate and screw constructs [20]. A provisional closed reduction is first achieved via either closed or limited percutaneous means. After reduction has been achieved, the proximal phalanx is flexed 90°, and a 1 cm incision is made over the dorsal aspect of the MCP joint allowing for creation of a small longitudinal split in the common digital extensor tendon. Under fluoroscopic guidance, the starting guidewire is placed slightly dorsal in the metacarpal head such that it is in-line with the center of the diaphysis on a lateral projection of the metacarpal. The guidewire is advanced across the fracture site to the subchondral bone of the metacarpal base. Using the appropriate sizing guides for the intramedullary fixation system selected, the appropriate screw length and diameter is selected. The appropriate screw length should account for recession of the screw at least 2 mm below the chondral surface of the metacarpal head. Careful attention should be paid to the inner diameter of the metacarpal isthmus, particularly in the ring finger metacarpal which often has the most narrow coronal plane intracortical diameter at the isthmus, and small finger which has the most narrow sagittal plane intracortical diameter at the isthmus [21, 22]. We prefer to template the screw over the skin under fluoroscopic guidance prior to implanting it to ensure appropriate canal fit.

Operative treatment of proximal and middle phalangeal fractures is accomplished by similar means to those described for the metacarpal. Fractures about the proximal phalangeal head or middle phalangeal base warrant careful scrutiny on radiographs to determine the congruency of the PIP joint, as fracture dislocations of the PIP sometimes require alternate treatment methods to those described here for fractures without associated joint dislocation [23]. Unicondylar and bicondylar fractures of the phalangeal head may be treated with smooth 0.035″ wires in either a parallel or crossing pattern, interfragmentary screw fixation, plate and screw constructs, or a combination of these strategies. Transverse and short oblique fractures of the proximal and middle phalanx can be treated with either retrograde or antegrade pinning with smooth 0.035″ or 0.045″ wires (Fig. 6.6a–d). Similar to that of the metacarpal, the authors' preference is to cut the wires below the skin and plan for removal in 3–6 weeks depending on the degree of healing present and fracture morphology. Plate and screw constructs may be employed for transverse, short oblique, or comminuted fractures (Fig. 6.7a, b). Plates may be placed on either the dorsal or lateral surfaces of the phalanx, with care taken to avoid irritation to the central slip or lateral bands

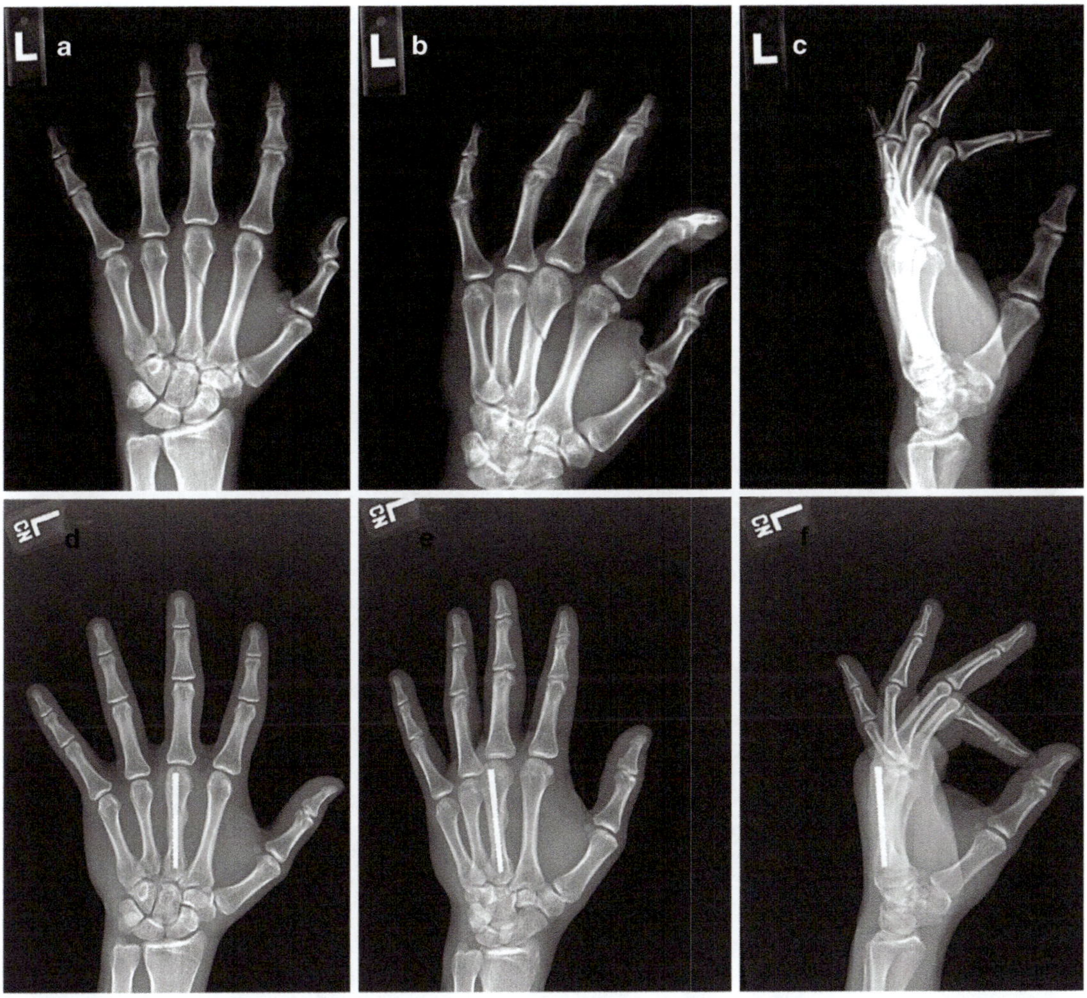

Fig. 6.5 (**a–f**) PA, oblique, and lateral radiographs of a left long finger distal metacarpal shaft fracture with significant clinical malrotation of the finger on examination (**a–c**). Six-week postoperative PA, oblique, and lateral radiographs demonstrate robust callous formation at the fracture site following intramedullary screw fixation (**d–f**)

of the dorsal apparatus. Retrograde or antegrade intramedullary screw fixation may also be considered for transverse and short oblique fractures of the proximal and middle phalanx and may allow for earlier return to activities (Fig. 6.8a–e). Spiral and long oblique fractures whose length measures at least two times the cortical diameter at the shaft are amenable to fixation with two or three interfragmentary lag screws. Occasionally, fractures of the proximal or middle phalangeal bases will require supplementary transarticular pinning of the PIP or MCP joints, or dorsal extension block pinning of either joint in order to maintain stable fracture reduction. Use of these modalities should be done with caution as this may result in a greater degree of motion loss that would be observed with non-transarticular fracture fixation.

Post-treatment Rehabilitation

Following most surgical treatment of metacarpal fractures, the athlete is immobilized in a radial gutter splint for the index and long finger metacarpals or an ulnar gutter splint for the ring and

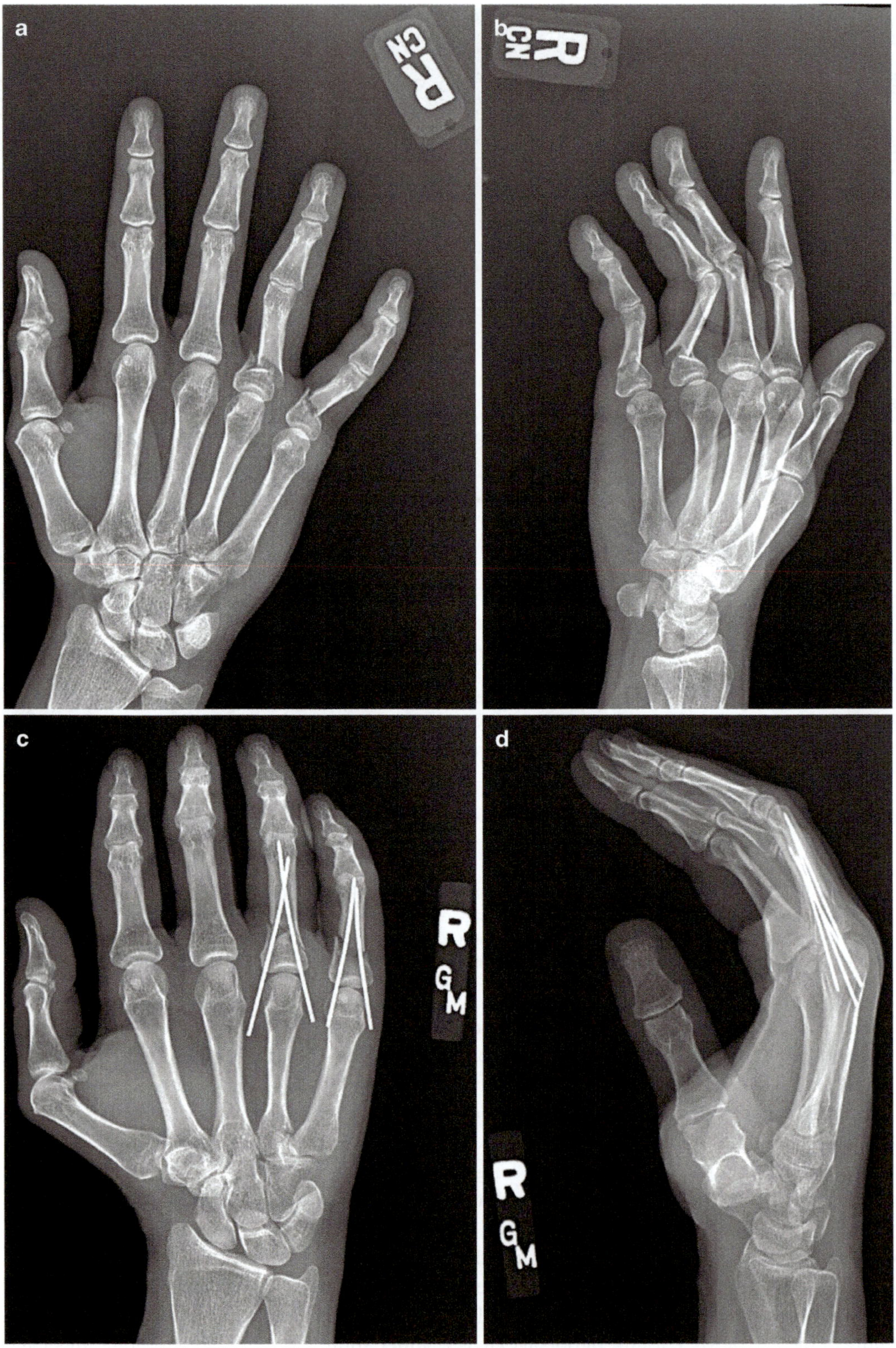

Fig. 6.6 (**a**–**d**) PA and lateral radiographs of transverse fractures of the right ring and small finger proximal phalangeal bases (**a**, **b**) treated with closed reduction and percutaneous pinning with 0.045″ smooth wire fixation (**c**, **d**)

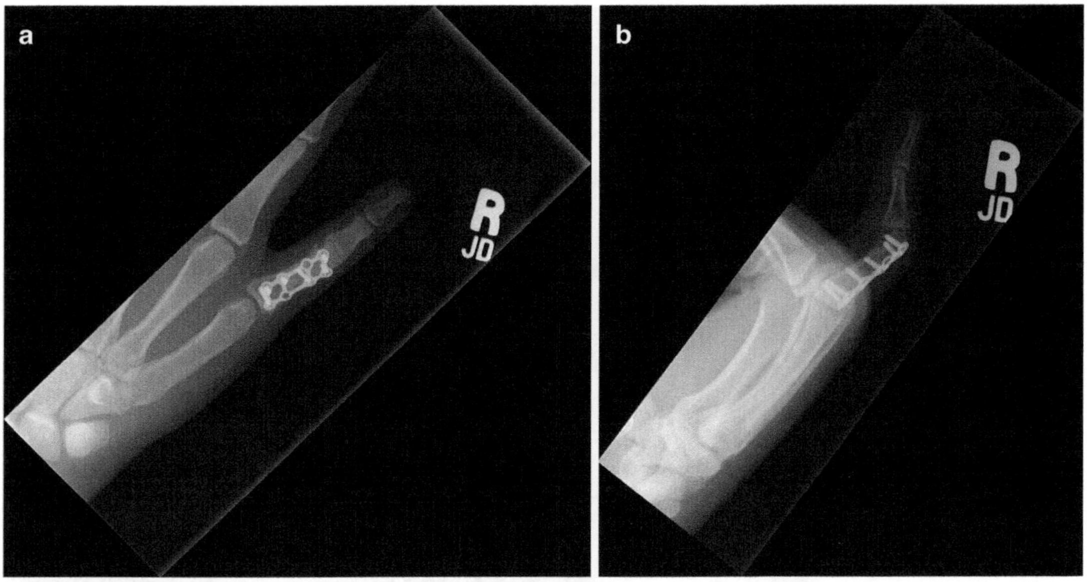

Fig. 6.7 (**a**, **b**) PA and lateral radiographs of a right small finger proximal phalanx fracture treated with open reduction and internal fixation with a plate and screw construct

small finger metacarpals. Active range of motion of the IP joints should be encouraged during the initial period of immobilization. Two weeks postoperatively, the patient is converted to a removable orthosis which blocks MCP motion but allows for continued free PIP and DIP motion. At 4 weeks, the player is converted to a hand-based radial or ulnar gutter splint for comfort and allowed to begin MCP range of motion. The immediate postoperative splint for those treated with intramedullary or transverse pinning should include the MCP joint in an intrinsic plus position with IP joints free. The player is subsequently converted to a removable orthosis to be worn as needed for comfort following suture removal at 2 weeks postoperatively. Following suture removal, the player is encouraged to return to conditioning activities as tolerated while adhering to the restrictions set forth for the operative hand. Players are allowed to begin full weightbearing activities once clinical and radiographic union are observed, generally at 6–8 weeks postoperatively. Athletes treated with rigid fixation including intramedullary screw, interfragmentary lag screw, or plate and screw constructs are allowed to return to early range of motion at the discretion of the treating surgeon, sometimes as early as 3–5 days postoperatively.

Rehabilitation following fixation of phalangeal fractures includes immobilization in a radial gutter splint with the digits in intrinsic plus position with the DIP joint free for proximal phalanx fractures of the index and long finger, or a similarly fashioned ulnar gutter splint for proximal phalanx fractures of the ring and small finger. Fractures of the middle phalanx are immobilized in a digital gutter splint incorporating the adjacent digit, with the MCP joint left free for range of motion. At 2 weeks, sutures (if present) are removed and the athlete is converted to removable orthosis similar to their immediate postoperative splint. The player is allowed to begin removing their splint for gentle ROM of all joints beginning at 3–4 weeks postoperatively if the fracture remains stable on follow-up radiographs. The removable orthosis is generally discontinued between 4 and 6 weeks postoperatively once the player has achieved pain-free range of motion. Players are allowed to begin full weightbearing activities once clinical and radiographic union are observed, generally at 6–8 weeks postoperatively.

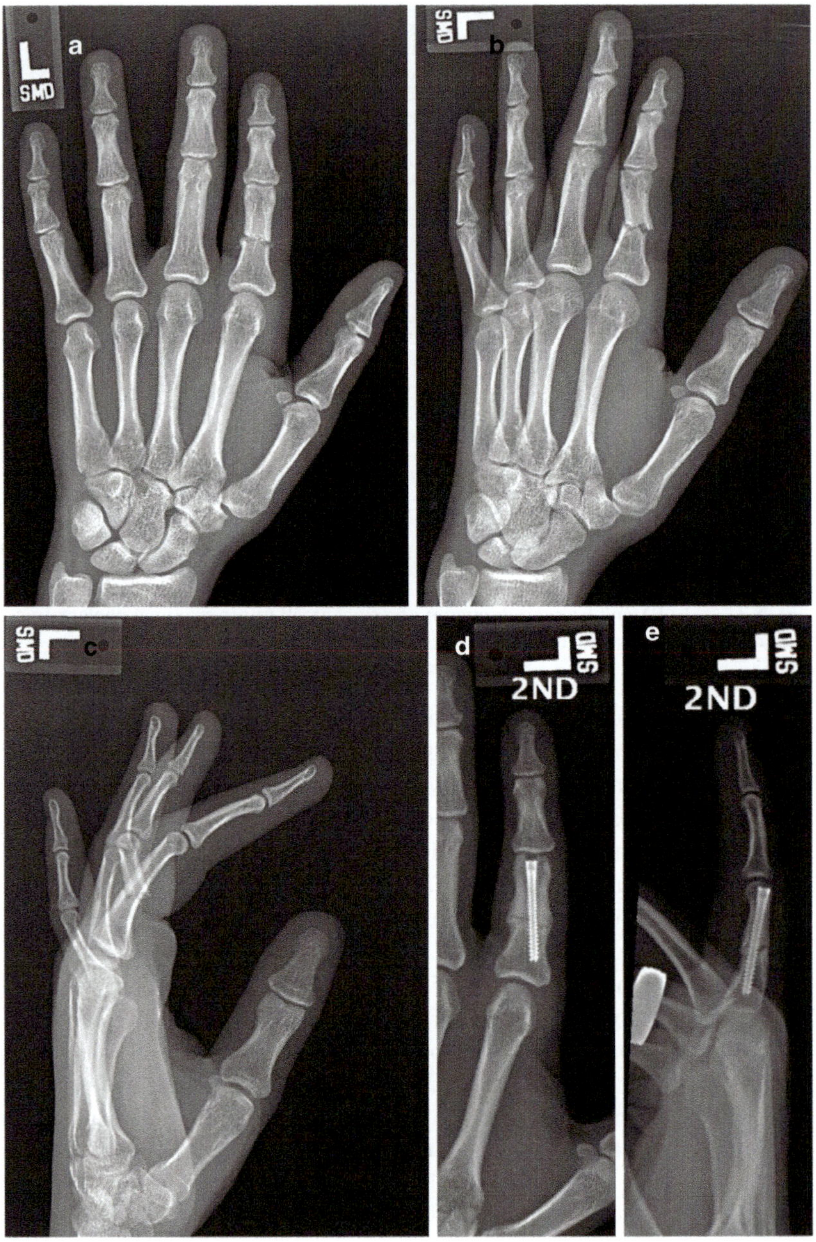

Fig. 6.8 (**a**–**e**) PA, oblique, and lateral radiographs of a transverse fracture of the index proximal phalanx (**a**–**c**) treated with retrograde intramedullary screw fixation (**d**, **e**)

Complications

Complications may occur as a result of both non-operative and operative treatment of metacarpal and phalangeal fractures. Patients treated with smooth wire fixation are at risk for pin-site irritation or pin-site infection. Superficial pin-site infections should be treated with 7–10 days of oral antibiotics, with close monitoring by the training room staff and treating surgeon to ensure resolution of the infection. Deep infection is rare with the described operative treatment modalities, but if present should be treated with prompt surgical debridement of the infection, removal or exchange of the hardware if possible, and appropriate antimicrobial therapy.

Smooth wire fixation may also result in wire breakage, which may complicate wire retrieval at the time of union or contribute to delayed union, nonunion, or malunion if occurring in the early postoperative period. Similarly, hardware failure has been observed with both interfragmentary screw and plate and screw constructs which may contribute to delayed union, nonunion, or malunion of the fracture. Malrotation of the digit following surgical fixation can be observed if careful attention is not directed to restoration of the normal digital flexion cascade intraoperatively. As little as 5° of malrotation can cause clinically significant digital overlap and may result in player dissatisfaction with the operation and limitations in performance. Shortening of the metacarpal may be poorly tolerated, as an extensor lag of 7° has previously been observed to result from every 2 mm of metacarpal shortening.

Postoperative stiffness is frequently observed following operative treatment of metacarpal and phalangeal fractures. Loss of motion may occur as a result of extensor tendon adhesion over the metacarpal, dorsal apparatus adhesions over the digit, collateral ligament contracture or tethering by fixation hardware, and capsular contracture. The degree to which stiffness occurs is often dependent upon the ability to effectively mobilize the athlete following surgery. The importance of edema control and early range of motion of the uninvolved joints cannot be overemphasized to the training staff and the athlete. Clinical examination by the treating surgeon at regular intervals postoperatively may allow for identification and early intervention for impending stiffness resulting in minimal lost time from competition. While removal of hardware for plate and screw constructs is not routinely indicated, this may be considered in players with postoperative stiffness and suspected tendinous adhesions undergoing an extensor tenolysis with or without concomitant dorsal capsulectomy.

Early Return to Play

The goal of both operative and nonoperative treatment of metacarpal and phalangeal fractures is to achieve clinical and radiographic fracture union and allow the athlete to return to competition as quickly and as safely as possible. In a survey of professional sports franchise hand consultants, it was noted that 38% favored immediate return to protected play for nondisplaced metacarpal fractures, while another 56.8% recommended return to protected play at 3–4 weeks (approximately the time of clinical union) [24]. In this same survey, unprotected play was allowed at 4–8 weeks by 73% of hand consultants. For players undergoing nonoperative treatment, we advocate for early edema, control, and initiation of range of motion of the unaffected adjacent joints to allow for early return to play. For patients with nondisplaced or minimally displaced metacarpal fractures amenable to nonoperative treatment, return to positional drills and batting practice may be allowed as early as 2 weeks if the patient is pain-free and has the requisite range of motion for each of these activities. Provided the player continues to progress with a focused return to play program under the supervision of the team's trainer, return to full competition may be allowed as early as 3 weeks (though it can take up to 6–8 weeks) without the need for formal orthosis wear. If early return to play is critically important due to any number of factors (scholarships, contractual implications, postseason, or championship competition), athletes may be counseled on the risks and benefits of intramedullary screw fixation of nondisplaced and minimally displaced fractures of the metacarpals and phalanges if it is felt this will allow for earlier return of range of motion and subsequent return to play. Players undergoing rigid intramedullary fixation of these fractures are often allowed to begin an early active range of motion as early as day 3 postoperatively, including MCP and PIP joint motion for metacarpal and proximal phalangeal joints, respectively. It is recommended that if players are to return to early baseball-related activities, the finger of the affected ray should be buddy taped to an adjacent digit to allow for assistance with range of motion and discourage malrotation of the involved digit.

References

1. Karl JW, Olson PR, Rosenwasser MP. The epidemiology of upper extremity fractures in the United States, 2009. J Orthop Trauma. 2015;29(8):e242–4.
2. Chung KC, Spilson SV. The frequency and epidemiology of hand and forearm fractures in the United States. J Hand Surg Am. 2001;26(5):908–15.
3. Rettig AC. Epidemiology of hand and wrist injuries in sports. Clin Sports Med. 1998;17(3):401–6.
4. Rettig AC. Athletic injuries of the wrist and hand. Part I: traumatic injuries of the wrist. Am J Sports Med. 2003;31(6):1038–48.
5. Aitken S, Court-Brown CM. The epidemiology of sports-related fractures of the hand. Injury. 2008;39(12):1377–83.
6. Lehman JD, Krishnan KR, Stepan JG, Nwachukwu BU. Prevalence and treatment outcomes of hand and wrist injuries in professional athletes: a systematic review. HSS J. 2020;16(3):280–7.
7. Collins CL, Comstock RD. Epidemiological features of high school baseball injuries in the United States, 2005-2007. Pediatrics. 2008;121(6):1181–7.
8. Posner M, Cameron KL, Wolf JM, Belmont PJ Jr, Owens BD. Epidemiology of Major League Baseball injuries. Am J Sports Med. 2011;39(8):1676–80.
9. Rhee PC, Camp CL, D'Angelo J, Desai VS, Shin SS, Sheridan D, et al. Epidemiology and impact of hand and wrist injuries in major and minor league baseball. Hand (N Y). 2019:1558944719864450.
10. Strickland JW. Considerations for the treatment of the injured athlete. Clin Sports Med. 1998;17(3): 397–400.
11. Nakamura K, Patterson RM, Viegas SF. The ligament and skeletal anatomy of the second through fifth carpometacarpal joints and adjacent structures. J Hand Surg Am. 2001;26(6):1016–29.
12. Chin SH, Vedder NB. MOC-PSSM CME article: metacarpal fractures. Plast Reconstr Surg. 2008;121(1 Suppl):1–13.
13. Panchal-Kildare S, Malone K. Skeletal anatomy of the hand. Hand Clin. 2013;29(4):459–71.
14. Fufa DT, Goldfarb CA. Fractures of the thumb and finger metacarpals in athletes. Hand Clin. 2012;28(3):379–88, x.
15. Gaston RG, Chadderdon C. Phalangeal fractures: displaced/nondisplaced. Hand Clin. 2012;28(3):395–401, x.
16. Camp CL, Wang D, Sinatro AS, D'Angelo J, Coleman SH, Dines JS, et al. Getting hit by pitch in professional baseball: analysis of injury patterns, risk factors, concussions, and days missed for batters. Am J Sports Med. 2018;46(8):1997–2003.
17. Goldfarb CA. Commentary metacarpal fracture in the professional baseball player. Hand Clin. 2012;28(3):389.
18. Shin SS. Phalangeal fractures in baseball: commentary. Hand Clin. 2012;28(3):403.
19. Johnson J, Fowler J, Costello J, Ruppert K, Kaufmann R. Optimal oblique radiographs to identify fifth carpometacarpal dorsal subluxations: a cadaveric study. J Hand Surg Am. 2018;43(12):1139 e1–5.
20. del Pinal F, Moraleda E, Ruas JS, de Piero GH, Cerezal L. Minimally invasive fixation of fractures of the phalanges and metacarpals with intramedullary cannulated headless compression screws. J Hand Surg Am. 2015;40(4):692–700.
21. Dunleavy ML, Candela X, Darowish M. Morphological analysis of metacarpal shafts with respect to retrograde intramedullary headless screw fixation. Hand (N Y). 2020:1558944720937362.
22. Hoang D, Vu CL, Jackson M, Huang JI. An anatomical study of metacarpal morphology utilizing CT scans: evaluating parameters for antegrade intramedullary compression screw fixation of metacarpal fractures. J Hand Surg Am. 2021;46(2):149 e1–8.
23. Shah CM, Sommerkamp TG. Fracture dislocation of the finger joints. J Hand Surg Am. 2014;39(4): 792–802.
24. Dy CJ, Khmelnitskaya E, Hearns KA, Carlson MG. Opinions regarding the management of hand and wrist injuries in elite athletes. Orthopedics. 2013;36(6):815–9.

Thumb Basilar Joint Injuries

7

Mia M. Qin, Chirag M. Shah, Thomas A. Wiedrich,
Joseph T. Labrum IV, and Douglas R. Weikert

Fractures

Introduction

Fractures of the base of the thumb metacarpal are common injuries in athletes. These injuries encompass extra-articular fractures and intra-articular fractures, including Bennett fractures and Rolando fractures. In the general population, fractures of the base of the thumb metacarpal are estimated to be 4% of all hand fractures [1]. The epidemiology of thumb basilar fractures has not been well defined in sports in general or in baseball specifically. Thumb basilar fractures do occur in baseball, however are much more common in contact sports such as basketball, football, and hockey [2].

Pertinent Anatomy

The thumb metacarpal lies in a pronated position relative to the other metacarpals. The trapeziometacarpal joint has a biconcave saddle articulation with the trapezium, providing the thumb motion in three planes: flexion/extension, abduction/adduction, and pronation/supination, which provides 40% of hand function [3–6]. The bony geometry of the joint, joint capsule, and surrounding ligaments impart stability to the joint. Understanding the complex relationship between these anatomic structures allows one to appreciate the behavior of these fractures.

M. M. Qin · C. M. Shah · T. A. Wiedrich (✉)
Department of Orthopaedic Surgery, Northwestern University Feinberg School of Medicine, Chicago, IL, USA
e-mail: douglas.weikert@vanderbilt.edu

J. T. Labrum IV · D. R. Weikert
Department of Orthopaedic Surgery, Vanderbilt Medical Center, Nashville, TN, USA

G. M. Lourie (ed.), *Hand and Wrist Injuries in Baseball*,
https://doi.org/10.1007/978-3-030-81659-9_7

Mechanism of Injury/History

In extra-articular base of thumb metacarpal fractures, the fracture deforms in a predictable fashion based on its particular attachments, resulting in apex dorsal angulation, adduction, and flexion of the distal fragment. The dorsal angulation is secondary to extension of the metacarpal base by the abductor pollicis longus and flexion of the distal shaft by the thenar muscles [2, 7].

Bennett fractures refer to two-part intra-articular fractures of the thumb metacarpal base with separation of the metacarpal from the volar-ulnar joint fragment. The volar-ulnar portion of the metacarpal base is stabilized to the trapezium by the anterior oblique ligament [2, 8, 9]. There is mounting evidence to suggest the dorsal radial ligament is a major stabilizer to the CMC joint of the thumb [10]. Because of the intact muscular attachments to the thumb metacarpal, the metacarpal shaft subluxes dorsally, proximally, and radially primarily by the abductor pollicis longus. The extensor pollicis longus, extensor pollicis brevis, and adductor pollicis also contribute to the deforming forces [11]. The size of the volar-ulnar fragment affects the degree of displacement owing to increased stability with a larger fragment [12].

Rolando fractures are classically described as T- or Y-shaped intra-articular fractures of the base of the thumb metacarpal, but today, the eponym describes any comminuted intra-articular fracture involving the base of the thumb metacarpal [2]. The anterior oblique ligament prevents displacement of the volar fragment, the adductor pollicis draws the distal diaphyseal fragment into adduction, and the abductor pollicis longus pulls the lateral epiphyseal fragment upward and outward [11].

The mechanism of injury for thumb basilar fractures can vary from falling onto an outstretched hand to direct blow from contact. The contact may be with another player or with sporting equipment, including ball, helmet, etc. Bennett and Rolando fractures occur by an axial load directed through a partially flexed metacarpal shaft [7].

Physical Exam

The initial management of thumb basilar fractures begins with an on- or off-field evaluation after injury. One should have a high index of suspicion for fracture in a baseball player with hand swelling following a fall or high injury impact. The hand should be evaluated for wounds suggestive of an open fracture, neurovascular status, gross deformity, crepitus with palpation, or instability if tolerated on exam. Lack of full motion or subtle angular deformity may suggest fracture or joint subluxation.

Imaging

Initial imaging should include posterior-anterior, lateral, and oblique radiographs. Additional views include a Roberts view, which is a true anterior-posterior view of the thumb. This is obtained with the arm in full pronation and the dorsum of the thumb on the X-ray cassette. A true lateral view is obtained with the hand pronated 20–30° and the beam angled 10–15° distally. CT is occasionally used for pre-surgical planning to determine the degree of intra-articular displacement and for highly comminuted fractures. This advanced imaging modality can often help with planning the type of fixation to be used in more complex fracture patterns. MRI has limited value in thumb basilar fractures.

Conservative Treatment

Conservative treatment in the form of thumb spica splint or cast is rarely recommended for extra-articular fractures and almost never recommended for intra-articular fractures in baseball players. A high degree of angulation, up to 30°, is well tolerated in extra-articular fractures owing to the large amount of motion at the thumb carpometacarpal joint. However, apex dorsal angulation beyond 30° will lead to thumb webspace narrowing and compensatory metacarpophalangeal joint hyperextension, which is poorly tolerated [2, 7].

Surgical Treatment

Extra-articular fractures can be treated surgically either with closed reduction and crossed K-wire fixation or with open reduction and plate/screw fixation (Figs. 7.1 and 7.2). Closed reduction is obtained using a combination of traction, extension, and pronation with direct pressure on the metacarpal base. Plate/screw fixation is often advocated for in baseball players, as it provides a more stable construct compared with K-wire fixation. This may allow for earlier range of motion [2, 7].

The surgical goal in intra-articular fractures is to obtain fracture reduction with a congruent joint. Bennett fractures in a non-athlete population are often treated with closed reduction and percutaneous pinning with K-wires (Figs. 7.3

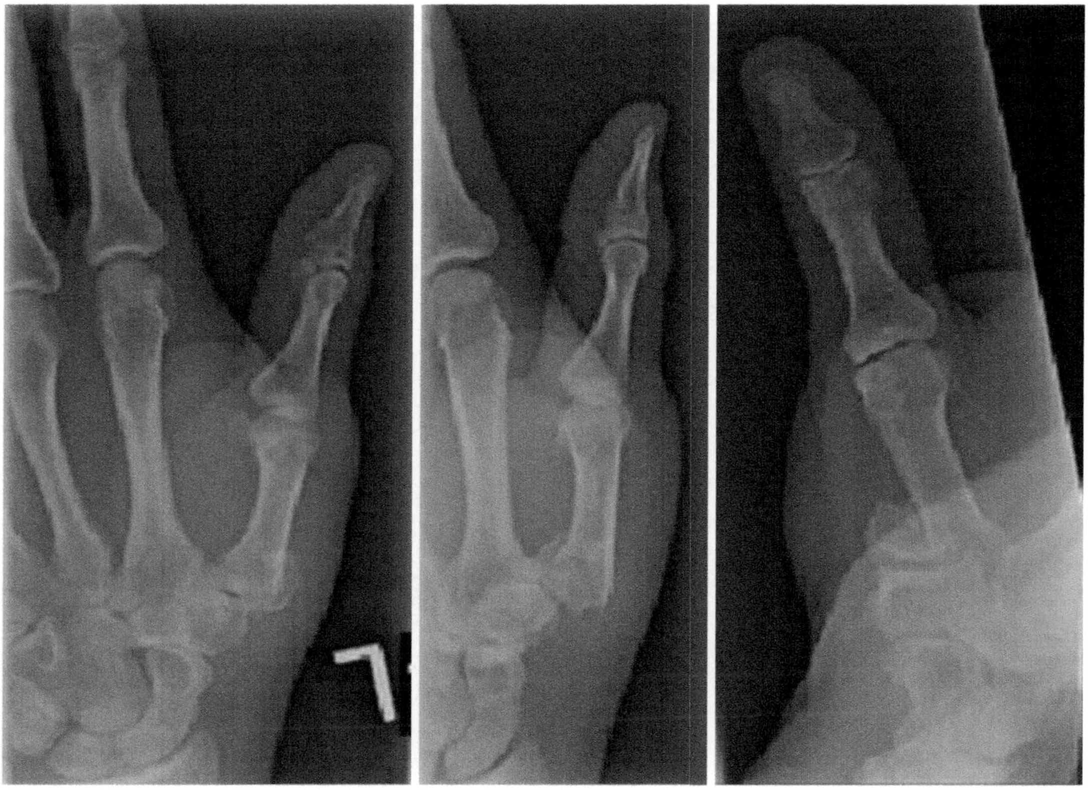

Fig. 7.1 Thumb metacarpal base fracture preoperative radiographs

and 7.4). One K-wire is placed from the metacarpal into the volar-ulnar fragment, and the second K-wire is placed from the base of the first metacarpal into either the trapezium or the base of the second metacarpal. Closed reduction and pinning in baseball players is reserved for those fractures with a fragment too small to capture with screws. In baseball players, open reduction and internal fixation is advocated to minimize immobilization and due to enhanced stability of the construct (Figs. 7.5 and 7.6). Using a Wagner approach, a 1.5–2.7 mm screw is used in the base of the metacarpal across the fracture. If there is a concern regarding stability with screw fixation alone, trans-articular pinning across the carpometacarpal joint can supplement fixation [2, 13].

Rolando fractures are best treated with open reduction and internal fixation with plate and screw construct (Figs. 7.7 and 7.8) [2, 4, 13]. The prognosis is best for simple T- or Y- shaped Rolando fractures where the volar-ulnar and dorsal articular fragments can be anatomically reduced. In more comminuted fractures, anatomic reduction may be impossible. Bone graft may be used to help fill metaphyseal voids. If there is significant comminution hindering open reduction and fixation, distraction and external fixation relying on ligamentotaxis may be required [12, 14, 15]. Fractures treated with external fixation may have detrimental effects on the athlete's season or possibly career [2, 7].

The length of postoperative immobilization in a thumb spica splint or cast varies based on the specific fracture characteristics and stability of fixation. Thumb spica immobilization should leave the thumb interphalangeal joint free to allow for immediate interphalangeal joint motion. If a trans-articular pin is placed, it is generally removed at 4 to 5 weeks postoperatively for initiation of range of motion.

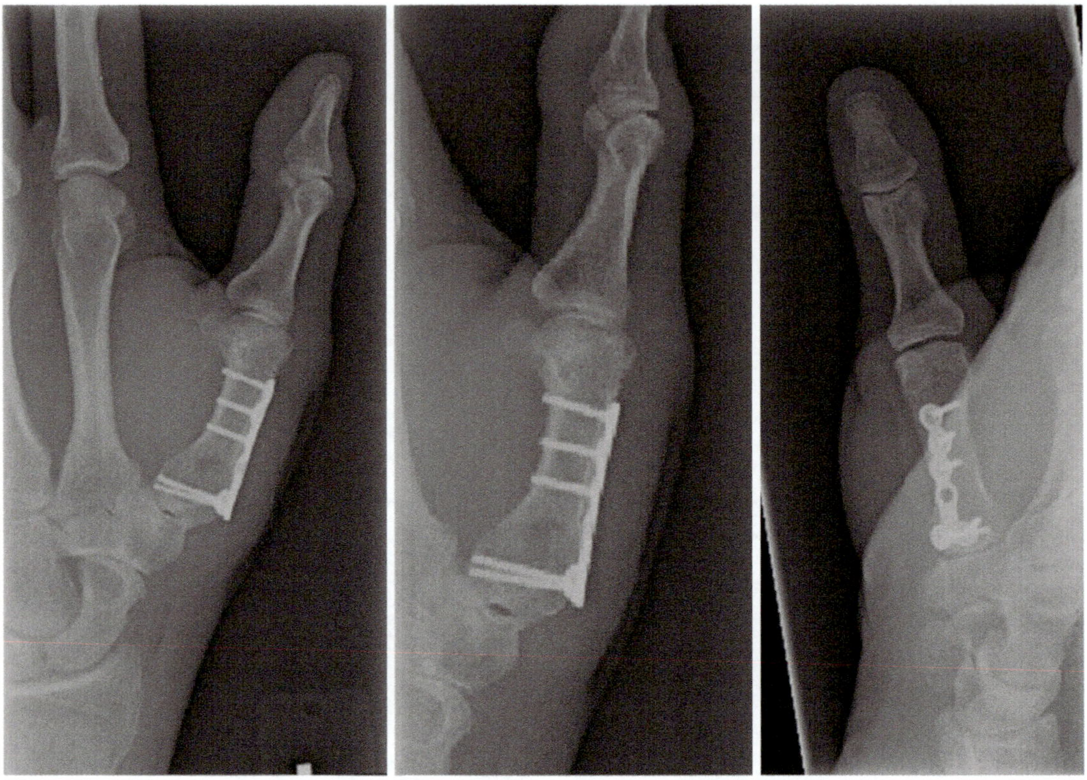

Fig. 7.2 Thumb metacarpal base open reduction and internal fixation postoperative radiographs

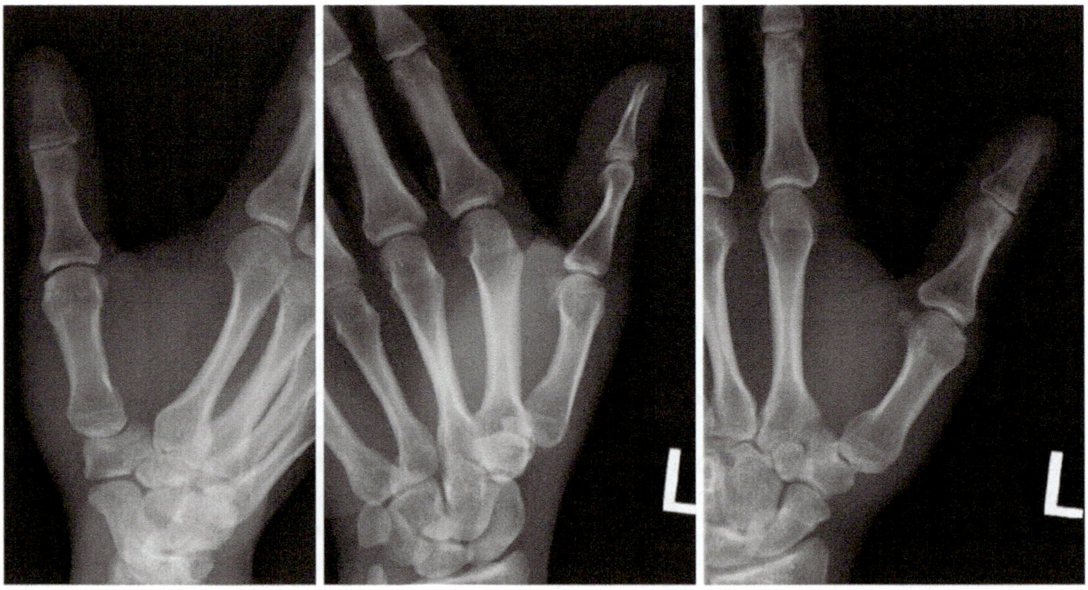

Fig. 7.3 Bennett fracture preoperative radiographs

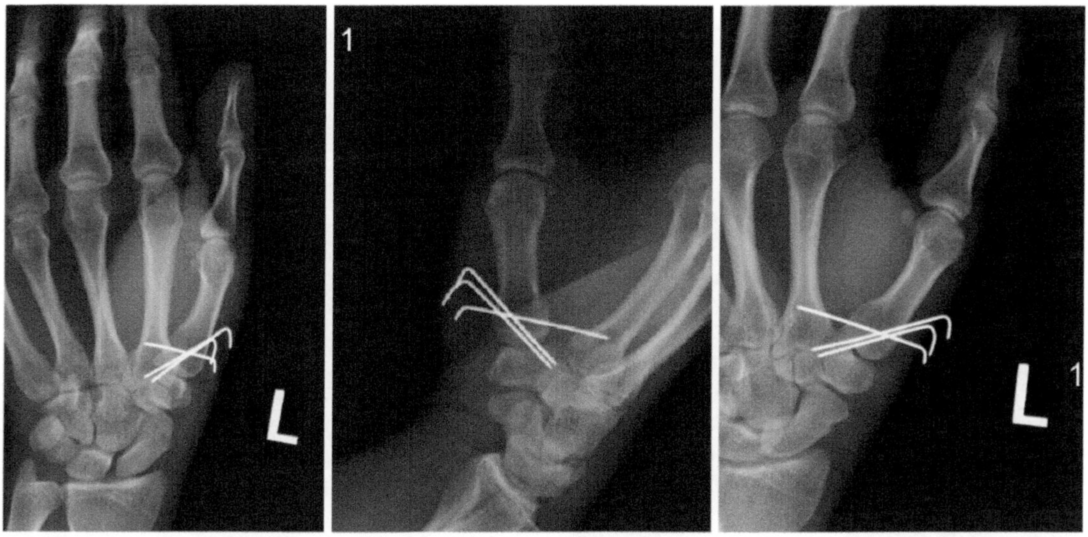

Fig. 7.4 Bennett fracture closed reduction and percutaneous pinning postoperative radiographs

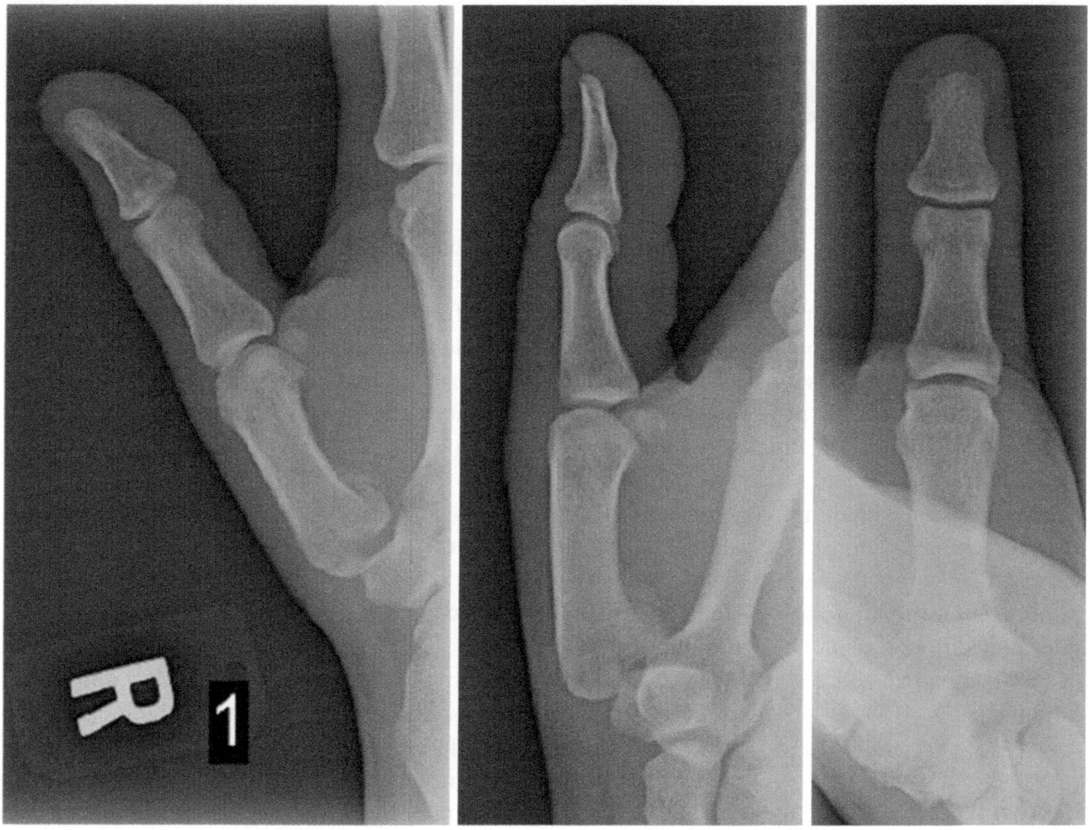

Fig. 7.5 Bennett fracture preoperative radiographs

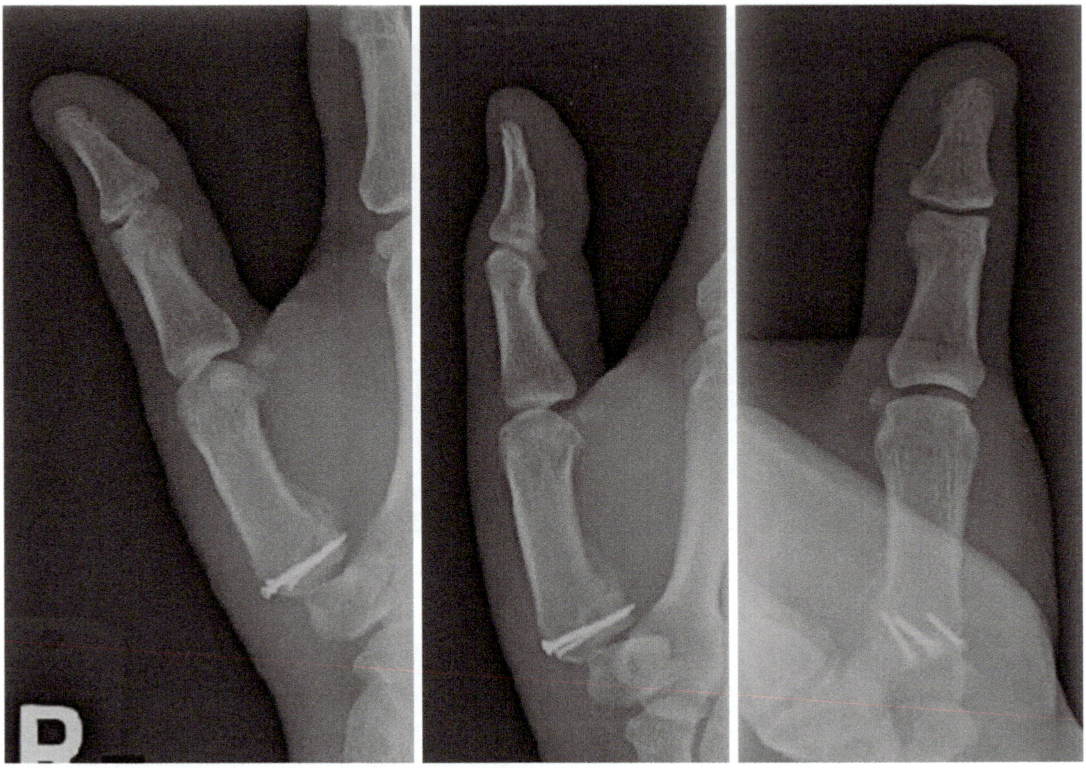

Fig. 7.6 Bennett fracture open reduction and internal fixation postoperative radiographs

Complications

There are many potential complications of thumb basilar fractures in baseball players. Due to the deforming forces, there is a risk of loss of reduction, which can lead to post-traumatic arthritis and joint instability. The surgical approach and internal fixation increases the risk of extensor tendon adhesions affecting range of motion and smooth tendon gliding. The superficial radial nerve can lie within the surgical field and must be protected to avoid injury and postoperative irritation. In addition to this, the subcutaneous nature of the fixation can cause symptomatic hardware prominence.

Return to Play

Due to the high stresses on the thumb, return to play is not advocated before clear bony healing is demonstrated at 6–10 weeks postoperatively [2, 7]. There is no protective splint or cast that can allow for earlier return to play prior to bony healing. Bone stimulators have been suggested to decrease time to healing; however, there is no evidence proving their utility in this clinical setting.

Dislocations

Introduction

Pure thumb carpometacarpal (CMC) joint dislocations, while rare, represent a significant baseball injury that can alter athletic performance and result in loss of playing time. Appropriate management of these injuries in baseball players can be challenging, with treatment focused on optimizing outcome and allowing return to previous level of sport in a timely fashion.

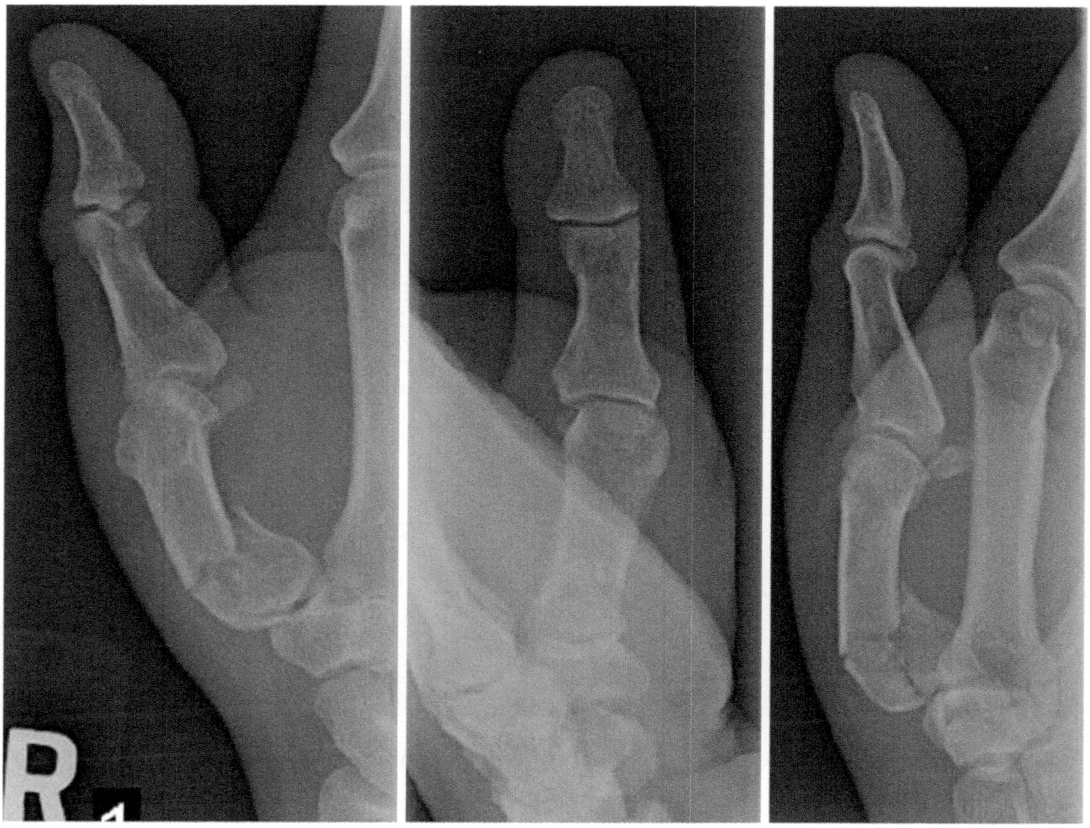

Fig. 7.7 Rolando fracture preoperative radiographs

Mechanism of Injury

Thumb carpometacarpal (CMC) joint dislocations classically result from axial loading of the thumb during partial thumb CMC flexion. This results in excessive loading of the dorsal joint capsule which ultimately fails, allowing dorsal dislocation of the first metacarpal with respect to the trapezium. These injuries are typically traumatic in nature [16, 17]. As a result, thumb CMC joint dislocations are more commonly seen in infielders and catchers as opposed to pitchers, as these position players are more likely to sustain direct trauma to the hand during batting, base running, or fielding [18]. Volar dislocation of the thumb CMC joint is exceedingly rare but has been reported [19].

Hand injuries resulting from baseball and softball injuries have been reported to comprise 2.2% of all emergency department visits [20]. Pure thumb CMC joint dislocations account for less than 1% of all hand injuries [21]. An epidemiological study of Major League Baseball players from 2010 to 2016 observed 231 hand injuries, constituting 14% of all upper extremity injuries sustained during the study period [19]. Of players sustaining hand injuries, infielders were the most likely to sustain a hand injury (62%), followed by pitchers (26%) and catchers (12%) [19]. Of the 231 hand injuries noted in the study period, 106 (46%) involved fractures and only 2 (0.9%) required operative intervention [19].

Pertinent Anatomy

The CMC joint of the thumb is a unique articulation that is vital to the athlete's hand function. The relatively incongruent saddle articulation between the thumb metacarpal base and

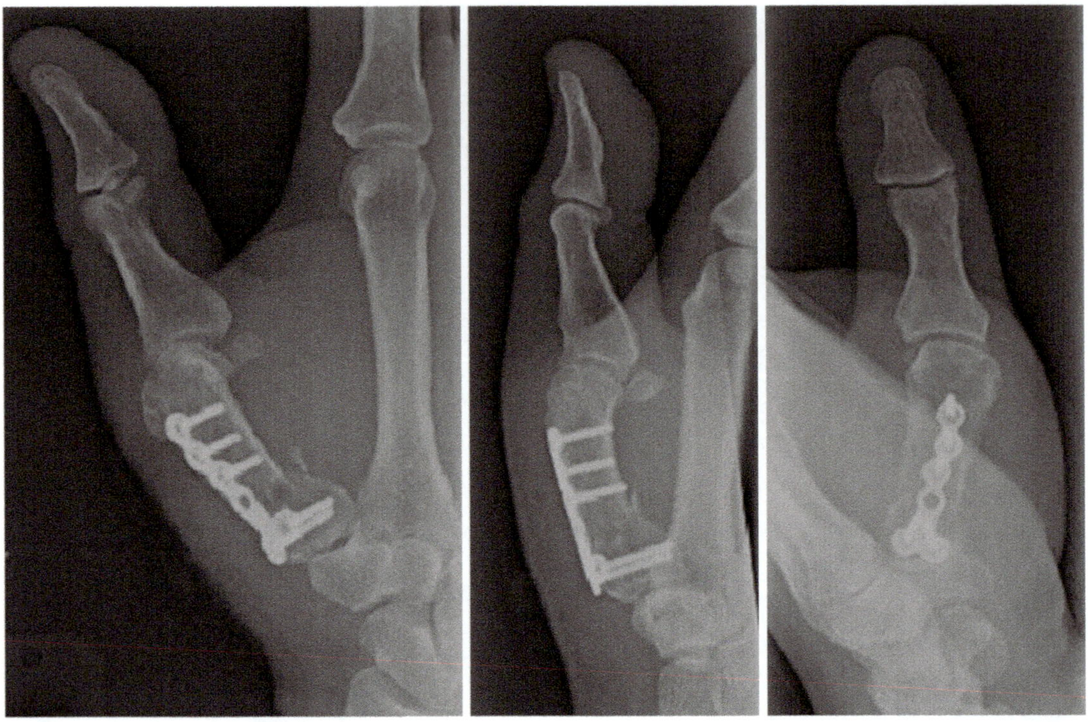

Fig. 7.8 Rolando fracture open reduction and internal fixation postoperative radiograph

trapezium represents a semi-constrained joint with little inherent bony stability. The trapezium functions as the base of the thumb CMC joint, with anchoring articulations to the scaphoid, trapezoid, and base of the index metacarpal (Komatsu et al.). As a result of a unique biaxial articulation, the thumb metacarpal is able to articulate on the trapezium with motion arcs of flexion and extension, adduction and abduction, as well as wide circumduction [22, 23]. The thumb trapeziometacarpal joint therefore contributes to thumb opposition and prehension, introducing dexterity that is vital to hand function. The thumb CMC joint does withstand significant forces during hand function. Joint reactive forces seen across the thumb CMC joint can reach 13 times the force seen at the tip of the finger during hand grasp and pinch [24].

Ligamentous structures surrounding the thumb CMC joint are crucial to its function, introducing static stability to an inherently unstable articulation [25]. Ladd et al. identified seven principal ligaments surrounding the thumb CMC joint in a cadaveric study of 30 hands [22]. These ligaments included three dorsal deltoid-shaped ligaments (dorsal radial, dorsal central, and posterior oblique), two volar ligaments (anterior oblique and ulnar collateral), and two ulnar ligaments (dorsal trapeziometacarpal and intermetacarpal). The dorsal ligament complex (dorsoradial) and the anterior oblique ligament are considered the most important stabilizers of the thumb trapeziometacarpal joint, with recent research suggesting the dorsal ligament complex as the primary stabilizer of the thumb trapeziometacarpal joint [22, 23, 26].

The dorsal ligament complex as a whole represents the strongest ligamentous structure surrounding the thumb CMC joint. This dorsal ligamentous complex is taut in thumb CMC flexion, with the dorsoradial ligament serving as the primary check rein for dorsal subluxation of the thumb metacarpal as can be seen in thumb CMC dislocation [27]. In cases of thumb CMC dislocation, there is often complete tearing of the dorsal ligament complex as well as the dorsal joint capsule.

Volarly, the thumb trapeziometacarpal joint is primarily stabilized by the anterior oblique ligament. The anterior oblique ligament, also referred to as the "beak ligament," originates on the volar edge of the trapezium (palmar tubercle) and inserts ulnar to abductor pollicis longus on the volar distal extension of the thumb metacarpal, stabilizing the thumb CMC joint against dorsoradial subluxation [22, 25].

History/Physical Exam

Prompt evaluation of acute hand injuries should be on field or in the dugout. The focus should be on identifying any deformity, open wound, soft tissue swelling, bruising, or tenderness. The player will usually exhibit pain and sometimes describe subluxation of the joint.

In the setting of dorsal thumb CMC dislocation, the athlete typically has significant swelling and deformity about the dorsoradial hand. The thumb metacarpal is held in a position of flexion and the athlete is unable to make a fist. There is often a prominence located over the thumb CMC joint as a result of the thumb metacarpal positioned dorsally with respect to the trapezium. Range of motion is significantly limited and attempts at passive range of motion elicit significant pain. Acute management should be focused on expeditious diagnosis and reduction.

When athletes present for evaluation on a subacute or delayed basis following closed reduction, examination should be focused on stability of the thumb CMC joint. Any subluxation of the thumb CMC joint noted on physical examination should serve as confirmation of an unstable thumb CMC joint that requires further radiographic evaluation and operative intervention. The thumb CMC joint can be stressed with axial loading while the thumb is held in slight flexion. In cases of residual instability, dorsal subluxation of the thumb metacarpal can be appreciated. It is also important to examine the ulnar collateral ligament in patients presenting with thumb CMC dislocation, as the UCL can also be completely torn or incompetent [28].

As with all acute hand injuries, imaging plays an important role in the initial evaluation. Anteroposterior, lateral, and oblique images of the hand are necessary to allow adequate radiographic evaluation of the injury [29].

Imaging

In the setting of presumed thumb CMC dislocation, ideally, radiographic evaluation should be carried out prior to attempts at reduction. Scrutiny of the thumb metacarpal base is warranted to rule out a Bennett fracture dislocation, which can have similar clinical presentation and represents a more common pathology in baseball-related hand trauma. This distinction is an important one as it affects acute management as well as surgical treatment.

Stress radiographs can be carried out following primary reduction to evaluate thumb CMC stability. These radiographs allow visualization of hypermobility of the thumb trapeziometacarpal joint with comparison to the contralateral side. They are executed by having the patient push the radial border of the affected thumb against the radial border of the contralateral thumb while keeping the hands parallel to the X-ray cassette. Instability will manifest as excessive radial subluxation of the thumb metacarpal base at the thumb CMC joint when compared to the unaffected side [30].

Additionally, fluoroscopic imaging serves as an excellent tool to acutely assess the injured hand both statically and dynamically. Fluoroscopy can confirm the clinical diagnosis of a thumb CMC dislocation and whether a concentric reduction has been achieved. Dynamically, the fluoroscope can demonstrate the degree of instability during stress testing of the CMC joint.

Conservative Treatment

Initial management of the dislocated thumb CMC joint consists of closed reduction and placing a thumb spica splint. This is usually accomplished with longitudinal traction and dorsal pressure over the thumb metacarpal. While an "easy" reduction is usually the case, this often implies instability and the need for addition means of stabilization. Once post-reduction instability has been demonstrated (physical exam, X-rays, fluoroscopy), surgical stabilization should be expected.

In athletes with a concentric and stable thumb CMC joint following pure thumb CMC dislocation, immobilization in a short thumb spica cast is typically employed for 4–6 weeks [17, 28, 31]. Stability must be assured based on imaging and physical examination before nonoperative management is undertaken. Rehabilitation and gradual return to play may take an additional 4–6 weeks after cast removal.

Surgical Treatment

Most thumb CMC dislocations will have residual instability and require operative intervention. Pure thumb CMC dislocations with residual instability, treated nonoperatively, will adversely affect the throwing athlete, resulting in painful grip, pinch, and diminished strength, significantly altering both batting and fielding performance. After the thumb CMC joint has been determined to be unstable, MRI may be considered for preoperative planning for further evaluation of the ligamentous injury surrounding the thumb CMC joint.

The operative treatment of choice of pure thumb CMC dislocations with residual instability remains controversial, but many support open primary repair of the dorsoradial ligament and/or dorsal ligament complex with capsulorrhaphy. Excellent outcomes have been reported following acute primary ligament repair [16, 17, 28, 32]. Previous reports of closed reduction with percutaneous fixation and immobilization have had mixed results with residual instability and need for revision surgery [32].

In cases of chronic thumb CMC joint instability where primary repair was insufficient or not possible, the reconstruction can be augmented with a slip of the flexor carpi radialis (FCR). This can be carried out via the Eaton-Littler technique, the modified Eaton-Littler technique, or ligament repair with FCR augmentation.

Following both primary repair and FCR reconstruction, patients are immobilized in a thumb spica cast or thumb spica splint for 4–6 weeks, followed by rehabilitation, strengthening, and gradual return to play. The entire process may take 8–10 weeks since protective bracing while playing is not usually possible.

In summary, pure thumb carpometacarpal (CMC) joint dislocations, while uncommon in baseball players, may represent a significant injury with extended loss of playing time. Most of these injuries are inherently unstable and require surgical intervention. Demonstrating a concentric reduction, appropriately repairing the soft tissue CMC stabilizers, and allowing enough time for soft tissue healing are all imperative in obtaining a desired outcome.

References

Fracture

1. Stanton JS, Dias JJ, Burke FD. Fractures of the tubular bones of the hand. J Hand Surg Eur Vol. 2007;32(6):626–36.
2. Fufa DT, Goldfarb CA. Fractures of the thumb and finger metacarpals in athletes. Hand Clin. 2012;28(3):379–88, x.
3. Panchal-Kildare S, Malone K. Skeletal anatomy of the hand. Hand Clin. 2013;29(4):459–71.
4. Chin SH, Vedder NB. MOC-PSSM CME article: metacarpal fractures. Plast Reconstr Surg. 2008;121(1 Suppl):1–13.
5. Cooney WP 3rd, Lucca MJ, Chao EY, Linscheid RL. The kinesiology of the thumb trapeziometacarpal joint. J Bone Joint Surg Am. 1981;63(9):1371–81.
6. Moran SL, Berger RA. Biomechanics and hand trauma: what you need. Hand Clin. 2003;19(1):17–31.
7. Kadow TR, Fowler JR. Thumb injuries in athletes. Hand Clin. 2017;33(1):161–73.
8. Bettinger PC, Berger RA. Functional ligamentous anatomy of the trapezium and trapeziometacarpal joint (gross and arthroscopic). Hand Clin. 2001;17(2):151–68, vii.
9. Bettinger PC, Linscheid RL, Berger RA, Cooney WP 3rd, An KN. An anatomic study of the stabilizing ligaments of the trapezium and trapeziometacarpal joint. J Hand Surg Am. 1999;24(4):786–98.

10. Kawanishi Y, Oka K, Tanaka H, Okada K, Sugamoto K, Murase T. In vivo 3-dimensional kinematics of thumb carpometacarpal joint during thumb opposition. J Hand Surg Am. 2018;43(2):182 e1–7.
11. Soyer AD. Fractures of the base of the first metacarpal: current treatment options. J Am Acad Orthop Surg. 1999;7(6):403–12.
12. Carlsen BT, Moran SL. Thumb trauma: Bennett fractures, Rolando fractures, and ulnar collateral ligament injuries. J Hand Surg Am. 2009;34(5):945–52.
13. Wahl EP, Richard MJ. Management of metacarpal and phalangeal fractures in the athlete. Clin Sports Med. 2020;39(2):401–22.
14. Gelberman RH, Vance RM, Zakaib GS. Fractures at the base of the thumb: treatment with oblique traction. J Bone Joint Surg Am. 1979;61(2):260–2.
15. Buchler U, McCollam SM, Oppikofer C. Comminuted fractures of the basilar joint of the thumb: combined treatment by external fixation, limited internal fixation, and bone grafting. J Hand Surg Am. 1991;16(3):556–60.

Dislocation

16. Fotiadis E, Svarnas T, Lyrtzis C, et al. Isolated thumb carpometacarpal joint dislocation: a case report and review of literature. Orthop Surg Res. 2010;5(1):16.
17. Bosmans B, Verhofstad MHJ, Gosens T. Traumatic thumb carpometacarpal joint dislocations. J Hand Surg Am. 2008;33(3):438–41.
18. Fares MY, Salhab HA, Khachfe H, et al. Upper limb injuries in Major League Baseball. Phys Ther Sport. 2020;41:49–54.
19. Sawalha S. Volar dislocation of the thumb carpometacarpal joint: a case report. Acta Orthop Traumatol Turc. 2017;51(4):352–4.
20. Dawson W, Pullos N. Baseball injuries to the hand. Ann Emerg Med. 1981;10:302–6.
21. Mueller JJ. Carpometacarpal dislocations: report of five cases and review of the literature. J Hand Surg. 1986;11A:184–8.
22. Ladd AL, Lee J, Hagert E. Macroscopic and microscopic analysis of the thumb carpometacarpal ligaments: a cadaveric study of ligament anatomy and histology. J Bone Joint Surg Am. 2012;94(16):1468–77.
23. Komatsu I, Lubahn JD. Anatomy and biomechanics of the thumb carpometacarpal joint. Oper Tech Orthop. 2018;28:1–5.
24. Berger AJ, Meals RA. Management of osteoarthrosis of the thumb joints. J Hand Surg Am. 2015;40(4):843–50.
25. McCann MR, Rust PA, Wallace R. The stabilising effect of the anterior oblique ligament to prevent directional subluxation at the trapeziometacarpal joint of the thumb: a biomechanical cadaveric study. Arch Bone Jt Surg. 2018;6(2):105–11.
26. Lin JD, Karl JW, Strauch RJ. Trapeziometacarpal joint stability: the evolving importance of the dorsal ligaments. Clin Orthop Relat Res. 2014;472(4):1138–45.
27. Bettinger PC, Linscheid RL, Berger RA, et al. An anatomic study of the stabilizing ligaments of the trapezium and trapeziometacarpal joint. J Hand Surg Am. 1999;24(4):786–98.
28. Lahijji F, Zandi R, Maleki A. First carpometacarpal joint dislocation and review of literatures. Arch Bone Jt Surg. 2015;3(4):300–3.
29. Sundaram N, Bosley J, Stacy GS. Conventional radiographic evaluation of athletic injuries to the hand. Radiol Clin N Am. 2013;51(2):239–55.
30. Wolf JM, Oren TW, Ferguson B, et al. The carpometacarpal stress view radiograph in the evaluation of trapeziometacarpal joint laxity. J Hand Surg Am. 2009;34(8):1402–6.
31. Khan AM, Ryan MG, Teplitz GA. Bilateral carpometacarpal dislocations of the thumb. Am J Orthop. 2003;32(1):38–41.
32. Annappa R, Kotian P, Aithala PJ, et al. Ligamentous reconstruction of traumatic dislocation of thumb carpometacarpal joint: case report and review of literature. J Orthop Case Rep. 2015;5(4):79–81.

8 Distal Tip Injuries and Blisters

Douglas Carlan

Distal fingertip injuries in baseball are common and can lead to significant losses of playing time. Injuries to the hand, fingers, and thumb make up 10% of musculoskeletal injuries in Major and Minor League Baseball [1]. Hand and finger injuries comprise up to 21.8% of hit by pitch injuries and result in mean of 14.39 playing days lost [2]. The fingertip is the most exposed area of the hand which leads to its high susceptibility to injury. Baseball activities provide several unique opportunities for injury to the fingertips of its participants, both amateur and professional. Traumatic fingertip injuries in baseball such as distal phalangeal fractures and nail bed injuries may occur during fielding balls, sliding into base, or hitting. Attritional injuries such as fingertip blisters and nail plate fractures occur in pitchers. This chapter will discuss injuries to the distal fingertip, including traumatic injuries such as distal phalangeal tuft fractures and nail bed injuries, as well as attritional friction blisters in throwers.

Evaluation of the injured fingertip begins with a thorough examination of the injured and uninjured digits. Neuromuscular status is quickly assessed. Open wounds and nail bed injuries are inspected for soft tissue defects and displacement as well as underlying bony involvement. Fingers should be evaluated for clinical alignment as well as for classic fracture signs of swelling, pain, and bony tenderness. Digital functions such as flexion and extension are assessed and deficits are noted. If clinical suspicion indicates, injuries of the distal fingertip are evaluated with X-ray. A standard finger X-ray series should include PA, lateral, and oblique views as some fractures are only visible on a single view.

Distal phalangeal fractures consist of fractures of the tuft and extraarticular shaft and intraarticular fractures of the distal interphalangeal joint which may include volar flexor digitorum profundus avulsions (Jersey finger) and dorsal terminal extensor avulsions (Mallet finger). This chapter will discuss fracture of the tuft and extraarticular shaft. Tendon avulsions of the DIP joint are discussed elsewhere in other chapters.

Fractures of the distal phalangeal shaft may be transverse, longitudinal, or oblique. They are often minimally displaced and stable. Displaced fractures may require closed reduction, which are often stable once reduced. Closed stable shaft fractures of the distal phalanx are typically treated with nonoperatively with splinting for 3–6 weeks followed by rapid mobilization [3]. Open or unstable fractures may require debridement and percutaneous pin or screw fixation [4]. Symptomatic nonunions are rare, but can be treated with percutaneous pinning with or without bone grafting [3]. Whether treated operatively or nonoperatively, splints should include the DIP joint, but avoid the PIP joint. Diligent mobilization

D. Carlan (✉)
Eaton Orthopaedics, LLC, St. Petersburg, FL, USA
e-mail: Dcarlan@eatonortho.com

G. M. Lourie (ed.), *Hand and Wrist Injuries in Baseball*,
https://doi.org/10.1007/978-3-030-81659-9_8

of all uninjured joints in the hand is encouraged. Return to play is a function of injury severity, healing, handedness, position, and timing of season. Once the injury/fracture is determined to be stable, one must assess player comfort and ability to perform. Protective devices such splints or guards can often be used on glove hand injuries in order to accelerate return to play.

Tuft fractures are the result of crushing or direct impact injuries to the flared distal aspect of the distal phalanx. In baseball, they are most associated with ball versus fingertip, such as hit by pitch or line drive versus fingertip. They are often associated with nail matrix injury or pulp lacerations. Painful subungual hematomas are often seen with closed fractures [3]. More significant injuries include displaced fractures and nail bed lacerations through the perionychium or eponychium.

Tuft fractures are often stable secondary to the generous fibrous network of the fingertip. Closed tuft fractures with intact nail plate are amenable to nonoperative treatment. The fingertip is splinted and large subungual hematomas are drained for pain relief. Drainage is performed with a heated paperclip or ophthalmic electrocautery. When the heated object contacts the pooled blood, it cools while leaving a large enough hole in the nail plate for ongoing drainage [5]. The fingertip and DIP joint are then splinted for comfort, typically 7–14 days [3]. The player will often transition to a sturdy nonrestrictive compressive wrap (athletic tape or a simple Band-Aid) for support once the pain has subsided. These often heal with symptomatic stable fibrous unions. Return to play is determined by tolerance to symptoms and ability to perform.

Open tuft fractures are often unstable and have associated lacerations through the pulp or nail bed. Treatment includes fracture debridement, stabilization, and laceration repair. Some fractures may be stabilized with acute nail bed repair and nail plate replacement alone [5]. More unstable or widely displaced fractures require longitudinal pinning for stabilization prior to nail bed repair. Lacerations of the perionychium and particularly the eponychium require nail plate removal and anatomical repair with a small (6-0 or 7-0) absorbable suture. The nail plate is then replaced to assist in maintenance of reduction.

Blisters

Friction blisters are common in athletics. These range in severity and are uniquely related to index and long fingertips, and occasionally the thumb of baseball pitchers, as the fingertip is the last point of contact as the ball is released. They are most common in the areas of the fingertip that contact the seam of the ball [6]. Fingertip blisters lead to pain, altered grip, and loss of pitching command. They often lead to loss of playing time.

Blisters occur in areas of the body where the stratum corneum and stratum granulosum are substantial, such as the palmar and plantar surfaces of the hands and feet. These layers transmit surface forces to the stratum spinosum, thus disrupting the spinosum layer and causing a blister. In areas with less robust strata, the corneum and granulosum, abrasion forms instead [7, 8]. By 48 h a new granulosum layer is formed and by 120 h a new corneum layer is formed [9, 10].

Frictional forces and number of cycles affect blister formation. Moist skin increases frictional forces, while dry skin reduces friction [7, 8, 11]. Baseball pitchers' distal pulp experiences frictional forces during release of the baseball as they use the index and long finger as well as the thumb to impart spin on the baseball. Frictional forces are higher leading to increased blister susceptibility in humid environments.

Methods of blister prevention are anecdotal and steeped in tradition. Prevention methods involve minimizing the added moisture from sweating and playing in humid environment. Antiperspirant sprays are often utilized by pitchers to reduce the added moisture from sweat [12]. This may need to be reapplied to the hand and fingers between innings. Other options include using a rosin bag and dry towel or placing the hand in a rice bucket between innings. The rice absorbs moisture and prevents pruning of the digits. Digital callouses may develop and lead to blistering. Callouses need to be maintained by trimming and contouring rough or loose edges that may lead to prevent blister formation.

Blister treatment is similarly anecdotal and is largely performed by the training staff. Blisters may be drained by using a sterile syringe to penetrate only the top layer of the blister. Drainage provides pain relief and allows apposition of the skin layers for quicker healing. If a player remains in the game after drainage, they must be carefully monitored for skin avulsion or secondary blistering underneath. Skin adhesives such as skin glues or super glue may be utilized, but often need to be reapplied throughout the game. Once removed from the game, treatment includes warm water Betadine soaks for disinfecting and toughening the surrounding skin [6]. Compounded creams and salves contain alum powder and tincture of benzoin may be utilized to promote blister healing. Antibiotic ointments that moisten and soften the skin should be avoided. Bandages that trap moisture against the skin are also discouraged.

Fingernail fractures are common in pitchers. Vertical or horizontal fractures typically occur in the long finger from the force of the ball as it is released from the fingertip. Playing time is rarely limited due to these injuries. Treatment is symptomatic only. To support the injured nail and avoid loss of playing time, a nail cast may be applied. A nail cast is fashioned out of Steri-Strips cut to fit the nail and placed perpendicular to the fracture. A second layer of Steri-Strips is cut and placed perpendicular to the first layer. Super glue is then applied to the Steri-Strips. It is allowed to dry the reapplied. A total of four layers of glue is preferred (Fig. 8.1). Once dry, the player may return to play as tolerated.

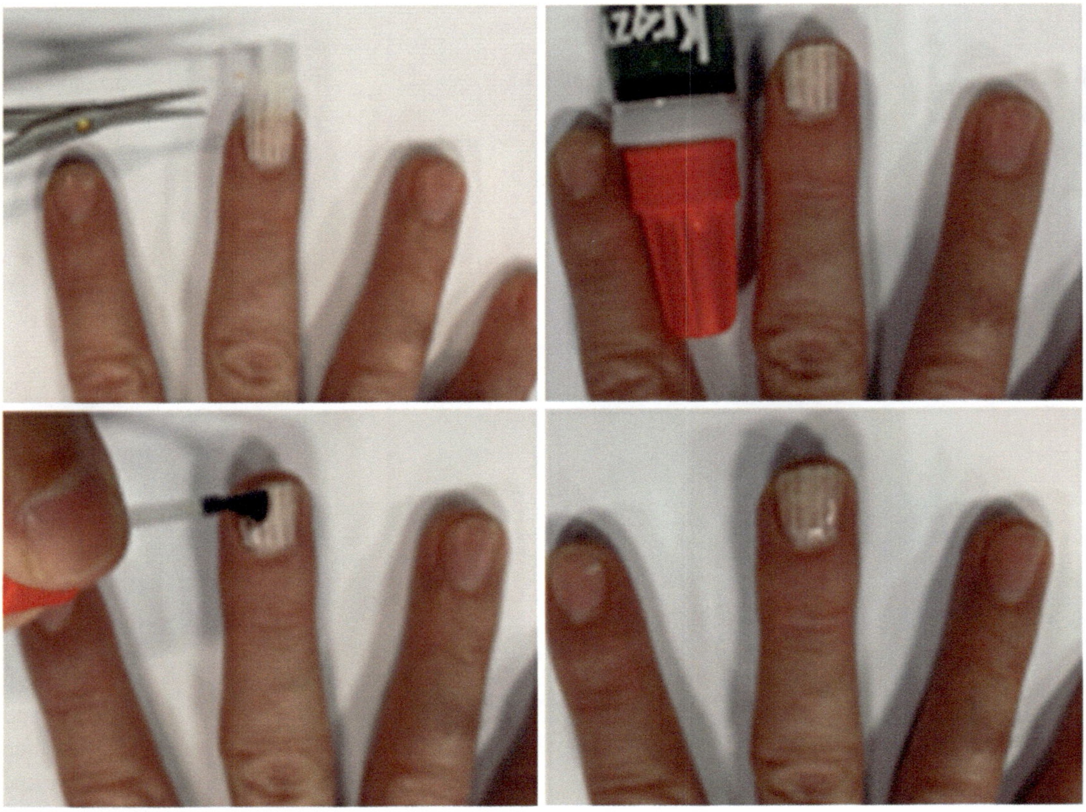

Fig. 8.1 Nail cast application

References

1. Camp CL, Dines JS, van der List JP, Conte S, Conway J, Altchek DW, et al. Summative report on time out of play for major and minor league baseball. Am J Sports Med. 2018;46(7):1727–32.
2. Camp CL, Wang D, Sinatro AS, D'Angelo J, Coleman SH, Dines JS, et al. Getting hit by pitch in professional baseball. Am J Sports Med. 2018;46(8):1997–2003.
3. Green DP, Hotchkiss RN, Peterson WC. Green's operative hand surgery, vol. 1. 4th ed. Churchill Livingstone; 1999. p. 732–3.
4. Trimble TE. Principles of hang surgery and therapy. 2001. p. 79–84.
5. Krull EA, Zook EG, Baron R, Haneke E. Nail surgery. A text and atlas. Philadelphia: Lippincott Williams & Wilkins; 2001. p. 91–109.
6. Vinson M. Tricks of the trade: finger care. Professional Baseball Athletic Trainers Society Blog. 2017.
7. Sulzberger MB, Cortese TA, Fishman L, Wiley HS. Studies on blisters produced by friction. I. Results of linear rubbing and twisting technics. J Invest Dermatol. 1966;47(5):456–65.
8. Naylor PD. Experimental friction blisters. Br J Dermatol. 1955;67(10):327–42.
9. Epstein WL, Fukuyama K, Cortese TA. Autographic study of friction blisters. RNA, DNA, and protein synthesis. Arch Dermatol. 1969;99(1):94–106.
10. Cortese TA Jr, Fukuyama K, Epstein W, Sulzberger MB. Treatment of friction blisters. An experimental study. Arch Dermatol. 1968;97(6):717–21.
11. Highley DR, Coomey M, DenBeste M, Wolfman LJ. Frictional properties of skin. J Invest Dermatol. 1977;69(3):303–5.
12. Reynolds K, Darrigrand A, Roberts D, Knapik J. Effects of an antiperspirant with emollients on foot-sweat accumulation and blister formation while walking in the heat. J Am Acad Dermatol. 1995;33:626–30.

Part II

Ligament Injuries of the Hand and Wist

Scapholunate Ligament Injuries in Baseball

9

Michael Sun and Steven S. Shin

Introduction

The intact scapholunate interosseous ligament (SLIL) acts as the primary stabilizer of the scapholunate (SL) joint. It is vital to stability of the carpus but also commonly injured [1, 2]. Injuries to the SLIL may be acute or chronic in nature and may consist of partial or complete tears. Acute traumatic complete injuries to the SLIL may result in SL dissociation [3]. Untreated, chronic injuries can set the wrist on a path of progressive instability, deformity, and arthritic degeneration, rendering the wrist severely painful and dysfunctional [2]. In baseball, injury to the SLIL has been observed to occur from collision with other players or the wall, or when diving for a ball. It has been postulated that during a fall on an outstretched hand that results in a SLIL tear, the wrist is in a position of extension, ulnar deviation, and carpal supination [4]. Some also believe that the torque placed on the wrist from the act of bat swinging may either create an SLIL injury or exacerbate an existing injury [5]. Due to the spectrum of pathology that can be associated with SLIL injury, treatment can be challenging even in the general population. In the competitive baseball player, additional considerations should be given.

Anatomy and Biomechanics

The SLIL is a C-shaped structure that binds together the scaphoid and lunate (Fig. 9.1). It is comprised of three distinct segments: dorsal, volar, and proximal [6]. The dorsal segment is the thickest and comprised of a collection of obliquely oriented fibers between the dorsal proximal pole of the scaphoid and the dorsal aspect of the lunate. It has an approximate thickness of 3 mm and length of 5 mm [1, 6]. The volar segment is comprised of even more obliquely oriented fibers between the volar scaphoid and volar aspect of the lunate and has an

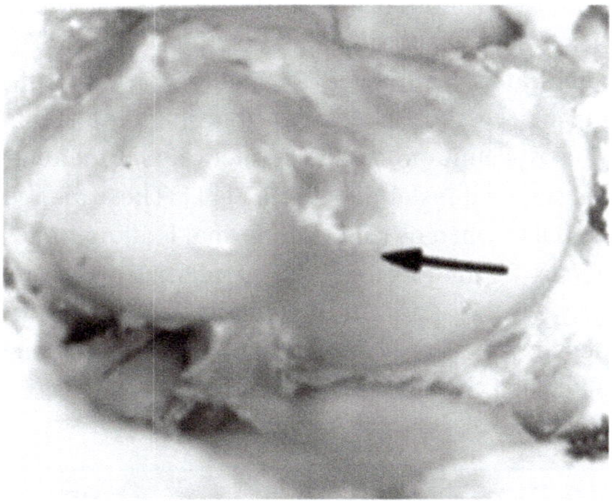

Fig. 9.1 The scapholunate interosseous ligament (black arrow) creates a seamless transition between the articular surfaces of the scaphoid and lunate. (With permission from Kuo et al. [16])

M. Sun (✉) · S. S. Shin
Department of Orthopaedic Surgery, Cedars-Sinai Medical Center, Los Angeles, CA, USA
e-mail: michael.sun@cshs.org; steven.shin@cshs.org

G. M. Lourie (ed.), *Hand and Wrist Injuries in Baseball*,
https://doi.org/10.1007/978-3-030-81659-9_9

approximate thickness of 1 mm and length of 5 mm [6]. The proximal segment of the SLIL is formed by fibrocartilaginous tissue that blends with the proximal articular cartilages of the scaphoid and lunate [1, 2, 6]. Near the junction of the volar and proximal segments, the SLIL blends with the radioscapholunate ligament [2, 6]. The dorsal segment of the SLIL has been found to be the strongest with a linear load to failure value of 260 N, followed by the volar segment with a value of 118 N, and finally the proximal segment with a value of 63 N [7].

While the SLIL, particularly the dorsal segment, is considered the primary stabilizer of the SL joint, several extrinsic ligaments act as secondary stabilizers. Dorsally, the dorsal radiocarpal and dorsal intercarpal ligaments help to stabilize the dorsal SL interval [8]. Volarly, the radioscaphocapitate, long radiolunate, and radioscapholunate ligaments are thought to further contribute to SL stability [1, 9]. These extrinsic ligaments may compensate to stabilize the SL joint when part of the SLIL is injured [10].

In the uninjured wrist, with flexion or radial deviation, the scaphoid and lunate flex in unison through the intact SLIL. Conversely, with wrist extension or ulnar deviation, the intact SLIL enables the scaphoid and lunate to extend in unison [1]. When the SLIL is injured, incongruous SL motion may result. As the scaphoid flexes, the lunate, if its association with the triquetrum is maintained through secondary ligaments, will be forced into abnormal extension. This dynamic process is termed dorsal intercarpal segment instability (DISI) [11]. These altered carpal mechanics lead to abnormal loading forces across the radiocarpal and intercarpal joints and may result long term in a predictable pattern of degenerative arthritis known as scapholunate advanced collapse (SLAC) [12].

Diagnosis

Clinical Presentation

Patients with symptomatic SLIL injuries will often present with poorly localized pain and tenderness in the periscaphoid region of the wrist [3]. If the injury is subacute, patients may report sensations of snapping or clicking with wrist motion, and the pain may be better localizable to the dorsal aspect of the SL interval [2, 3]. Players may report that these symptoms began after an event of sudden axial force on an outstretched hand, such as diving for a ball or collision with another player on the field [5].

On physical examination, the affected wrist should be compared to the contralateral uninjured wrist. The injured wrist will demonstrate decreased grip strength and range of motion [2, 3]. The Watson scaphoid shift test may be useful to detect scaphoid instability [13]. In this maneuver, the examiner's thumb applies a dorsally directed pressure over the patient's scaphoid tubercle as the patient's wrist is then passively ranged from a position of ulnar deviation and slight extension to radial deviation and slight flexion. In a positive test, this maneuver will elicit pain and cause the proximal pole of the scaphoid to subluxate out of the scaphoid fossa and onto the dorsal rim of the radius. When the examiner releases the applied pressure from the scaphoid tubercle, the patient's scaphoid will spontaneously reduce with an apparent "clunk." While the scaphoid shift test has been demonstrated to give a false positive result in up to one-third of individuals, in a patient with a positive result compared to the contralateral wrist and an appropriate history, it may still be a useful maneuver to aid in diagnosis of an SLIL injury [14, 15].

Imaging

Patients with suspected SLIL injuries should have high-quality posteroanterior (PA), lateral, and anteroposterior (AP) clenched fist radiographs of their wrist obtained [16]. Contralateral radiographs of the uninjured wrist should be obtained for comparison. Radiographic findings can vary immensely from completely normal to showing overt instability.

On PA radiographs, a widened SL interval may be suggestive of an SLIL injury. However,

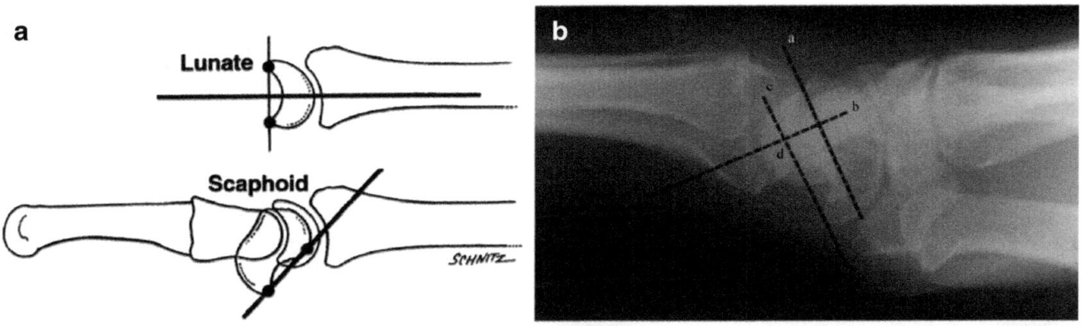

Fig. 9.2 (**a**) The lunate axis is perpendicular to the lunate tangent, a line that connects the dorsal and volar lips of the lunate. The scaphoid tangent is a line connecting the proximal and distal volar cortices of the scaphoid. (**b**) (a) Lunate tangent, (b) lunate axis, (c) scaphoid tangent, (d) a SL angle of 90°. (With permission from Kuo et al. [16])

this finding alone must be approached cautiously as there is significant variability in the literature on the definition of an abnormal SL distance. A SL interval >2.5 mm has been found to be 60% sensitive and 75% specific and confer a 2.41 positive likelihood ratio for an SLIL lesion [17]. Other signs of instability include the appearance of a shortened scaphoid and the "cortical ring sign," whereby flexion of the scaphoid causes it to be superimposed upon itself on the AP radiograph [18].

On lateral wrist radiographs, the SL angle can be measured, and a value outside of normal (range 30–60°) may be indicative of SL instability [2]. The SL angle is the angle between the scaphoid tangent and a line perpendicular to the lunate tangent (Fig. 9.2). The scaphoid tangent is a line that is drawn tangential to the volar cortices of the scaphoid. The lunate tangent is a line that is drawn connecting the volar and dorsal lips of the lunate. When the SLIL is injured and the scaphoid flexes and lunate extends uninhibited, the SL angle increases, and a SL angle >70° is suggestive of instability. A SL angle >63° has been found to be 43% sensitive and 93% specific and confer a 7.30 positive likelihood ratio for a SLIL injury [17].

When static radiographs appear normal but clinical suspicion for SLIL injury remains high, stress radiographs can be helpful to exacerbate SL widening and demonstrate dynamic instability. While multiple positions to obtain stress views have been described, the AP clenched fist view is used most frequently and has been shown in cadaveric models to produce the largest SL gap (Fig. 9.3) [19]. This view is obtained with the patients' forearms pronated, fists clenched, and wrists positioned at approximately 30° ulnar deviation. Patients can be asked to clench a pencil in their fists to facilitate positioning.

Arthrography was previously a popular imaging modality in assessing for SLIL injuries, but it is less commonly performed today. When performed, contrast is injected into the radiocarpal, midcarpal, and radioulnar joints, and the wrist is brought through range of motion to facilitate diffusion of the contrast through the SLIL defect. However, studies have demonstrated a high prevalence of bilaterally positive arthrograms in patients with unilateral wrist pain, bringing into the question the utility of this imaging modality [20, 21].

Magnetic resonance imaging (MRI) is now commonly utilized in the assessment of SLIL injuries (Fig. 9.4). With a 1.5-T wrist coil, MRI has been shown to be 38–88% sensitive and 46–100% specific in the diagnosis of SLIL injuries [2, 3]. MRI with a 3-T coil has been reported to be 89% sensitive and 100% specific [22]. High-resolution MRI has the additional benefit of providing detailed information on the location (volar or dorsal) and size of the injury, and information on other pathologies such as additional ligamentous lesions or tendonitis.

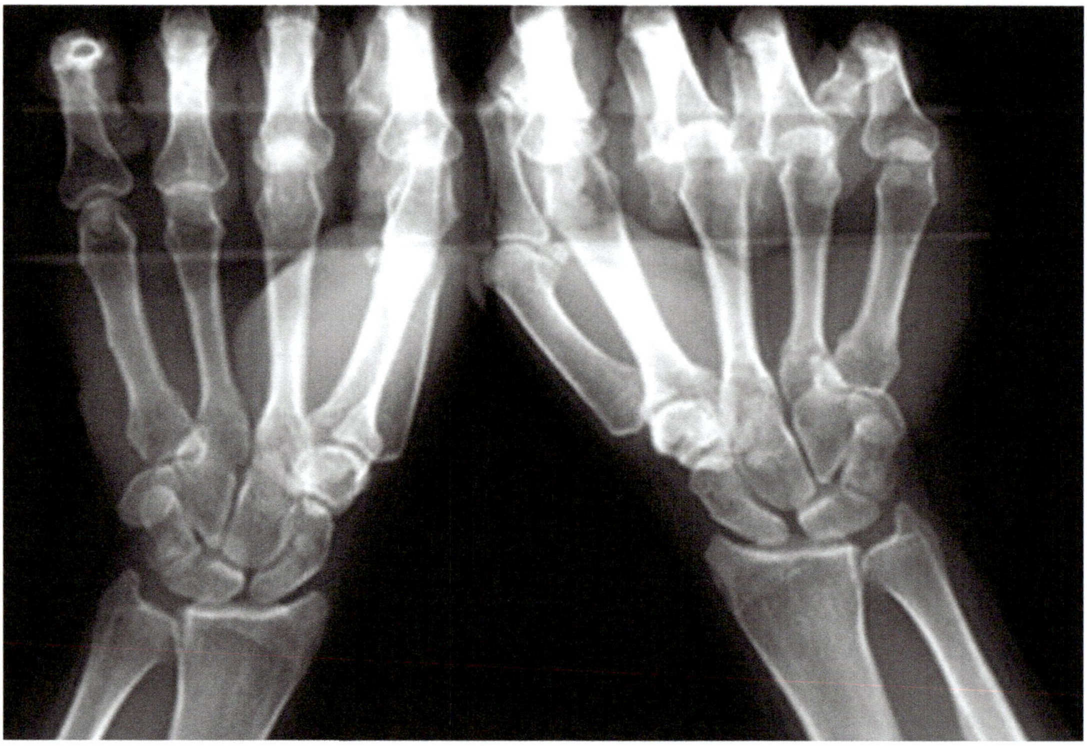

Fig. 9.3 Radiograph of bilateral clenched fist stress view showing asymmetrical SL gapping. (With permission from Lee et al. [19])

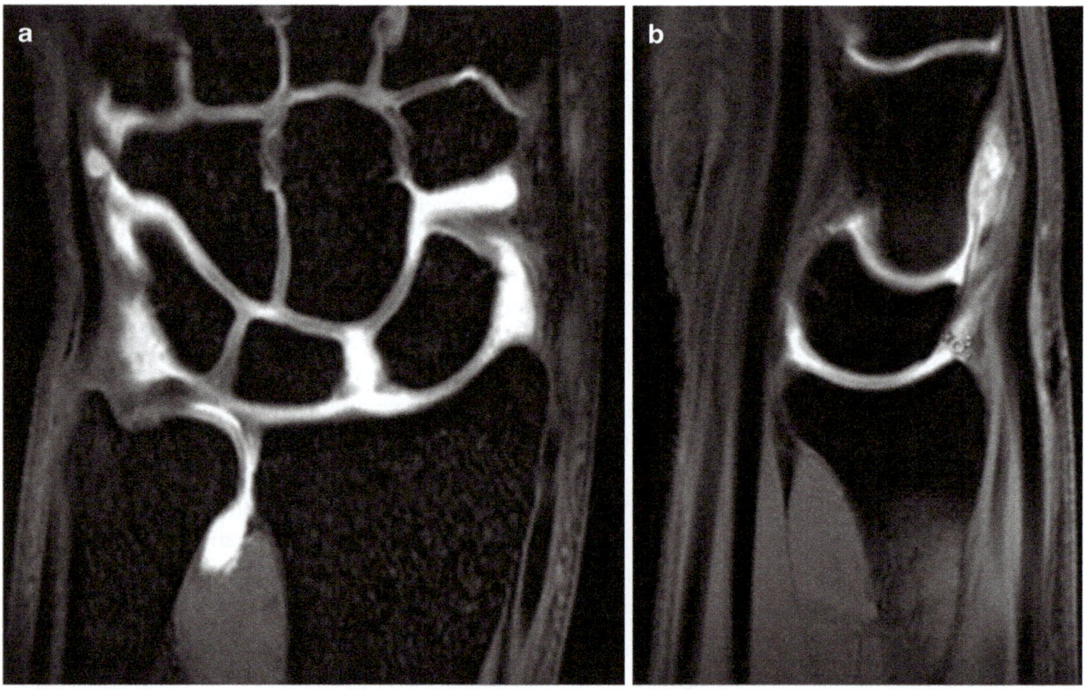

Fig. 9.4 (a) Coronal cut of MR arthrogram demonstrating complete SLIL tear with gapping. (b) Sagittal cut of MR arthrogram demonstrating extended lunate

Diagnostic Arthroscopy

Wrist arthroscopy is a useful modality that allows surgeons to definitively diagnose and, in some cases, simultaneously treat SLIL injuries [23]. Small partial tears that are undetectable by other imaging modalities may be easily identifiable arthroscopically.

The SLIL is best visualized in the radiocarpal space through the 3–4 portal where it should appear as a slight concave structure confluent with the scaphoid and lunate [23]. If difficult to identify, gentle probing will reveal the SLIL to be softer than the osseous structures around it. The arthroscope is then transitioned to the midcarpal radial (MCR) portal where it should appear in the midcarpal space taut, congruent, and without step-offs. When torn, fibers of the SLIL hanging into the radiocarpal space can block visualization through the 3–4 portal, in which case visualization may be improved by transitioning the arthroscope to the 6R portal. As the severity of SLIL injury and subsequent incongruous motion between the scaphoid and lunate increases, the SLIL becomes better evaluated in the midcarpal space.

Treatment

Treatment of symptomatic tears of the SLIL is controversial. The chronicity of the injury can also dictate the type of treatment rendered [2]. Regardless of the treatment given, the player is counseled about the seriousness of the injury including the lack of treatments that produce universally good results. During the season, partial tears are preferably treated nonoperatively to avoid a lengthy postoperative absence. The classification and definition of partial tears can be confusing but usually describes the thickness or location of the tear [2, 24]. For example, a player may have a "partial-thickness tear of the volar band of the SL ligament," or he may have a "full-thickness tear of the dorsal and central bands of the SL ligament"; both are partial tears of the ligament. Nonoperative treatments of these partial tears include rest, use of a wrist brace, anti-inflammatory or steroid medications, and/or cortisone injections [2]. Ideally, the player's symptoms will abate during the first few weeks after injury and the initiation of treatment. If there is not sufficient improvement in the player's symptoms, then consideration should be given to operative treatment. Options for operative treatment are arthroscopic debridement and open repair versus reconstruction [2, 23].

Arthroscopic debridement is reserved for partial tears of the ligament as described above. The loose, unstable portions of the ligament are removed with the goal of decreasing irritation and pain at the joint [23]. Debridement can be accompanied by thermal shrinkage, which can act to further stabilize as well as denervate the torn area [25, 26]. The goal of denervation is to decrease the painful stimulus emanating from the tear [25]. Although thermal shrinkage has not been shown to be effective in treating shoulder instability, this has not borne out in the wrist [25–29]. While ligament debridement may decrease the player's pain, it does not restore ligament tissue nor normal biomechanics or kinematics at the scapholunate joint.

If arthroscopic debridement is unsuccessful and the partial tear is a full-thickness tear of the dorsal band, we recommend reconstruction of the dorsal band with a free palmaris graft tendon augmented with suture tape and secured with interference anchors, also known as internal brace augmentation. More recently, we have been performing reconstruction with a 2 mm suture tape (FiberTape, Arthrex, Naples, FL) alone with good results. A cadaveric biomechanical study found that a two-anchor FiberTape reconstruction was about three times stronger than a suture anchor repair alone but still significantly weaker than the entire ligament [30]. The strength of a three-anchor FiberTape construct is being studied presently and is described below.

If the SLIL tear is complete, open repair or reconstruction of the ligament should be considered. Although capsulodesis or ligamentodesis has been described as an alternative to reconstruction to counteract hyperflexion of the scaphoid, it is our preference to proceed directly to reconstruction if arthroscopic debridement is unsuccessful at relieving the player's symptoms [31]. The first described technique of an open repair utilized small drill holes in both the scaphoid and lunate through which suture was passed and used to repair the ligament back to either bone [32]. Supplemental K-wires are placed for 2 to 3 months to maintain the joint in a reduced position. These wires are later removed, and therapy is begun. If the ligament quality has degraded to the point where a repair is no longer possible, reconstruction of the ligament should be considered.

Various graft options have been proposed for reconstruction. One of the original reconstruction techniques utilizes a distally attached strip of the flexor carpi radialis (FCR) tendon [33, 34]. The tendon strip is passed through a retrograde drill hole in the scaphoid, exiting dorsally at the proximal pole. It is passed ulnarly under the dorsal radiocarpal (DRC) ligament and then back to the dorsal lunate, where it is secured back to itself. In another technique described by Ross et al., the same tendon graft is tunneled from the scaphoid into the lunate and triquetrum, secured with inference screws, then back to itself [35]. Other described techniques use a free palmaris graft and suture anchors, bone-ligament-bone or bone-retinaculum-bone autograft, and synthetic augmentation or reconstruction with suture tape [36–39]. Currently, our preference for surgical treatment of complete tears of the SLIL is a three-anchor FiberTape-only reconstruction. Our rationale is as follows: collagen-based reconstructions, like tendon weaves, have not been universally successful and often stretch over time, especially in more chronic cases [40]. A synthetic reconstruction using a material like FiberTape does not stretch over time like collagen does [41]. Although we do not yet have long-term results using this type of reconstruction, preliminary results have been very encouraging. The senior author has also recently been inserting nonabsorbable suture into the holes and grasping the dorsal capsule with these sutures, essentially performing a capsulodesis and adding biology to the reconstruction. Additionally, small drill holes are made in the area of the ligament attachments to the scaphoid and lunate to encourage bleeding and fibrous healing.

We now describe the technique for the three-anchor FiberTape-only reconstruction (Fig. 9.5).

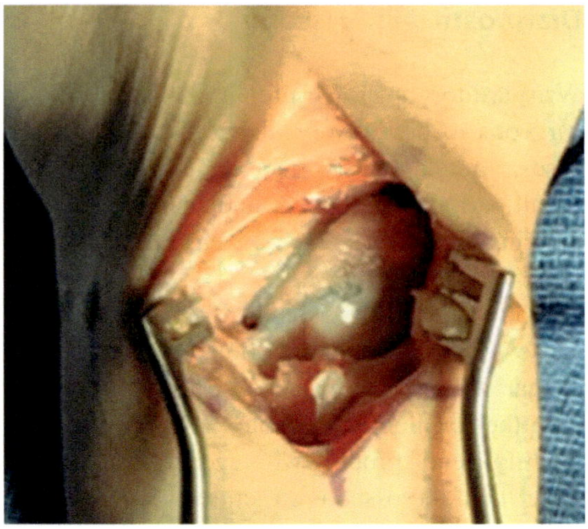

Fig. 9.5 Dorsal view of a three-anchor FiberTape-only reconstruction of the SLIL

A longitudinal incision is made over the mid-dorsal wrist. The extensor pollicis longus tendon is released from the third dorsal compartment, and the extensor tendons are retracted radially and ulnarly. A dorsal radially based capsule-sparing capsulotomy is made, and the capsule is reflected radially to reveal the underlying complete scapholunate ligament tear [42]. The radiocarpal and midcarpal joints are inspected to rule out the presence of arthrosis. 0.062 inch joystick K-wires are placed into the scaphoid and lunate away from the planned drill holes for the interference anchors. A 3.0 mm drill hole is made at the dorsal aspect of the scaphoid proximal pole, about 3 mm radial to the joint space, using the drill bit from the 3.5 mm SwiveLock drill kit (Arthrex, Naples, FL). A FiberTape is placed around the SwiveLock fork tip and inserted into the bottom of the hole. The anchor body is then inserted into the hole, securing the tape through interference fit. Another 3.0 mm hole is made at the dorsal aspect of the lunate through the mid-body, and, with the joint reduced, the tape is inserted into this second hole and secured again with a second SwiveLock anchor. At this point, the joint is examined to ensure that the gap has narrowed. The free limb of the FiberTape is then brought back over the dorsal scapholunate joint (but not over the midcarpal joint) and inserted into a third 3.0 mm hole at the radial-dorsal aspect of the scaphoid, where it is secured with a third SwiveLock anchor. Extraneous tape is excised sharply with a knife. Fluoroscopy is used to examine placement of the holes in the scaphoid and lunate and joint reduction. In more chronic cases, the SL angle may not be completely corrected, but the gap is often narrowed. If sutures were placed into the holes along with the tape, they are now passed dorsally through the capsular flap and tied, adding a dorsal capsulodesis to the synthetic reconstruction. We are cognizant of the fact that the strong volar band of the ligament is not addressed in this technique and volar gapping will most likely occur with wrist extension; however, we are not aware of the significance of this clinically. The wound is irrigated copiously with normal saline solution and then closed in layers. A plaster wrist splint is applied leaving the thumb and fingers free for early active motion postoperatively.

Rehabilitation

We will describe the postoperative course of therapy we utilize for all of our patients who have undergone the three-anchor FiberTape-only reconstruction of the SLIL. After suture removal at 7–10 days postoperatively, the wrist is placed into a molded, waterproof brace, leaving the thumb and fingers free for continued active motion. Active motion is initiated at 6 weeks postoperatively and passive motion at 8 weeks postoperatively. Strengthening is initiated at 10 weeks postoperatively. Consideration is given to beginning sports-specific activities at the 12-week postoperative mark and return to competitive play at the 4- to 6-month mark, depending on the player's clinical progress and follow-up radiographs demonstrating maintenance of SL joint reduction (Fig. 9.6).

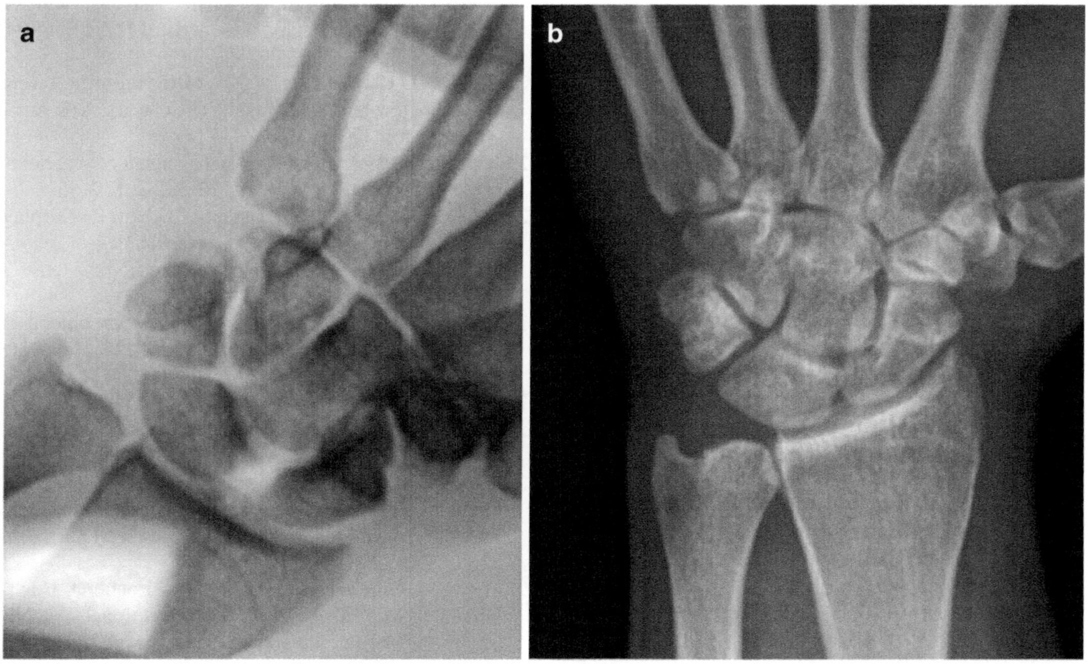

Fig. 9.6 (**a**) Intraoperative fluoroscopy of the wrist showing SL joint widening. (**b**) Radiograph of the wrist 6 months after three-anchor FiberTape-only reconstruction of the SLIL. Note the absence of SL joint widening

Summary

Diagnosis and treatment of SLIL injuries can be challenging because of the spectrum of pathologies that can exist. For patients both in the general population and those who are competitive athletes, a thoughtful approach is essential while navigating these injuries. For the competitive baseball player, management decisions must consider not only the injury chronicity, severity, and available treatment options but also the timing within the competitive season and within the player's overall professional career. Keeping these factors in mind is critical toward achieving the best possible outcome.

References

1. Rajan PV, Day CS. Scapholunate interosseous ligament anatomy and biomechanics. J Hand Surg Am. 2015;40(8):1692–702.
2. White NJ, Rollick NC. Injuries of the scapholunate Interosseous ligament: an update. J Am Acad Orthop Surg. 2015;23(11):691–703.
3. Kitay A, Wolfe SW. Scapholunate instability: current concepts in diagnosis and management. J Hand Surg Am. 2012;37(10):2175–96.
4. Cohen MS. Ligamentous injuries of the wrist in the athlete. Clin Sports Med. 1998;17(3):533–52.
5. Graham TJ. Perspective on scapholunate ligament injuries in baseball players. Hand Clin. 2012;28(3):261–4.
6. Berger RA. The gross and histologic anatomy of the scapholunate interosseous ligament. J Hand Surg Am. 1996;21(2):170–8.
7. Berger RA, Imeada T, Berglund L, An KN. Constraint and material properties of the subregions of the scapholunate interosseous ligament. J Hand Surg Am. 1999;24(5):953–62.
8. Viegas SF, Yamaguchi S, Boyd NL, Patterson RM. The dorsal ligaments of the wrist: anatomy, mechanical properties, and function. J Hand Surg Am. 1999;24(3):456–68.
9. Berger RA. The anatomy of the ligaments of the wrist and distal radioulnar joints. Clin Orthop Relat Res. 2001;383:32–40.
10. Crawford K, Owusu-Sarpong N, Day C, Iorio M. Scapholunate ligament reconstruction: a critical analysis review. JBJS Rev. 2016;4(4):e41–8.
11. Garcia-Elias M. The treatment of wrist instability. J Bone Joint Surg Br. 1997;79(4):684–90.
12. Weiss KE, Rodner CM. Osteoarthritis of the wrist. J Hand Surg Am. 2007;32(5):725–46.
13. Watson HK, Ashmead D, Makhlouf MV. Examination of the scaphoid. J Hand Surg Am. 1988;13(5):657–60.
14. Watson H, Ottoni L, Pitts EC, Handal AG. Rotary subluxation of the scaphoid: a spectrum of instability. J Hand Surg Br. 1993;18(1):62–4.
15. Wolfe SW, Gupta A, Crisco JJ 3rd. Kinematics of the scaphoid shift test. J Hand Surg Am. 1997;22(5):801–6.
16. Kuo CE, Wolfe SW. Scapholunate instability: current concepts in diagnosis and management. J Hand Surg Am. 2008;33(6):998–1013.
17. Megerle K, Pohlmann S, Kloeters O, Germann G, Sauerbier M. The significance of conventional radiographic parameters in the diagnosis of scapholunate ligament lesions. Eur Radiol. 2011;21(1):176–81.
18. Cautilli GP, Wehbé MA. Scapho-lunate distance and cortical ring sign. J Hand Surg Am. 1991;16(3):501–3.
19. Lee SK, Desai H, Silver B, Dhaliwal G, Paksima N. Comparison of radiographic stress views for scapholunate dynamic instability in a cadaver model. J Hand Surg Am. 2011;36(7):1149–57.
20. Cantor RM, Stern PJ, Wyrick JD, Michaels SE. The relevance of ligament tears or perforations in the diagnosis of wrist pain: an arthrographic study. J Hand Surg Am. 1994;19(6):945–53.
21. Herbert TJ, Faithfull RG, McCann DJ, Ireland J. Bilateral arthrography of the wrist. J Hand Surg Br. 1990;15(2):233–5.
22. Magee T. Comparison of 3-T MRI and arthroscopy of intrinsic wrist ligament and TFCC tears. AJR Am J Roentgenol. 2009;192(1):80–5.
23. Geissler WB. Arthroscopic management of scapholunate instability. J Wrist Surg. 2013;2(2):129–35.
24. Messina JC, Van Overstraeten L, Luchetti R, Fairplay T, Mathoulin CL. The EWAS classification of scapholunate tears: an anatomical arthroscopic study. J Wrist Surg. 2013;2(2):105–9.
25. Burn MB, Sarkissian EJ, Yao J. Long-term outcomes for arthroscopic thermal treatment for scapholunate ligament injuries. J Wrist Surg. 2020;9(1):22–8.
26. Danoff JR, Karl JW, Birman MV, Rosenwasser MP. The use of thermal shrinkage for scapholunate instability. Hand Clin. 2011;27(3):309–17.
27. Darlis NA, Weiser RW, Sotereanos DG. Partial scapholunate ligament injuries treated with arthroscopic debridement and thermal shrinkage. J Hand Surg Am. 2005;30(5):908–14.
28. Longo UG, Rizzello G, Loppini M, Locher J, Buchmann S, Maffulli N, et al. Multidirectional instability of the shoulder: a systematic review. Arthroscopy. 2015;31(12):2431–43.
29. Miniaci A, McBirnie J. Thermal capsular shrinkage for treatment of multidirectional instability of the shoulder. J Bone Joint Surg Am. 2003;85(12):2283–7.
30. Park IJ, Maniglio M, Shin SS, Lim D, McGarry MH, Lee TQ. Internal bracing augmentation for scapholunate interosseous ligament repair: a cadaveric biomechanical study. J Hand Surg Am. 2020;45(10):985-e1.

31. Moran SL, Cooney WP, Berger RA, Strickland J. Capsulodesis for the treatment of chronic scapholunate instability. J Hand Surg Am. 2005;30(1):16–23.
32. Lavernia CJ, Cohen MS, Taleisnik J. Treatment of scapholunate dissociation by ligamentous repair and capsulodesis. J Hand Surg Am. 1992;17(2):354–9.
33. Brunelli GA, Brunelli GR. A new technique to correct carpal instability with scaphoid rotary subluxation: a preliminary report. J Hand Surg Am. 1995;20(3 Pt 2):S82–5.
34. Van Den Abbeele KL, Loh YC, Stanley JK, Trail IA. Early results of a modified Brunelli procedure for scapholunate instability. J Hand Surg Br. 1998;23(2):258–61.
35. Ross M, Loveridge J, Cutbush K, Couzens G. Scapholunate ligament reconstruction. J Wrist Surg. 2013;2(2):110–5.
36. Cuenod P, Charriere E, Papaloizos MY. A mechanical comparison of bone-ligament-bone autografts from the wrist for replacement of the scapholunate ligament. J Hand Surg Am. 2002;27(6):985–90.
37. Ho PC, Wong CW, Tse WL. Arthroscopic-assisted combined dorsal and volar scapholunate ligament reconstruction with tendon graft for chronic SL instability. J Wrist Surg. 2015;4(4):252–63.
38. Morrell NT, Weiss AP. Bone-retinaculum-bone autografts for scapholunate interosseous ligament reconstruction. Hand Clin. 2015;31(3):451–6.
39. Weiss AP. Scapholunate ligament reconstruction using a bone-retinaculum-bone autograft. J Hand Surg Am. 1998;23(2):205–15.
40. Anderson SR, Youssefzadeh KA, Limpisvasti O. Anterior cruciate ligament reconstruction with suture tape augmentation: a surgical technique. Arthrosc Tech. 2019;8(12):e1579–e82.
41. Coetzee JC, Ellington JK, Ronan JA, Stone RM. Functional results of open Broström ankle ligament repair augmented with a suture tape. Foot Ankle Int. 2018;39(3):304–10.
42. Berger RA, Bishop AT. A fiber-splitting capsulotomy technique for dorsal exposure of the wrist. Tech Hand Up Extrem Surg. 1997;1(1):2–10.

Thumb Metacarpophalangeal Joint Collateral Ligament Injury

10

Adriana M. Urruela and Michelle G. Carlson

Thumb Ulnar Collateral Ligament

The ulnar collateral ligament (UCL) tear is the most common injury to the thumb metacarpophalangeal (MCP) joint. In a study evaluating 1000 injuries to the thumb MCP, the UCL was involved in 86% of the injuries [1]. Acute injuries have been characterized in multiple sports including baseball. Even in their partial form, participation in athletics can be compromised by pain and weakness.

Injury to the thumb ulnar collateral ligament was initially described by Campbell as an occupational injury on observation of chronic laxity of gamekeepers' thumbs in Scotland. The gamekeepers placed the necks of wounded rabbits in between the thumb and index finger webspace. They snapped the neck of the rabbit in a sudden movement that placed a large radial-directed stress on the UCL, which resulted in chronic laxity of the UCL [2]. Later in Europe, in the 1960s, publications referencing acute ruptures of the thumb UCL appeared with higher frequency. Investigators often described acute traumatic ruptures of UCLs in downhill skiers, coining the condition skier's thumb [3]. The skiing injury usually occurred after a fall on an outstretched hand strapped to the handle of a ski pole. Since these initial descriptions, this injury has been described in almost every sport, particularly ball-handling, racquet-wielding, and stick-wielding sports.

Anatomy and Mechanism of Injury

The thumb MCP joint is a diarthrodial joint with little intrinsic osseous stability [4]. Range of motion varies between individuals with respect to flexion-extension arcs and degree of valgus laxity [5]. Stability of the MCP joint is a result of static and dynamic stabilizers. The static stabilizers are the proper collateral ligament, accessory collateral ligament, volar plate, and dorsal capsule. The dynamic stabilizers include the extrinsic (extensor pollicis longus [EPL], extensor pollicis brevis [EPB], flexor pollicis longus [FPL]) and intrinsic muscles of the thumb (adductor pollicis and flexor pollicis brevis [FBP]).

Of the static stabilizers, the collateral ligaments are the key constraints to radial-directed and ulnar-directed forces [6, 7]. The UCL is a thick band that measures 4–8 mm in width and 12–14 mm in length, and it is comprised of two distinct structures: the proper and accessory UCL. The proper UCL extends from slightly dorsal to the mid-axis of the metacarpal head to the volar aspect of the proximal phalanx (Fig. 10.1) [8]. This structure is tighter in flexion and looser in extension, serving as the primary restraint to

A. M. Urruela · M. G. Carlson (✉)
Hospital for Special Surgery, New York, NY, USA
e-mail: urruelaa@HSS.EDU; carlsonm@hss.edu

G. M. Lourie (ed.), *Hand and Wrist Injuries in Baseball*,
https://doi.org/10.1007/978-3-030-81659-9_10

valgus stress with the thumb MCP joint in flexion [9]. The accessory UCL originates slightly more volar on the metacarpal head and inserts onto the volar plate and ulnar sesamoid. Unlike the proper UCL, this structure is tighter in extension and looser in flexion, serving as the primary restraint to valgus stress with the MCP joint in extension (Fig. 10.2) [8, 10]. An anatomic study of the UCL has determined center of origin to be 4.2 mm from the dorsal surface and 5.3 mm proximal to the articular surface of the metacarpal head and inserting 2.8 mm from the volar surface and 3.4 mm distal to the phalangeal base [11].

Of the dynamic stabilizers, the adductor pollicis is particularly important. The adductor pollicis inserts on the proximal phalanx and ulnar sesamoid at a 48° angle and lies volar to the MCP axis of rotation [12]. The adductor mechanism consists of an aponeurosis superficial to the MCP capsule and UCL. In 1962, Stener [8] described a lesion observed in complete avulsions of the distal insertion of the UCL in which the ligament lies superficial and proximal to the adductor aponeurosis. In traumatic severe radial deviation of the MCP joint, the avulsed distal end of the UCL comes to lie on top of the distally displaced adductor aponeurosis. The aponeurosis then prevents apposition of the ligament back to the proximal phalanx. Stener predicted that the lack on contact at the site of ligament rupture would result in failure of ligament healing. This situation occurred in 25 out of 39 cases (64%) and all necessitated surgical intervention.

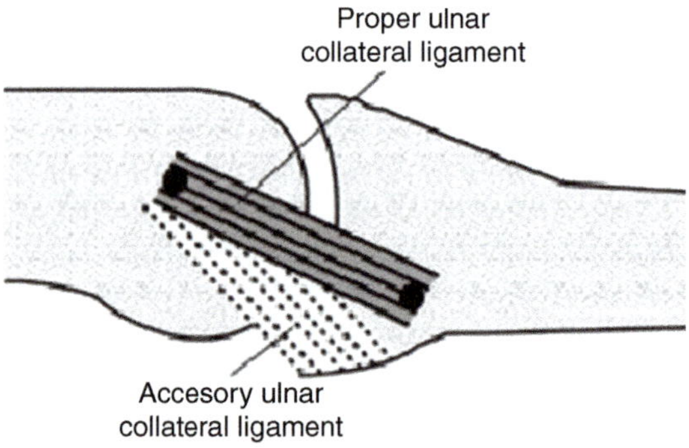

Fig. 10.1 Anatomic origin and insertion of ulnar collateral proper and accessory ligaments. (From Bean et al. [8]; with permission)

The mechanism of injury is usually from a valgus-directed or radial-directed load that produces a hyperabduction moment about the thumb MCP joint and leads to UCL injury. The most common acute mechanism is a fall onto an abducted thumb. This most commonly occurs when sliding into a base. Feet first sliding decreases but does not completely eliminate the incidence of UCL injuries. Protective gloves that keep the thumb adducted to the hand can prevent this injury. Similarly, a ball that strikes the ulnar side of the thumb can generate forces to the UCL that supersedes the measured failure load of the intact ligament of 294N [13]. Injury can result in partial or complete tear of the ligament, but can also involve injury to the dorsal capsule and volar plate stretching the adductor expansion.

Diagnosis: History and Clinical Exam

The evaluation begins with an accurate history and physical examination. Patients usually describe a valgus injury to the thumb, although

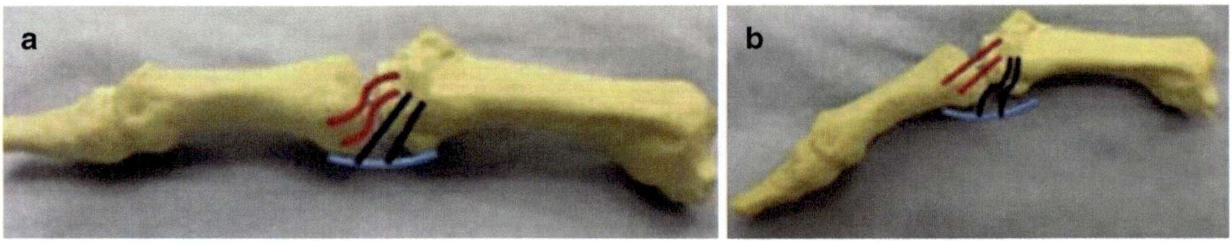

Fig. 10.2 Ulnar collateral ligaments (accessory and proper). (**a**) Thumb MCP joint in extension (**b**) Thumb MCP joint in extension. The proper collateral ligament is shown as lax in extension (wavy lines) and tight in flexion (straight lines). The accessory ligament is tight in extension (straight lines) and lax in flexion (wavy lines). (Reproduced with permission and copyright of Elsevier. From Avery et al. [10])

the exact mechanism may not be remembered. Pain, swelling, and ecchymosis are typically noted. Deformities such as radial deviation or palmar subluxation of the proximal phalanx on the metacarpal may be noted depending on the extent of the injury. Tenderness to palpation is encountered over the ulnar aspect of the MCP joint. Ulnar-sided deep scar tissue or a palpable bump can sometimes denote a Stener lesion [8]. However, the absence of both does not necessarily rule out a Stener lesion [5].

The most important aspect of the physical exam is stress testing of the thumb MCP with comparison to the contralateral side. To properly examine the thumb UCL, the metacarpal neck should be stabilized while producing a radial-directed force on the proximal phalanx; careful control of rotation is necessary (Fig. 10.3). Parameters of importance are the degrees of valgus laxity in full extension and 30° of flexion, injured and contralateral thumb, and presence of an endpoint. Instability or laxity is characterized as greater than 30° of radial deviation with radial-directed stress; greater than 15° of increased radial deviation compared with the contralateral, uninjured thumb; and lack of an endpoint [5]. In patients who show profound guarding, a local anesthetic injection can help with stress testing. With the MCP joint in 30° of flexion, greater than 30° of valgus laxity indicates rupture of the proper collateral ligament. At 0° of extension, the accessory collateral ligament is taut. If there is greater than 30° of valgus laxity at 0° extension, rupture of both accessory and proper collateral ligaments has likely occurred.

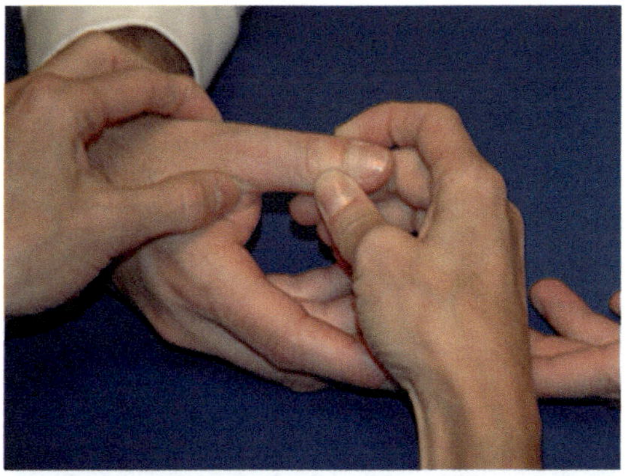

Fig. 10.3 Proper examination of the UCL requires stabilization of the metacarpal neck while producing a radial-directed force on the proximal phalanx; careful control of rotation is necessary

The importance of clinical diagnosis is stressed because there exist cases in which nondisplaced fractures of the ulnar base of the proximal phalanx can be associated with displaced UCL tears [14, 15]. Kaplan [14] argued that if the endpoint after radial stressing is 30° greater than the contralateral side, surgical exploration is warranted regardless of radiographic appearance. It is important to note that a stress examination will not displace a nondisplaced fracture that did not displace with the force of the initial injury.

Radiographic Examination

Imaging for suspected UCL tears of the thumb MCP joint should begin with posteroanterior and lateral radiographs of the thumb. Radiographic radial deviation or palmar subluxation strongly suggests instability. A supination deformity relative to the metacarpal head called the "sag sign" can also suggest instability [16]. Associated injuries include avulsion fractures at the base of the proximal phalanx and metacarpal head or neck fractures as well as MCP joint fracture dislocations and carpometacarpal joint subluxations.

Stress radiographs are controversial [17]. Proponents contend that stress radiographs can differentiate between tears of the proper UCL alone and those with accessory UCL tears. In a cadaveric study published in 2013, McKeon et al. showed that while varus angulation increases with proper UCL and accessory UCL transection, only radial translation of the proximal phalanx on the metacarpal head was seen in combined proper and accessory UCL transection [18].

Other diagnostic tests commonly utilized are magnetic resonance imaging (MRI) and ultrasonography (US). Ultrasound imaging is a noninvasive and cost-effective technique, which has been used in several centers with great success [19–22]. However, US results have varied widely with accuracy of 40–92%; this is likely dependent on the examiner's skill and technique [23].

MRI studies have been performed on a larger scale and results are more consistent [24–26]. Coronal imaging through the thumb MCP joint provides clear confirmation of full-thickness avulsions of the UCL (or RCL). A study published in 1995 [19] compared US and MRI showing 100% sensitivity and specificity of MRI compared to 88% sensitivity and 83% specificity using US (Fig. 10.4).

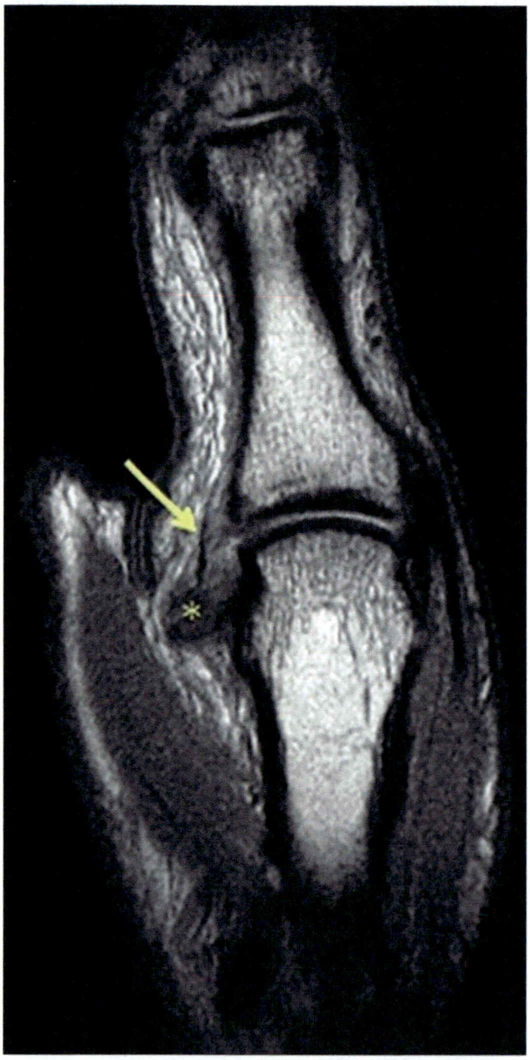

Fig. 10.4 Coronal MRI of the thumb metacarpophalangeal joint showing an avulsion of the UCL from the base of the proximal phalanx, with a Stener lesion (asterisk). The UCL is proximal to the adductor aponeurosis (yellow arrow). (Reproduced from Avery et al. [71])

Classification

The most widely used description of collateral ligament tears is a three-tier classification system based on stability. Grade 1 injury is a sprain associated with pain but no joint instability. Grade 2 is a partial tear with asymmetric laxity on side-to-side comparison but there is a firm endpoint. Grade 3 injuries involve a complete tear with laxity and no discernable endpoint.

Conservative Treatment

Treatment is largely dependent on whether the tear is partial or complete. Whereas a complete tear of the UCL (grade 3 injuries) indicates surgical treatment, grade 1 and 2 injuries can be treated nonoperatively [4]. Partial UCL injuries do well without residual pain or disability when treated conservatively. As the treating physician, one should be familiar with local and sport-specific regulations when choosing the style of immobilization, because the thumb should be protected from radial-directed forced. In nonoperative treatment, the patient is fitted for a hand-based thumb spica cast or splint (Fig. 10.5). The splint should be worn at all times for a period of 4–6 weeks followed by mobilization and strengthening by 6–8 weeks. When returning to baseball, a playing splint can be applied and taped to the athlete's hand as shown in Fig. 10.6.

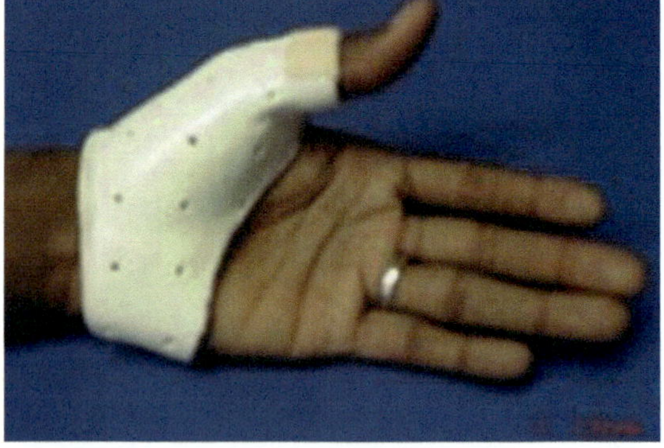

Fig. 10.5 Hand-based thumb spica splint

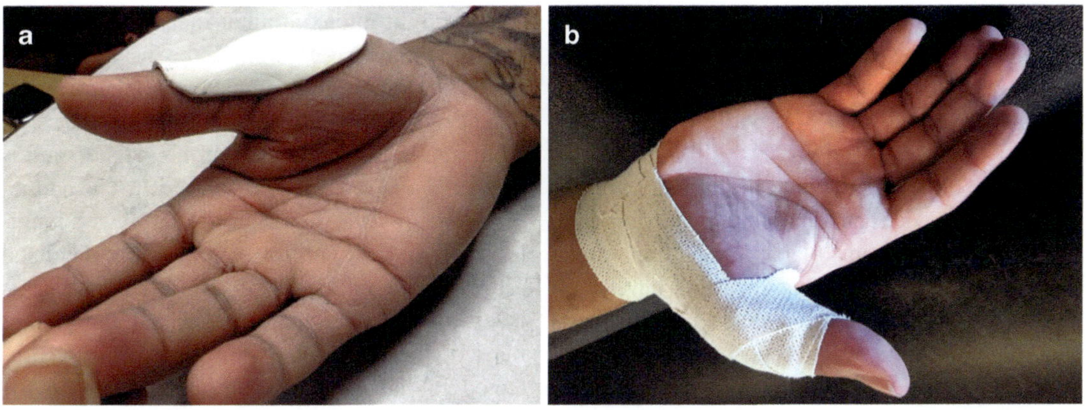

Fig. 10.6 Playing splint (**a**). Playing splint taped to athlete's hand (**b**)

In general grade 3 tears are commonly treated with surgery, but there have been reports of grade 3 tears treated successfully with nonoperative management [27, 28]. The presence of a Stener lesion denotes a complete tear in which the distal aspect of the ligament is trapped proximal to the adductor aponeurosis and there is a low likelihood to achieve healing and stability with nonoperative management.

A point of controversy with respect to the elite athlete involves treatment of avulsion fractures of the ulnar base of the thumb proximal phalanx. In a study involving 30 patients with bony lesions treated with thumb spica casts or splints, Kuz [29] reported that all patients were satisfied with nonoperative treatment despite a 25% nonunion rate. Similarly, Sorene and Goodwin [30] retrospectively reported on 28 thumbs treated nonoperatively with no instability at 2.5 years' follow-up, despite a 60% nonunion rate. Conversely, Dinowitz et al. [31] reported nine failures of minimally displaced UCL avulsion fractures that were treated nonoperatively. All nine patients, after being treated with 6 weeks of immobilization in a cast, presented with persistent thumb pain and disability with activities requiring strong pinch. With open reduction internal fixation, pinch strength increased from 36% to 89% contralateral side and grip increased from 77% to 93%. The investigators stated that minimally displaced UCL avulsion fractures frequently involve rotation of the articular segment toward the fracture site, preventing successful fracture healing. Often when fracture fragments are small, excision of the bony fragment and repair of the ligament to the fracture site on the proximal phalanx with a suture anchor is the most reliable approach.

Surgical Treatment

Acute UCL Repairs

In high-level athletes such as baseball players, acute complete tears of the UCL should be repaired to provide MCP joint stability, restore pinch strength, and return athletes to play. Timing of surgical treatment is also important. Often, even with a Stener lesion, the ligament can be repaired up to 3 months after injury, to allow the player to finish the season. If more than 3 months of the season remains and the player has a Stener lesion, then repair should be performed immediately. If no Stener lesion is seen on MRI, then later repair of the ligament is possible.

Many techniques have been described for repair of acute UCL tears including transosseous nonabsorbable sutures, suture buttons [32], direct periosteal closure [33–36], suture anchors [37–42], interference docking screws [43], condylar shaving with suture anchors [44], and arthroscopic repair [45]. In a study published in 2008, Katolik et al. compared two groups of 30 patients treated with pull-out sutures with bone tunnels and suture anchors. They reported decreased tourniquet times, better range of motion, and increased pinch strength in patients treated with suture anchors at an average 29-month follow-up. Additionally, the overall cost per patient was lower with suture anchors [46].

Despite the surgical technique used, the objective is to provide an anatomic reduction and repair of the ligament to bone. When anatomic reduction is achieved, clinical results have consistently shown favorable results in pain reduction, range of motion, and return to strength and stability. Additionally, biomechanical studies have shown that nonanatomic reconstruction of the UCL alters MCP biomechanics and joint motion [7]. Careful review of preoperative imaging and familiarity with the various ways the ruptured ligament displaces should be considered when approaching surgical repair. Often, the formation of granulation tissue and early scarring make the identification of the proper and accessory ligaments difficult. It is important to identify the proper and accessory collateral ligaments to avoid a malreduction of the native ligament.

Suture Augmentation Technique [47]

Recently, suture tape augmentation for repair of the thumb UCL has been described in competitive athletes. The goal of suture tape augmentation is to add strength to the repair at time zero. A biomechanical study comparing the strength of a traditional suture anchor repair to repair augmented with suture tape found that the augmented repair was at least five times stronger than the suture anchor repair [48]. In a study published in 2020, Gibbs and Shin described a cohort of 18 competitive athletes with acute UCL ruptures treated with repair and suture tape augmentation [49]. All athletes returned to the same level of play, and those attempting to return in-season returned to the same level of play at a mean of just under 5 weeks. They state that augmenting the repair with suture tape may prevent prolonged immobilization, expedite thumb motion, and improve postoperative recovery.

The senior author prefers to use two SwiveLock anchors (Arthrex) augmented with SutureTape (Arthrex) for repair of the thumb UCL.

A straight midaxial ulnar incision is centered over the thumb MCP joint. As the dissection continues by isolating the adductor aponeurosis, the dorsal cutaneous branch of the radial nerve is identified in the dorsal half of the incision and is protected and retracted dorsally [50]. The adductor aponeurosis is then incised sharply and longitudinally in line with the skin incision; the distal aspect is left intact with a 2 mm cuff along its insertion for later repair. The dorsal and palmar flaps of the aponeurosis are also carefully protected for later repair. The palmar aponeurosis flap is mobilized to determine the integrity of the accessory collateral ligament at the deepest aspect of the dissection. The junction of the dorsal capsule and proper UCL is incised sharply to create a dorsoulnar oblique longitudinal capsulotomy. This inside-out view allows for visualization of the displaced native ligament as well as confirmation of site of rupture, either from the metacarpal head or base of the proximal phalanx. The ligament is then carefully dissected and the site of repair prepared with a small curette or #69 blade to promote bone to ligament healing.

A 3.5 mm SwiveLock anchor (Arthrex) loaded with SutureTape (Arthrex) and two 2-0 Ethibond sutures is inserted into the volar-ulnar base of the proximal phalanx, at the anatomic footprint of the native UCL (Fig. 10.7). The native UCL is repaired back to the distal footprint using the preloaded Ethibond sutures. The suture tape tails are then held taut and brought proximally in line with the ligament to the ulnar aspect of the metacarpal

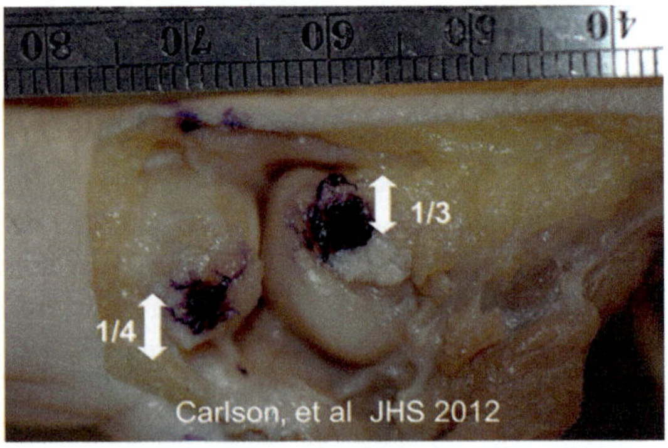

Fig. 10.7 Gross specimen showing the center of the UCL footprint on the metacarpal head (right side) and base of the proximal phalanx (left side) (Carlson et al. [11])

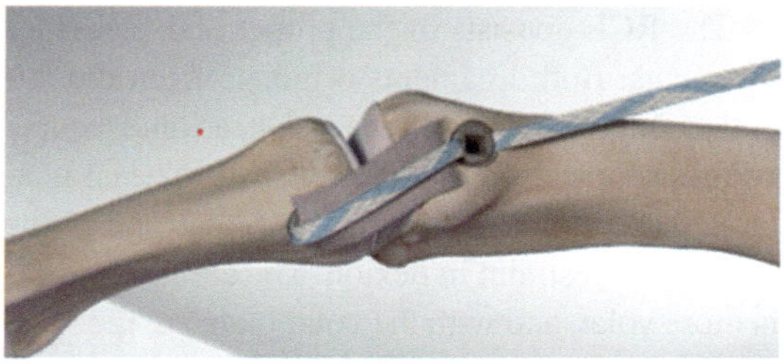

Fig. 10.8 Suture tape augmentation for UCL repair

head. The MCP joint is then held in 30° of flexion, and the suture tape tails are anchored at the normal anatomic location of the proximal UCL footprint using a second 3.5 mm SwiveLock anchor (Arthrex) (Fig. 10.8) The thumb MCP joint is then examined to confirm resistance to radial-directed stress and maintenance of full MCP motion. The capsule is then reapproximated with 4-0 Mersilene suture. The adductor tendon is reapproximated with 4-0 Mersilene suture and skin is closed with 4-0 subcuticular quill suture.

Postoperative Rehabilitation

Postoperative protocol for acute repair requires 6 weeks of immobilization in a hand-based thumb spica splint with the interphalangeal (IP) joint free (see Figs. 10.5 and 10.6). Finger and IP joint motion is encouraged immediately after the surgery. Active thumb MCP motion is allowed at 6 weeks and the need for hand therapy is rare. Players return to play at 6 weeks wearing a glove that keeps the thumb adducted to protect them while running bases.

Chronic UCL Reconstructions

Acute repair of an in season elite athlete may not be feasible, and immobilization and protection of the thumb MCP joint may allow for continued participation. Most subacute UCL injuries with Stener lesions can be repaired 3–4 months after injury. After 4 months, UCL tears are generally considered chronic. Instability associated with chronic UCL tears may cause significant disability with pain and weakness in pinch and grip. In chronic injuries, primary repairs have not been shown to have the same success as acute injuries. In a systematic review published in 2013, Samora et al. showed that UCL reconstruction for chronic injuries has similar good outcomes seen after acute repairs [51].

Several reconstructions for the thumb UCL have been described involving dynamic transfers, ligament reconstruction with transosseous tunnels, and bone tendon grafts. In 1971, Neviaser et al. reported a series of stable, pain-free thumbs after MCP capsulorrhaphy with adductor aponeurosis advancement to the base of the proximal phalanx [52]. Additionally, McCue et al. described an adductor advancement with ligament reattachment in 25 athletes allowing eventual return to sport participation for all patients [53]. In 1993, Glickel et al. described a technique using free tendon graft passed through two gouge tracks in the proximal phalanx and one in the metacarpal [54]. Over a mean follow-up of 4.5 years, 92% of patient's regained stability, all patient were relieved of pain, postoperative key pinch was 95% of the contralateral side, and 85% arc of motion was maintained.

Multiple tendon grafts have been used for reconstruction including palmaris longus, split EPB [33], full-thickness EPB [55], slip of abductor pollicis longus [56], second extensor compartment retinaculum [57], and fourth toe extensor digitorum [58]. Additionally, multiple techniques of reconstruction have been described including figure of eight weaves and fixation through bone tunnels and biointerference screws.

Technique

The senior author prefers to use a ligament reconstruction technique with 3.5 SwiveLock anchors (Arthrex) for fixation. Dissection is done similar to that of an acute repair, but in chronic injuries, the ligament is scarred and must be debrided fully to visualize the anatomic footprints on the metacarpal head and proximal phalanx. A palmaris longus autograft is harvested and cut to 4 cm in length. Whip-stitches passing suture is used and the graft is loaded into two 3.5 SwiveLock anchors (Arthrex). The graft is first secured to the proximal phalanx with one SwiveLock anchor. The joint is then reduced at 30° of flexion, and the graft is tensioned as tight as possible and secured with a second SwiveLock anchor in the metacarpal. The reconstructed ligament is then sutured to the volar plate using a 4-0 nonabsorbable suture. A layered closure is then performed as described previously. The MP joint is held in 20° of flexion with a 0.045 Kirschner wire to protect the reconstruction.

Postoperative Rehabilitation

Postoperative rehabilitation for chronic reconstruction is similar to that of acute repairs. Protection in a hand-based thumb spica splint is utilized for 8 weeks. Digital and thumb IP motion is encouraged immediately. At 8 weeks, MCP motion is initiated after k-wire removal. As in acute repairs, splint wear should be continued during sports for at least 3 months.

Thumb Radial Collateral Ligament

Thumb MCP radial collateral ligament injuries of the thumb are far less common than UCL injuries. They constitute approximately 10–42% of collateral ligament injuries of the thumb [59, 60]. These injuries occur in sporting events when a ball or player imparts a sudden ulnar-directed force to the thumb distal phalanx. The anatomy on the radial side of the thumb MCP joint is not the mirror image of the ulnar side and therefore warrants a separate discussion.

Anatomy and Mechanism of Injury

The musculotendinous insertions on the radial side are weaker than their ulnar counterparts. There are three main musculotendinous insertions on the radial side of the MCP joint: the two heads of the flexor pollicis brevis (FPB) and the abductor pollicis brevis (APB). The deep head of the FPB inserts onto the volar plate and lateral sesamoid. The superficial head of the FPB inserts into the volar aspect of the proximal phalanx. The abductor pollicis brevis (APB) is the most superficial layer on the radial side; it is situated more dorsally and inserts more distally than the FPB insertions. The APB aponeurosis is also broader than the adductor aponeurosis, which serves as the rationale as to why Stener-type lesions are rare on the radial aspect of the MCP joint [61].

The RCL consists of the proper and accessory ligaments. Both ligaments originate from the lateral condyle of the metacarpal head and course volarly to insert on the base of the proximal phalanx. The proper RCL is more dorsal and is the main static restraint in flexion. The accessory RCL is more volar, and with the volar plate are the main static restraints to the MCP in extension. The RCL is 4–8 mm wide and 12–14 mm long. Its insertion is wider than its origin, which may explain why proximal tears occur more frequently than distal tears [62]. An anatomic study defined the center of the RCL origin at the metacarpal as 3.5 mm from the dorsal surface and 3.3 mm from the articular surface, with the center of the RCL insertion on the proximal phalanx as 2.8 mm from the volar surface and 2.6 mm from the articular surface.

The dorsal capsule is an important structure in RCL tears. When the RCL tears, the MCP joint is often translated ulnar and volar [9]. The translation is a result of the more palmar situated adductor insertion, which serves as a strong volar and ulnar deforming force.

Injury Diagnosis: History and Clinical Exam

Like UCL injuries, RCL injuries are common in the elite athlete and a complete history is key to diagnosis. The mechanism of injury is usually an ulnarly directed force on the MCP joint of the thumb through a fall or object striking the thumb. Patients complain of pain, swelling, and stiffness. Unlike UCL injuries, instability is not common. In acute tears, patients often show ecchymosis over the dorsal radial MCP joint. Occasionally, there is an excessive dorsoradial prominence in chronic RCL injuries. The prominence of the radial metacarpal condyle as the distal thumb is adducted and palmarly subluxated.

Physical examination should assess for tenderness over the radial aspect of the thumb MCP, tenderness over the dorsal radial capsule, range of motion, stability in flexion, and stability in extension. If necessary, an anesthetic injection can be used to assist with stability testing. The joint should also be assessed with an anterior and posterior drawer to check for palmar subluxation, because dorsal capsular tears are associated with RCL injuries. Then examining the thumb MCP joint, the examiner must stabilize the metacarpal neck while providing an ulnar-directed force to the proximal phalanx in both full extension (to test the accessory RCL) and 30° of flexion (to test the proper RCL). The injured thumb should always be compared with the noninjured contralateral thumb. Palmar subluxation greater than 3 mm, instability greater than 30°, or instability greater than 15° compared with the uninjured side is indicative of a complete tear.

Imaging

Standard AP and lateral radiographs should be obtained to assess for avulsion injuries, associated fractures, and volar MCP subluxation. In the chronic setting, MCP arthritis may be present as well. Stress dynamic fluoroscopy may also be useful but is controversial.

Advanced imaging with ultrasonography (US) or MRI may be useful (Fig. 10.9). In certain centers, dynamic ultrasound can be used to test for both static and dynamic stability. As with UCL injuries, MRI scans are the most reliable way of assessing the integrity of the ligament [63].

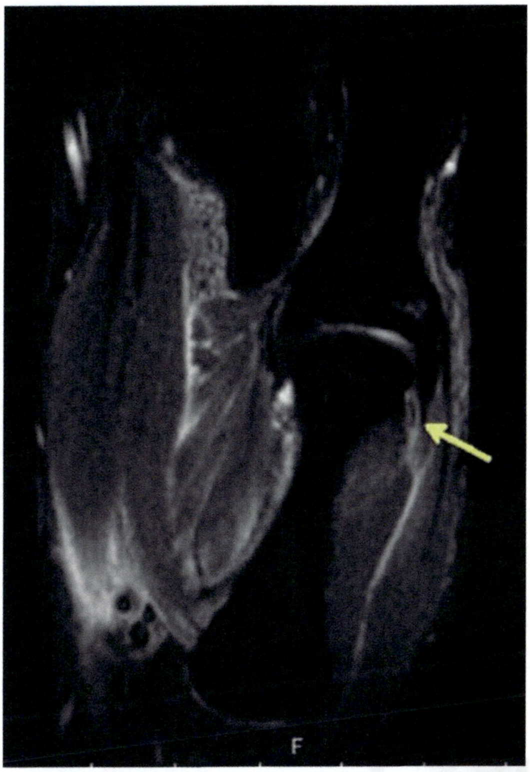

Fig. 10.9 T2-weighted coronal MRI of the thumb MP joint demonstrating a tear of the radial collateral ligament off the metacarpal head

Classification

As with thumb UCL injuries, the classic ligament injury grading system is applied to RCL injuries. Grade 1 tears are incomplete with no instability on examination. Grade 2 tears are partial tears with laxity but a firm endpoint. Grade 3 tears are complete tears with instability and no identifiable endpoint.

Conservative Treatment

As in UCL injuries, the treatment of grade 1 and 2 partial tears of the RCL is immobilization [4, 11, 31]. A hand-based thumb spica splint is recommended for 5–6 weeks. Most investigators recommend surgical treatment of grade 3 complete tears, but this is controversial. Proponents of nonoperative treatment of grade 3 tears contend that there is no interposing aponeurosis that interferes with ligament healing [64], and to date, there have only been two reports of Stener-like lesions with RCL tears [65].

Advocates for surgical repair of grade 3 tears state that acute unstable injuries may lead to symptomatic instability and degenerative joint disease of the thumb MCP. The volar and ulnar pull of the adductor as well as the ulnar pull of the EPL may prevent the ligament from healing, or force the ligament to heal in an elongated position [66, 67].

Surgical Treatment

Acute and Chronic Repair

The literature surrounding thumb RCL repairs is heterogenous and largely consists of comparisons between various acute and chronic techniques. Smith et al. [35] used 3 weeks as the cutoff between acute and chronic injuries and advocated for primary repair in all acute injuries and reconstruction in all chronic injuries.

Durham et al. compared results between repairs of acute and chronic RCL injuries in 18 patients [68]. Six patients underwent acute ligament repairs which included midsubstance tear suture repairs, reattachment to bony metacarpal origin for proximal ruptures, and distal avulsion fracture pinnings. Twelve patients underwent chronic repair which included APB advancement, distal RCL advancement, distal RCL reattachments with abductor advancement, imbrication of RCL in a pants-over-vest fashion, imbrication with abductor advancement, and reconstruction with a palmaris graft. At mean 6-year follow-up, there was a 94% subjective satisfaction rate, no patient had significant pain, and none was limited in their activities of daily living or avocational activities. There was no significant difference between pinch and grip strength in the groups treated acutely or late. There was a slight loss of MCP joint motion in both groups; the acute repair group had an 11% decrease in range of motion of the MCP joint compared with a 23% decrease in the chronic repair cohort.

In 2006, Horch et al. [69] described treatment of nine patients with chronic (over 15 days) RCL injuries with dorsal redirection of the APB tendon with fixation with an intraosseous suture anchor. Of the nine patients that underwent this procedure, none reported loss of MCP, IP, or thumb abduction motion. The majority of patients were satisfied with their surgery at an average of 39 months of follow-up. The authors concluded that APB-plasty is a safe and effective treatment for RCL instability.

In one of the largest case series for RCL repairs, Coyle [61] treated 38 patients with soft tissue sleeve advancement and bony reattachment tied over a button. Postoperatively, the MCP joint was immobilized with a k-wire and a thumb spica for 6 weeks for protection of the repair. At mean follow-up of 3.8 years, 87% were asymptomatic, 92% had normal pinch and grip strength, 79% had full range of motion of the thumb MCP joint, and all patients had normal IP range of motion. No patients reported symptomatic MCP volar instability, but 8% had mild asymptomatic MCP volar subluxation.

In 2006, Catalano et al. [67] published a study that compared 16 acute repairs to 10 reconstructions for grade 3 RCL injuries. Acute injuries were treated 2.5 weeks from trauma, whereas chronic injuries were treated 7 months after index trauma. Primary repair was carried out with direct suture repair for midsubstance tears or suture anchor repair for distal or proximal tears. Chronic injuries were reconstructed with palmaris or flexor carpi radialis grafts anchored inn bone tunnels. The study reported no significant differences in objective measurements between the acute repairs and late reconstructions at average follow-up of 59 months. There was no significant difference in MCP and IP range of motion, or any difference in grip or pinch strength, or MCP joint stability. Overall satisfaction was excellent in both groups [67].

In 1998, McDermott and Levin described five cases of chronic (greater than 2 months) RCL injuries treated with a Mitek suture anchor to anatomically reattach the ligament to the bone. All patients returned to activities within 2 to 3.5 months. Grip strength, pinch strength, and range of motion were normal by 6 months. At 2-year follow-up, all patients were satisfied and had clinically stable MCP joints [70].

Surgical Technique

The authors prefer suture anchor repair of the RCL with 2 3.5 mm SwiveLock anchors (Arthrex). A straight radial midaxial incision is centered over the thumb MCP joint. The abductor aponeurosis is defined and the radial-sided dorsal cutaneous branch is identified. The abductor aponeurosis is broader and more dorsal that the ulnar-sided adductor aponeurosis. The abductor aponeurosis is incised longitudinally in line with the skin incision. Dorsal and palmar flaps of the aponeurosis are carefully protected for later repair. A dorsoradial longitudinal capsulotomy is performed that allows an inside-out view of the proper and accessory collateral ligaments. Typically, the tear is off the metacarpal condyle. The site of repair is exposed carefully and denuded with a curette or #69 blade to promote bone to ligament healing.

A double-loaded 3.5 mm SwiveLock anchor (Arthrex) is used for fixation. The priority in radial-sided repairs is to advance the palmarly displaced ligament to a more dorsal anatomic position. The suture anchor is placed in the anatomic origin of the ligament on the metacarpal condyle. Repair of the ligament helps to prevent palmar subluxation of the proximal phalanx. Accessory collateral ligament tears off the volar plate are evaluated, and if present, they are repaired with 4-0 nonabsorbable suture. At this point, the MCP should be tested for an improvement in the clinical endpoint with an ulnar-directed stress. The capsule and the abductor aponeurosis are closed in separate layers with 4-0 nonabsorbable suture.

Postoperative Rehabilitation

Postoperative protocols include 6 weeks of immobilization in a hand-based thumb spica splint with the IP joint free. IP joint motion is encouraged immediately after the surgery. Active range of motion is initiated at 6 weeks and hand therapy is rarely necessary.

References

1. Moutet F, Guinard D, Lebrun C, et al. Metacarpophalangeal thumb sprains based on experience with more than 1,000 cases. Ann Chir Main. 1989;8(2):99–109.
2. Campbell CS. Gamekeeper's thumb. J Bone Joint Surg Br. 1955;37(1):148–9.
3. Gerber C, Senn E, Matter P. Skier's thumb. Surgical treatment of recent injuries to the ulnar collateral ligament of the thumb's metacarpophalangeal joint. Am J Sports Med. 1981;9(3):171–7.
4. Carlson MG, Warner KK, Meyers KN, et al. Mechanics of an anatomical reconstruction for the thumb metacarpophalangeal collateral ligaments. J Hand Surg Am. 2013;38:117–23.
5. Coonrad RW, Goldner JL. A study of the pathologic findings and treatment in soft-tissue injury of the thumb metacarpophalangeal joint, with a clinical study of the normal range of motion in one thousand thumbs and a study of post mortem findings of ligamentous structures in relation to function. J Bone Joint Surg Am. 1968;50(3):439–51.
6. Heyman P, Gelberman RH, Duncan K, et al. Injuries of the ulnar collateral ligament of the thumb metacarpophalangeal joint. Biomechanical and prospective clinical studies on the usefulness of valgus stress testing. Clin Orthop Relat Res. 1993;292:165–71.
7. Minami A, An KN, Coonay WP 3rd, et al. Ligament stability of the metacarpophalangeal joint: a biomechanical study. J Hand Surg Am. 1985;10(2):255–60.
8. Bean CH, Tencer AF, Trumble TE. The effect of thumb metacarpophalangeal ulnar collateral ligament attachment site on site on joint range of motion: an in vitro study. J Hand Surg Am. 1999;24(2):283–7.
9. Stener B. Displacement of the ruptured ulnar collateral ligament of the metacarpo-phalangeal joint of the thumb. J Bone Joint Surg Br. 1962;44(4):869–79.
10. Avery DM 3rd, Caggiano NM, Matullo KS. Ulnar collateral ligament injuries of the thumb: a comprehensive review. Orthop Clin North Am. 2015;46:281–92.
11. Carlson MG, Warner KK, Meyers KN, et al. The anatomy of the thumb metacarpophalangeal ulnar and radial collateral ligaments. J Hand Surg Am. 2012;37:2021–6.
12. Melone CP Jr, Beldner S, Basuk RS. Thumb collateral ligament injuries. An anatomic basis for treatment. Hand Clin. 2000;16(3):345–57.
13. Firoozbakhsh K, Yi IS, Moneim MS, et al. A study of ulnar collateral ligament of the thumb metacarpophalangeal joint. Clin Orthop Relat Res. 2002;403:240–7.
14. Kaplan SJ. The Stener lesion revisited: a case report. J Hand Surg Am. 1998;23(5):833–6.
15. Giele H, Martin J. The two-level ulnar collateral ligament injury of the metacarpophalangeal joint of the thumb. J Hand Surg Br. 2003;28(1):92–3.
16. Gurdezi S, Mok D. "Sag Sign" -- a simple radiological sign for detecting injury to the thumb ulnar collateral ligament. J Inj. 2008;39:191.
17. Noszian IM, Dinkhauser LM, Straub GM, et al. Ulnar collateral ligament injuries of the thumb. Dislocation caused by stress radiography in 2 cases. Acta Orthop Scand. 1995;66(2):156–7.
18. Mckeon KE, Gelberman RH, Calfee RP. Ulnar collateral ligament injuries of the thumb: phalangeal translation during valgus stress in human cadaver. Bone Joint Surg Am. 2013;95:881–7.
19. Hergan K, Mittler C. Sonography of the injured ulnar collateral ligament of the thumb. J Bone Joint Surg Br. 1995;77(1):77–83.
20. Bronstein AJ, Koniuch MP, von Holsbeeck M. Ultrasonographic detection of thumb ulnar collateral ligament injuries: a cadaveric study. J Hand Surg Am. 1994;19(2):304–12.

21. Noszian IM, Dinkhauser LM, Orthner E, et al. Ulnar collateral ligament: differentiation of displaced and nondisplaced tears with US. Radiology. 1995;194(1):61–3.
22. O'Callaghan BI, Kohut G, Hoogewoud HM. Gamekeeper thumb: identification of the Stener lesion with US. Radiology. 1994;192(2):477–80.
23. Hergan K, Mittler C, Oser W. Pitfalls in sonography of the gamekeeper's thumb. Eur Radiol. 1997;7(1):65–9.
24. Louis DS, Buckwalter KA. Magnetic resonance imaging of the collateral ligaments of the thumb. J Hand Surg Am. 1989;14(4):739–41.
25. Speath HJ, Abrams RA, Bock GW, et al. Gamekeepers thumb: differentiation of nondisplaced and displaced tears of the ulnar collateral ligament with MR imaging. Work in progress. Radiology. 1993;188(2): 553–6.
26. Hinke DH, Erickson SJ, Chamoy L, et al. Ulnar collateral ligament of the thumb: MR findings if cadavers, volunteers, and patients with ligamentous injury (gamekeeper's thumb). AJR Am J Roentgenol. 1994;163(6):1431–4.
27. Landsman JC, Seitz WH Jr, Froimson AI, Leb RB, Bachner EJ. Splint immobilization of gamekeeper's thumb. Orthopaedics. 1995;18:1161–5.
28. Pichora DR, McMurtry RY, Bell MJ. Gamekeepers Thumb: a prospective study of functional bracing. J Hand Surg [Am]. 1989;14:567–73.
29. Kuz JE, Husband JB, Tokar N, et al. Outcome of avulsion fractures of the ulnar base of the proximal phalanx of the thumb treated nonsurgically. J Hand Surg Am. 1999;24(2):275–82.
30. Sorene ED, Goodwin DR. Non-operative treatment of displaced avulsion fractures of the ulnar base of the proximal phalanx of the thumb. Scand J Plast Reconstr Surg Hand Surg. 2003;37(4):225–7.
31. Dinowitz M, Trumble T, Hanel D, et al. Failure of cast immobilization for thumb ulnar collateral ligament avulsion fractures. J Hand Surg Am. 1997;22(6):1057–63.
32. Wilppula E, Nummi J. Surgical treatment of ruptured ulnar collateral ligament of the metacarpophalangeal joint of the thumb. Injury. 1970;2(1):69–72.
33. Strandell G. Total rupture of the ulnar collateral ligament of the metacarpophalangeal joint of the thumb: results of surgery in 35 cases. Acta Chir Scand. 1959;118:72–80.
34. Kaplan EB. The pathology and treatment of radial subluxation of the thumb with ulnar displacement of the head of the first metacarpal. J Bone Joint Surg Am. 1961;43:541–6.
35. Smith MA. The mechanism of acute ulnar instability of the metacarpophalangeal joint of the thumb. Hand. 1980;12(3):225–30.
36. Downey DJ, Monheim MS, Omer GE Jr. Acute gamekeeper's thumb. Quantitative outcome of surgical repair. Am J Sports Med. 1995;23(2):222–6.
37. Derkash RS, Matyas JR, Weaver JK, et al. Acute surgical repair of skier's thumb. Clin Orthop Relat Res. 1987;216:29–33.
38. Abrahamsson SO, Sollerman C, Lundborg G, et al. Diagnosis of displaced ulnar collateral ligament of the metacarpophalangeal joint of the thumb. J Hand Surg Am. 1990;15(3):457–60.
39. Zeman C, Hunter RE, Freeman JR, et al. Acute skier's thumb repaired with a proximal phalanx suture anchor. Am J Sports Med. 1998;26(5):644–50.
40. Kozin SH. Treatment of thumb ulnar collateral ligament ruptures with the Mitek bone anchor. Ann Plast Surg. 1995;35(1):1–5.
41. Kato H, Minami A, Takahara M, et al. Surgical repair of acute collateral ligament injuries in digits with the Mitek bone suture anchor. J Hand Surg Br. 1999;24(1):70–5.
42. Weiland AJ, Berner SH, Hotchkiss RN, et al. Repair of acute ulnar collateral ligament injuries of the thumb metacarpophalangeal joint with an intraosseous suture anchor. J Hand Surg Am. 1997;22(4):585–91.
43. Rettig A, Rettig L, Welsch M. Anatomic reconstruction of thumb metacarpophalangeal joint ulnar collateral ligament using an interference screw docking technique. Tech Hand Up Extrem Surg. 2009;13: 7–10.
44. Haddock NT, Beasley RW, Sharma S. Thumb metacarpophalangeal joint ulnar collateral ligament repair with condylar shaving. Tech Hand Up Extrem Surg. 2009;13:199–201.
45. Ryu J, Faggan R. Arthroscopic treatment of acute complete thumb metacarpophalangeal ulnar collateral ligament tears. J Hand Surg Am. 1995;20:1037–42.
46. Katolik LI, Friedrich J, Trumble TE. Repair of acute ulnar collateral ligament injuries of the thumb metacarpophalangeal joint: a retrospective comparison of pull-out sutures and bone anchor techniques. Plast Reconstr Surg. 2008;122(5):1451–6.
47. De Giacomo AF, Shin SS. Repair of the thumb ulnar collateral ligament with suture tape augmentation. Tech Hand Up Extrem Surg. 2017;21(4):164–6.
48. Shin SS, van Eck CF, Uquillas C. Suture tape augmentation of the thumb ulnar collateral ligament repair: a biomechanical study. J Hand Surg Am. 2018;43(9):868.e1–86.e6.
49. Gibbs DB, Shin SS. Return to play in athletes after thumb ulnar collateral ligament repair with suture tape augmentation. Ortho J Sports Med. 2020;8(7): 1–5.
50. Osterman AL, Hayken GD, Bora FW Jr. A quantitative evaluation of thumb function after ulnar collateral ligament repair and reconstruction. J Trauma. 1981;21(10):854–61.
51. Samora JB, Harris JD, Griesser MJ, et al. Outcomes after injury to the thumb ulnar collateral ligament – a systematic review. Clin J Sports Med. 2013;23:247–54.
52. Neviaser RJ, Wilson JN, Lievano A. Rupture of the ulnar collateral ligament of the thumb (gamekeeper's thumb). Correction by dynamic repair. J Bone Joint Surg Am. 1971;53(7):1357–65.
53. McCue FC 3rd, Hakala MW, Andrews JR, et al. Ulnar collateral ligament injuries of the thumb in athletes. J Sports Med. 1974;2:70–80.

54. Glickel SZ, Malerich M, Pearce SM, et al. Ligament replacement for chronic instability of the ulnar collateral ligament of the metacarpophalangeal joint of the thumb. J Hand Surg Am. 1993;18(5):930–41.
55. Fairhurst M, Hansen L. Treatment of "Gamekeeper's Thumb" by reconstruction of the ulnar collateral liagment. J Hand Surg (Br). 2002;27:542–5.
56. Frykman G, Johansson O. Surgical repair of rupture of the ulnar collateral ligament of the metacarpophalangeal joint of the thumb. Acta Chir Scand. 1956;112(1):58–64.
57. Guelmi K, Thebaud A, Werther JR, et al. Bone-retinaculum-bone reconstruction for chronic posttraumatic instability of the metacarpophalangeal joint of the thumb. J Hand Surg Am. 2003;28:685–95.
58. Alldred AJ. Rupture of the collateral ligament of the metacarpophalangeal joint of the thumb. J Bone Joint Surg Br. 1955;37:443–5.
59. Edelstein DM, Kardashian G, Lee SK. Radial collateral ligament injuries of the thumb. J Hand Surg Am. 2008;33(5):760–70.
60. Tang P. Collateral ligament injuries of the thumb metacarpophalangeal joint. J Am Acad Orthop Surg. 2011;19(5):287–96.
61. Coyle MP Jr. Grade III radial collateral ligament injuries of the thumb metacarpophalangeal joint: treatment by soft tissue advancement and bony reattachment. J Hand Surg Am. 2003;28(1):14–20.
62. Lyons RP, Kozin SH, Failla JM, et al. The anatomy of the radial side of the thumb: static restraints in preventing subluxation and rotation after injury. Am J Orthop (Belle Mead NJ). 1998;27(11):759–63.
63. Schroeder NS, Goldfarb CA. Thumb ulnar collateral and radial collateral ligament injuries. Clin Sports Med. 2015;34:117–26.
64. Camp RA, Weatherwax RJ, Miller EB. Chronic post-traumatic radial instability of the thumb metacarpophalangeal joint. J Hand Surg Am. 1980;5(3):221–5.
65. Doty JF, Rudd JN, Jemison M. Radial collateral ligament injury of the thumb with a Stener-like lesion. Orthopaedics. 2010;33(12):925.
66. Posner MA, Retaillaud JL. Metacarpophalangeal joint injuries of the thumb. Hand Clin. 1992;8(4):713–32.
67. Catalano LW 3rd, Cardon L, Patenaude N, et al. Results of surgical treatment of acute and chronic grade 3 tears of the radial collateral ligament of the thumb metacarpophalangeal joint. J Hand Surg Am. 2006;31(1):68–75.
68. Durham JW, Khuri S, Kim MH. Acute and late radial collateral ligament injuries of the thumb metacarpophalangeal joint. J Hand Surg Am. 1993;18(2):232–7.
69. Horch RE, Dragu A, Polykandriotis E, et al. Radial collateral ligament repair of the thumb metacarpophalangeal joint using the abductor pollicis brevis tendon. Plast Reconstr Surg. 2006;117(2):491–6.
70. McDermott TP, Levin LS. Suture anchor repair of chronic radial ligament injuries of the metacarpophalangeal joint of the thumb. J Hand Surg Br. 1998;23(2):271–4.
71. Avery DM, Inkellis ER, Carlson MG. Thumb collateral ligament injuries in the athlete. Curr Rev Musculoskelet Med. 2017;10:28–37.

Collateral Ligament Injuries of the Fingers in Baseball Players

11

Caroline H. Hu and Jeffrey B. Husband

Introduction

Hand and wrist injuries in baseball players represent a significant cause of morbidity and days away from play. An evaluation of a collegiate baseball team over 3 seasons documented that 17% of orthopedic injuries occurred to the hand and wrist. Rhee et al. reported on hand and wrist injuries sustained by major league and minor league baseball players documented by the Major League Baseball's Health and Injury Tracking System (HITS) [1]. They identified 4478 hand and 1748 wrist injuries with a total of 105,246 lost days of play. The majority of the reported injuries occurred due to contact with the ball, the ground, the wall, another player, or with a bat (95%); 40% of injuries occurred when batting, 30% when fielding, 13% when pitching, and 11% while sliding. Among all the injuries, 4.7% were sprains of the proximal interphalangeal joint, 2.6% were sprains of the metacarpophalangeal joint, and 1.9% were sprains of the distal interphalangeal joint. Each of these injuries averaged 11.6, and 14 days of missed play for each injury, respectively. The frequency of surgery was very low for each of these injuries (2.4% for PIP, 1.7% for MP, and 0% for DIP injuries).

The literature on collateral ligament injuries in the fingers is scant. Most reports relate to rock climbers who most commonly sustain injuries to the PIP joint secondary to high forces generated by hook and crimp style grip during climbing [2]. In a study of 42 elite rock climbers, 40% were diagnosed with acute or chronic sprains of the collateral ligaments of the PIP joint [3]. Similar to the forces generated during rock climbing, pitchers may experience significant stress to the fingers when throwing a baseball. Pitchers are at risk for sustaining collateral ligament injuries of the fingers due to the high torque, repetitive movement associated with throwing a baseball. Kinoshita et al. used an instrumented baseball to measure finger forces that occurred when throwing a fast ball. They found that the peak reaction force exceeded 80% of the maximum finger strength measured for each digit [4].

Anatomy and Physiology of the Collateral Ligaments

The metacarpophalangeal and interphalangeal joints of the fingers are complex diarthrodial joints that function to allow for reach, pinch, and grasp that are also crucial for throwing and catch-

C. H. Hu
Department of Orthopaedic Surgery, University of Minnesota, Minneapolis, MN, USA
e-mail: chhu@umn.edu

J. B. Husband (✉)
Hand Surgery, TRIA Orthopedic Center, Minneapolis, MN, USA
e-mail: Jeffrey.Husband@tria.com

G. M. Lourie (ed.), *Hand and Wrist Injuries in Baseball*,
https://doi.org/10.1007/978-3-030-81659-9_11

ing. Advances in our understanding of the anatomy and physiology of the collateral ligaments have helped us to better understand their function.

The metacarpophalangeal joint is multiplanar and functions in flexion, extension, abduction, adduction, and circumduction as compared to the interphalangeal joints which allow only for flexion and extension. The principal axis of motion of the MP joints is in flexion and extension, with up to 90° of flexion and 20–30° of extension. Additionally, there are 10–40° of abduction and adduction which varies from finger to finger [5].

The metacarpal head is ellipsoidal in the sagittal plane and trapezoidal in the coronal plane with greater width on the palmar aspect [6]. The articular surface of the base of the proximal phalanx is concave and shallow similar to the glenoid in relation to the articular surface of the metacarpal head [5]. The articular anatomy along with the oblique course of the collateral ligaments creates a "cam effect," which results in increased stability of the MP joint in flexion as the collateral ligaments tighten [6, 7]. Accordingly, abduction and adduction are greatest in full extension of the joint [8].

The dynamic stabilizers of the MP joint include the intrinsic and extrinsic muscles and tendons, while the static stabilizers are the capsule, palmar plate, sagittal bands, deep transverse intermetacarpal ligaments, corner ligaments of the interosseous fascia, and the proper and accessory collateral ligaments [5]. The proper collateral ligaments originate on the dorsoradial and dorsoulnar aspects of the metacarpal head and insert on the **volar** palmar aspect of the base of the proximal phalanx. The ulnar collateral ligament (UCL) is less oblique, thinner, and narrower than the radial collateral ligament [9]. Using biplanar radiography, Minami et al. determined that the ulnar collateral ligament originates from a slightly more palmar and proximal position, approximately 1/3 from the dorsal border of the metacarpal head, inserting approximately 1/4 away from the palmar border of the proximal phalanx. More recently, using different methodology, Dy et al. determined that the center of origin of the radial collateral ligament (RCL) lies 40% volar from the dorsal border of the metacarpal head, whereas the center of insertion lies 46% dorsal from the palmar border of the proximal phalanx [10]. The accessory collateral ligaments are fan-shaped and increase in thickness from proximal to distal and originate slightly palmar and proximal to the origin of the proper collateral ligaments. They spread out to insert along the lateral border of the palmar plate [9]. The proper collateral ligaments are taut in MP joint flexion, while the accessory collateral ligaments are lax. The accessory collateral ligaments function antagonistically with the proper collateral ligaments as a reciprocal force couple to provide lateral stabilization of the MP joint [5].

Understanding the kinematics of the collateral ligaments is essential to understanding function of the joints. The collateral ligaments stabilize the joint and protect it from abduction and adduction stress. The finger MP joints are able to stabilize each other due to their proximity to one another and the deep transverse metacarpal ligaments. The MP joint is lax in extension and stable flexion to assist with grasp. The tautness of the collateral ligaments in flexion and laxity in extension has significant implications for the management of collateral ligament injuries in that immobilization in extension may lead to difficulty regaining MP joint flexion due to shortening of the collateral ligaments.

Pathophysiology of Injury

Experimental ligament rupture models have contributed to our understanding of the patterns of collateral ligament injury. Minamikawa et al. conducted serial sectioning of cadaver collateral ligaments at the PIP joint and found that lateral angulation greater than 10° in extension and 20° in flexion indicated loss of collateral ligament injury or complete proper collateral ligament rupture [11]. The PIP joint was not destabilized until at least half of the PCL and the accessory stabilizing structures were sectioned. Another cadaver model noted four distinct patterns of PIP joint ligament rupture: midsubstance tear, proximal detachment, distal detachment, and bony avulsion fracture [12]. These injury patterns varied according to the speed at which the strain was applied. Higher speed injuries caused distal tears, tears at the junction between the PCL and ACL and avulsion fractures at the insertion of the palmar plate, whereas low-speed injuries caused midsubstance tears. Low-speed injuries allowed the ligament to stretch prior to rupture and required higher forces. A rapidly applied force, moreover, is more likely to be a mechanism of the injury in the injured baseball player.

The frequency of injury to each finger has varied among case series and might differ based on several variables. In a 2-year period, Delaere et al. reported that 39% of MP joint collateral ligament injuries presenting to an emergency department involved digits other than the thumb [13]. The index finger MP joint is most susceptible to injury as it is a border digit and is more likely to be subjected to trauma. The index MP joint lacks a deep transverse metacarpal ligament on the radial side, but it is protected by the ulnar three fingers [14]. It is also stabilized by the first dorsal interosseous muscle. The small finger is also a border digit, and some studies have suggested that it has the highest occurrence of collateral ligament injury compared with the other fingers [15, 16]. Other reports found the highest frequency of collateral ligament injuries of the MP joint to involve the middle finger [13]. The index finger was more likely to have ulnar collateral ligament injuries at the MP joint, whereas the ring and small finger were more likely to involve the radial collateral ligaments [17]. Ulnar collateral ligament injuries are more common than radial collateral ligament injuries in every finger; however, the ratio of radial collateral ligament injuries to ulnar collateral ligament injuries is highest in the index finger [16]. Collateral ligament injuries to the DIP joint are less common, perhaps due to a shorter lever arm [18].

Throwing a baseball places palmar and ulnar stress on the PIP joints [19]. This stress may cause chronic injury to the collateral ligament over time. Conversely, acute collateral ligament injuries are more likely to be caused from traumatic high-speed injuries, such as being hit by a ball, sliding, or contact with another player. Sliding head first with the hand outstretched in front of the player places the fingers, hand, and wrist at a high risk for injury. This has led to the use of sliding gloves to protect the hand. Direct impact by a ballplayer against a wall on an extended finger can result in a significant force to the digit, leading to injury ranging from a minor sprain to a fracture dislocation.

Clinical Evaluation

Clinical History

A careful and detailed history remains important in assessing injuries to the fingers in baseball players. This includes evaluation of symptoms as well as exacerbating movements and the mechanism of a specific traumatic event. It is important to note at what point pain occurs during the throwing phase in pitchers. Other important history includes age, level of play, and position. There may be a history of a gradual and insidious onset of finger pain with throwing over a prolonged period. This may lead to chronic pain in the collateral ligament, possibly associated with instability [3]. The clinician should elicit a history of whether or not the symptoms are associated with any change in the frequency or type of training or throwing mechanism. In most instances, the player will report a single, significant traumatic injury.

The symptoms of injury to the collateral ligament include pain and swelling with impaired function at the injured joint. There may be difficulty with grip and throwing, catching, and batting.

Physical Examination

Physical examination involves a systematic evaluation of the hand and fingers, including inspection, range of motion, palpation for point tenderness, neurovascular status, measurement of strength, stress testing, and provocative tests for ligamentous instability. Inspection includes assessment of the resting posture, observing for angular malalignment. If this does occur, it suggests the presence of a complete collateral ligament injury. This would include scissoring of the digits during finger flexion, such as pronation of the index finger with scissoring under the middle finger with complete rupture of the radial collateral ligament of the MP joint [5]. The finger may deviate away from the site of the injury with a complete rupture. Acutely, there may be ecchymosis, swelling, and limited motion. Tenderness is present in acute and chronic injuries.

The collateral ligaments of the injured joint should be tested for instability. In certain instances, this may be very painful, and local anesthesia may be required to allow for complete evaluation.

Varus and valgus stress to the joint should be applied in full extension and at 30° of flexion. Testing in full flexion evaluates the integrity of the proper collateral ligaments, whereas testing in full extension evaluates the integrity of the accessory collateral ligaments. Testing in extension and at 30° of flexion is somewhat analogous to varus and valgus stress testing at the knee joint, where 30° of flexion decreases the stabilizing influence of the posterior capsular structures, which contribute to lateral stability in extension [11]. Stress testing should evaluate for both pain and laxity and to determine if there is an endpoint to instability. Proper collateral ligament laxity should decrease with flexion, and an increase of laxity or no change with flexion indicates a proper collateral ligament injury [8]. At the MP joint, the proper collateral ligaments have been traditionally tested at 30° of flexion; however, Wong et al. found variable differences in laxity at full extension and 30° of flexion, concluding that laxity should be tested in extension and 90° of flexion [8]. It should be remembered that the proper collateral ligament is lax at 0° of extension in the normal ligament and should not be interpreted as abnormal. The contralateral side hand should be used as control in measurement of range of motion and stress testing.

When evaluating the PIP joint for laxity, greater than 20° of lateral deviation with stress at 30° of flexion suggests complete rupture of the proper collateral ligament, whereas greater than 15° of lateral deviation in extension and/or greater than 30° in flexion suggests a rupture of the accessory collateral ligament as well [11].

Imaging

Plain radiographs including posterior-anterior, lateral, and oblique views should be obtained with any injury. Radiographs should be performed prior to any stress testing since the radiographs may reveal joint subluxation due to complete collateral ligament rupture or avulsion fracture. A Brewerton view may demonstrate a fracture of the metacarpal head. Stress views, in the absence of any fractures, may reveal joint instability when compared with nonstress views of the affected joint. In the setting of isolated ligamentous injury, however, radiographs rarely are helpful. In most cases, additional imaging is not required.

Ultrasound evaluation may assist in the diagnosis of collateral ligament injuries in challenging cases and allows for dynamic evaluation of each ligament. Ultrasound has been found to have 76% sensitivity and 81% specificity for complete tears of the collateral ligaments of the MP joints [20]. The collateral ligaments appear as thick echoic bands. With an acute sprain, the ligament has focal hypoechoic thickening due to hemorrhage and edema. Complete disruption of ligament continuity and surrounding soft tissue hyperemia will be seen with an acute full-thickness tear. There is thickening and elongation and a lack of soft tissue hyperemia with a chronic sprain [21]. Stress testing during a dynamic ultrasound evaluation may reveal joint space widening or an increased gap between the ends of the torn ligament. It should be remembered that there may be potential problems with diagnostic ultrasound in that the quality of the ultrasound is operator-dependent and that transducer position and the anatomic plane need to be properly oriented in order to adequately visualize the collateral ligaments [21]. The proper collateral and accessory collateral ligaments cannot be differentiated with ultrasound evaluation. Furthermore, concomitant injuries may demonstrate similar features of thickening and hypoechoic regions and may be mistaken for the collateral ligaments [22]. Arthrography has been used in the past to successfully diagnose collateral ligament injuries, but have generally been found not to be necessary to confirm the diagnosis [5, 13]. Magnetic resonance imaging has a 75% sensitivity and 98% specificity for collateral ligament tears of the MP joints [23]. An MRI may be helpful in differentiating between complete tears of the ligament versus partial tears and may help distinguish the site of injury or concomitant injuries to surrounding structures [14].

Grading Collateral Ligament Injuries

Gaston et al. classified a series of metacarpophalangeal joint radial collateral ligament injuries into four grades as a guide to treatment. Grade 1 injuries were defined as those with tenderness to palpation without laxity [5]. Grade 2 injuries were tender to palpation with laxity compared to the contralateral finger but with a definite endpoint. Grade 3 injuries had laxity without an endpoint.

Bowers et al. classified collateral ligament injuries of the PIP joint into three grades [24]. Similar to the metacarpophalangeal joint, grade 1 injuries of the proximal interphalangeal joint are associated with swelling and tenderness over the collateral ligament with no instability. Grade 2 injuries demonstrated a definite endpoint with less than 20° of deviation. Grade 3 PIP joint collateral ligament injuries included not only complete rupture of the collateral ligament but also the volar plate. There were greater than 20° of laxity with no definite endpoint.

Management of Collateral Ligament Injuries

The demands of baseball, including throwing, need to be considered when managing injuries to the collateral ligament of the fingers. Greater forces are involved in throwing a baseball than in performing normal everyday activities. In particular, the radial collateral ligament of the MP joint of the index finger is a crucial primary stabilizer for pinch. Proper grading of the injury is useful in determining the management of collateral ligament injuries. Treatment data are based on case series and small retrospective and prospective case studies. In almost all instances, these studies have shown that nonoperative management with rest, a short period of immobilization, and appropriate rehabilitation are optimal treatments for grade 1 or 2 injuries [5]. Gaston et al. recommended the following nonoperative treatment protocol for injuries to the radial collateral ligament of the MP joint. Grade 1 injuries are treated with splinting for 3 weeks with the MP joint in 30–45° of flexion to prevent an extension contracture, followed by buddy taping alone for 3 weeks [5, 13]. During the period of immobilization, patients removed the splint for flexion and extension exercises three times a day using buddy tapes. Grade 2 injuries are treated with 3 weeks of immobilization followed by 3 weeks of splinting. Patient is to begin range-of-motion exercises after transition to splinting with strengthening starting at 8 weeks and unrestricted return to activities at 12 weeks [5].

Grade 1 or 2 injuries of the collateral ligaments of the proximal interphalangeal joint are managed conservatively with a finger splint at 0° of extension followed by buddy taping with range of motion as pain decreases. The maximum volume of the PIP joint is in a position of approximately 30° of flexion. Un-splinted, the PIP joint tends to lie in this position and may lead to a flexion contracture. Therefore, splinting at 0° of extension helps reduce the risk of developing a flexion contracture and, generally, it is not difficult to regain flexion.

Recognizing that joint motion has a beneficial effect on ligament healing, immobilization is indicated for only a few days to allow for subsidence of pain and swelling. Furthermore, immobilization contributes to adhesion formation which reduces motion and to the production of disorganized collagen fibers which are biomechanically inferior to collagen found in normal ligament.

Elevation and ice followed by early protected motion with buddy tapes and the use of an appropriate orthosis allow for earlier recovery and return to play.

Nonsteroidal anti-inflammatory medications have been traditionally used extensively in the management of soft tissue injuries but should be used judiciously due to their adverse effect on ligament healing. Similarly, even though corticosteroid injections may reduce the pain and inflammation of acute ligament injuries, they should be avoided due to their potential to limit healing and cause collagen breakdown through the suppression of cytokine production which is required to promote healing.

Complete collateral ligament disruption resulting in joint instability, in many instances, requires surgical treatment, although evidenced by the low incidence of surgical repair documented in the literature, this appears to be very uncommon, possibly due to intact secondary joint stabilizers. Acute repair can be accomplished either directly or more commonly with the use of suture anchors, biotenodesis screws, or more rarely with a pull-out button. Patients with chronic pain and instability may be unable to return to play without surgical management. This relates to difficulty with pinch and grasp and may necessitate surgical reconstruction. Stiffness may also result following a non-treatment or inappropriate treatment for injuries to the PIP joints [25]. In the metacarpophalangeal joint, the injured finger may rotate and scissor beneath an adjacent finger [5].

Multiple surgical options are available including direct repair, direct suture to bone with a pull-out suture, direct repair to bone using suture anchors, interference screws, and ligament reconstruction with a tendon graft [5, 14, 16, 26, 27]. An acute intrasubstance tear may be amenable to direct repair. Pull-out sutures or suture anchors may be used as fixation for ligament avulsions. It may be necessary to remove small avulsed bony fragments from the ligament stump prior to fixation. Alternatively, a large bony fragment might be amenable to fixation with a Kirschner wire or mini screw [5]. Associated dorsal interosseous muscle avulsions from the proximal phalangeal insertion have been reported and should be repaired [13, 15]. Chronic tears may require ligament reconstruction using a donor tendon such as palmaris longus or with a distal slip of the flexor digitorum superficialis tendon for the PIP joint [5, 25, 28]. In situations where the collateral ligament is not robust enough for primary repair, a ligament reconstruction may be required. In some instances, a transarticular Kirschner wire may be used for noncompliant patients or tenuous repairs [5].

Postoperative Rehabilitation

Rehabilitation following repairs of the collateral ligaments of the MP joints vary according to author, but all involve a period of 2–3 weeks of immobilization with a hand-based splint with the MP joints in 30–45° of flexion. At the 2–3-week period, range of motion is begun out of the splint using buddy tapes. Strengthening is generally started at approximately 10 weeks [5, 13, 14, 16].

Following repair of the collateral ligament of the proximal interphalangeal joint, immobilization continues for 2–3 weeks with a finger splint with the PIP and DIP joints in full extension with active range-of-motion exercises with buddy tapes afterward. A night splint may be used up to 12 weeks following surgery.

Outcomes

Overall, patients appear to do well following collateral ligament repair, although there are no published data on outcome specifically in baseball players. Outcomes for collateral ligament repairs and reconstruction have been based on case reports and small case studies.

Acute collateral ligament repairs of the metacarpophalangeal joint tend to do well whereas repairs for chronic injuries have had less reliable results. Kang et al. reported on 12 patients with repairs of the radial collateral ligament of the MP joint using suture anchors. All patients had resolution of pain, return to activities of daily living, and no extensor lag or stress instability. Grips and lateral pinch strength exceeded that of the contralateral hand [14]. Delaere et al. performed collateral ligament repairs of the MP joints with direct suture, barbed wire, and screws for osteochondral avulsion fractures on 12 patients and all were asymptomatic at 2-year follow-up, without residual instability or pain [13]. Riederer et al. performed reconstruction of the radial collateral ligament of the MP joints with tendon grafts in 20 patients. Sixteen patients had excellent or good results with 93% recovery in grip strength and 92% pinch strength; however, 4 patients had poor results including 2 patients with residual marked instability [29]. In the largest reviewed study, Waxweiler et al. evaluated 46 patients with grade 3 injury of the metacarpophalangeal joint collateral ligament either acute or chronic who underwent repair with reinsertion at the base of the proximal phalanx or metacarpal head using a suture anchor. There were excellent outcomes at a meeting of 7 months postoperatively with 88.5% grip strength compared to the contralateral hand and a mean QuickDASH score of 9.56 (with 100 being full disability) [16]. Gaston et al. evaluated 14 patients with index MP joint radial collateral ligament injuries and found a difference in outcome between acute (<4 weeks) and chronic injuries. Four acute grade 1 or 2 injuries were treated nonoperatively and had excellent results with normal range of motion, stable pinch, and resolution of pain. Of the 10 patients with grade 3 injuries, 2 presented early and underwent repair with suture anchors with good results. Eight patients who presented late had fair or poor results, regardless of whether they were treated nonoperatively, with surgical repair or reconstruction [5]. The author suggested that persistent pain and instability with degenerative changes might benefit from fusion of the metacarpophalangeal joint.

Outcomes for repair of the collateral ligaments of the PIP joint are more limited. Lee et al. evaluated outcomes between nonoperative and operative treatment for grade 3 collateral ligament tears with 7 undergoing conservative treatment and 10 undergoing direct repair or repair with suture anchors. Range of motion improved more quickly and patients had less deformity and pain in the operative group; however, there was no lateral instability or significant difference in range of motion in either group [30]. Kato et al. performed PIP collateral ligament repairs using suture anchors in 12 patients and all returned to work or sport within 7 weeks of surgery [31]. No patient had any lateral instability of the PIP joint or pain at final follow-up.

References

1. Rhee PC, Camp CL, D'Angelo J, Desai VS, Shin SS, Sheridan D, Conte S. Epidemiology and impact of hand and wrist injuries in major and minor league baseball. Hand (N Y). 2019; https://doi.org/10.1177/1558944719864450.
2. Rooks MD, Johnston RB 3rd, Ensor CD, McIntosh B, James S. Injury patterns in recreational rock climbers. Am J Sports Med. 1995;23(6):683–5.
3. Rohrbough JT, Mudge MK, Schilling RC. Overuse injuries in the elite rock climber. Med Sci Sports Exerc. 2000;32(8):1369–72.
4. Kinoshita H, Obata S, Nasu D, Kadota K, Matsuo T, Fleisig GS. Finger forces in fastball baseball pitching. Hum Mov Sci. 2017;54:172–81.
5. Gaston RG, Lourie GM, Peljovich AR. Radial collateral ligament injury of the index metacarpophalangeal joint: an underreported but important injury. J Hand Surg Am. 2006;31(6):1355–61.
6. Tamai K, Ryu J, An K, Linscheid RL, Conney WP, Chao EY. Three-dimensional geometric analysis of the metacarpophalangeal joint. J Hand Surg Am. 1988;13(4):521–9.
7. Schultz RJ, Storace A, Krishnamurthy S. Metacarpophalangeal joint motion and the role of the collateral ligaments. Int Orthop. 1987;11:149–55.
8. Wong JC, Lutsky KF, Beredjiklian PK. Outcomes after repair of subacute-to-chronic grade III metacarpophalangeal joint collateral ligament injuries in fingers are suboptimal. Hand (N Y). 2014;9:322–8.
9. Minami A, An K-N, Cooney WP, Linscheid RL, Chao EYS. Ligamentous structures of the metacarpophalangeal joint: a quantitative anatomic study. J Orthop Res. 1984;1(4):361–8.
10. Dy CJ, Tucker SM, Kok PL, Hearns KA, Carlson MG. Anatomy of the radial collateral ligament of the index metacarpophalangeal joint. J Hand Surg Am. 2013;38(1):124–8.
11. Minamikawa Y, Horii E, Amadio PC, Cooney WP, Linscheid RL, An KN. Stability and constraint of the proximal interphalangeal joint. J Hand Surg Am. 1993;18(2):198–204.

12. Rhee RY, Reading G, Wray RC. A biomechanical study of the collateral ligaments of the proximal interphalangeal joint. J Hand Surg Am. 1992;17(1):157–63.
13. Delaere OP, Suttor PM, Degolla R, et al. Early surgical treatment for collateral ligament rupture of metacarpophalangeal joints of the fingers. J Hand Surg Am. 2003;28:309–15.
14. Kang L, Rosen A, Potter HG, Weiland AJ. Rupture of the radial collateral ligament of the index metacarpophalangeal joint: diagnosis and surgical treatment. J Hand Surg Am. 2007;32(6):789–94.
15. Ishizuki M. Injury to collateral ligament of the metacarpophalangeal joint of a finger. J Hand Surg Am. 1988;13(3):444–8.
16. Waxweiler C, Cuylits N, Lumens D, Van Hoonacker P, Drossos K, Lejeune A, Chahidi N. Surgical fixation of metacarpophalangeal collateral ligament rupture of the fingers. Plast Reconstr Surg. 2019;143:1421–8.
17. Prucz RB, Friedrich JB. Finger joint injuries. Clin Sports Med. 2015;34(1):99–116.
18. Carruthers KH, Skie M, Jain M. Jam injuries of the finger: diagnosis and management of injuries to the interphalangeal joints across multiple sports and levels of experience. Sports Health. 2016;8(5):469–78.
19. Matsuo T, Jinji T, Hirayama D, Nasu D, Ozaki H, Kumagawa D. Middle finger and ball movements around ball release during baseball fastball pitching. Sports Biomech. 2018;17(2):180–91.
20. Melville D, Jacobson JA, Haas ES, Brandon C, Brigido MK, Fessell D. Ultrasound of displaced ulnar collateral ligament tears of the thumb: the Stener lesion revisited. Skelet Radiol. 2013;42(5):667–73.
21. Draghi F, Gitto S, Bianchi S. Injuries to the collateral ligaments of the metacarpophalangeal and interphalangeal joints: sonographic appearance. J Ultrasound Med. 2018;37(9):2117–33.
22. Chiavaras MM, Jacobson JA, Yablon CM, Brigido MK, Girish G. Pit-falls in wrist and hand ultrasound. AJR Am J Roentgenol. 2014;203:531–40.
23. Hergan K, Mittler C, Oser W. Ulnar collateral ligament: differentiation of displaced and nondisplaced tears with US and MR imaging. Radiology. 1995;194(1):65–71.
24. Bowers WH. The anatomy of the interphalangeal joints. In: Bowers WH, editor. The hand and upper limb. Vol 1. The interphalangeal joints. Edinburgh: Churchill Livingstone; 1987. p. 2–13.
25. Carlo J, Dell PC, Matthias R, Wright TW. Collateral ligament reconstruction of the proximal interphalangeal joint. J Hand Surg Am. 2016;41(1):129–32.
26. Kato H, Minami A, Takahara M, Oshio I, Hirachi K, Kotaki H. Surgical repair of acute collateral ligament injuries in digits with the Mitek bone suture anchor. J Hand Surg Br. 1999;24(1):70–5.
27. Dy CJ, Tucker SM, Hearns KA, Carlson MG. Comparison of in vitro motion and stability between techniques for index metacarpophalangeal joint radial collateral ligament reconstruction. J Hand Surg Am. 2013;38(7):1324–30.
28. Lee JI, Jeon WJ, Suh DH, Park JH, Lee JM, Park JW. Anatomical collateral ligament reconstruction in the hand using intraosseous suture anchors and a free tendon graft. J Hand Surg Eur. 2012;37(9):832–8.
29. Riederer S, Nagy L, Büchler U. Chronic post-traumatic radial instability of the metacarpophalangeal joint of the finger: long-term results of ligament reconstruction. J Hand Surg Br. 1998;23:503–6.
30. Lee SJ, Lee JH, Hwang IC, Kim JK, Lee JI. Clinical outcomes of operative repair of complete rupture of the proximal interphalangeal joint collateral ligament: comparison with non-operative treatment. Acta Orthop Traumatol Turc. 2017;51(1):44–8.
31. Kato N, Nemoto K, Nakajima H, Motosuneya T, Fujikawa K. Primary repair of the collateral ligament of the proximal interphalangeal joint using a suture anchor. Scand J Plast Reconstr Surg Hand Surg. 2003;37(2):117–20.

Triangular Fibrocartilage Complex Injury

12

Keith G. Whitlock and David S. Ruch

Define the Specific Injury Your Chapter Will Address

The triangular fibrocartilage complex (TFCC) is a collection of ligamentous and fibrocartilaginous structures at the ulnar wrist which suspends the ulnar carpus, cushions load transmission across the ulnocarpal joint, and acts as the primary stabilizer of the distal radioulnar joint (DRUJ) [1]. The components of the TFCC are susceptible to injury in nearly all sports. From excessive impact and load bearing in gymnastics and martial arts, to chronic overuse and repetitive loading in racquet and throwing sports, the TFCC is a common source of ulnar-sided wrist pain in athletes. Regardless of the cause of injury as acute or chronic, the principles of management of the recreational and elite baseball player are often different than the general population. It is essential that the treating physician seek to understand the competitive level of the athlete and their intrinsic and extrinsic motivations for performance in order to tailor a unique treatment plan that balances adequate healing, return to sport, and long-term well-being [2–4]. The goal of this chapter will be to describe the relevant anatomy and functional implications of TFCC injuries and summarize evidence-based strategies for diagnosis, treatment, and rehabilitation of the competitive baseball player.

K. G. Whitlock (✉) · D. S. Ruch
Department of Orthopaedic Surgery, Duke University Medical Center, Durham, NC, USA
e-mail: keith.whitlock@duke.edu; d.ruch@duke.edu

Incidence and Uniqueness to Baseball

Injuries to the TFCC are a common cause of ulnar-sided wrist pain in athletes, and often present with significant disability resulting in time away from competition. Athletes from a wide range of sports are susceptible to these injuries including gymnastics, martial arts, wrestling, American football, rugby, hockey, basketball, golf, tennis, and baseball [3, 5–8]. Although the general incidence of TFCC injuries in sports is not well defined, the epidemiology of sports-related injuries to the hand and wrist has been estimated between 3% and 25% of all sports-related injuries [4, 9].

In a 10-year study of athletes at the Olympic training center in Colorado Springs, Rettig and colleagues found that 8.7% of the 8311 documented injuries suffered across 36 sports involved the hand or wrist. Incidence varied by sport, with roller hockey accounting for 30%, baseball 25%, boxing 17%, basketball 17%, and volleyball 13%. By their review of the literature in 1998, they determined that between 3% and 9% of all athletic injuries involve the hand or wrist [4].

G. M. Lourie (ed.), *Hand and Wrist Injuries in Baseball*,
https://doi.org/10.1007/978-3-030-81659-9_12

A recent study published by Fares and colleagues in 2020 reviewed the epidemiology of upper extremity injuries in major league baseball during the 2010 to 2016 seasons. They found that 49% (1609) of all documented injuries involved the upper extremity, with 7% of upper extremity cases involving the wrist. Injuries to the shoulder and elbow were most common, representing 35% and 31% of upper extremity injuries, respectively. Interestingly, injuries of the wrist were more commonly seen in fielders (5.6%) than pitchers (0.6%) and catchers (0.7%). Additionally, just 4.5% of wrist injuries underwent surgical intervention during the time period, compared to 11% of shoulder and 32% of elbow injuries [10].

While pain-free function of the ulnar side of the wrist is important to nearly all athletes, the unique physical demands required for high-level performance in baseball depend heavily on the function of the TFCC, namely, the dynamic pronosupination and power grip necessary for throwing and swinging place repetitive loads across the structures of the TFCC [11]. The baseball swing itself creates force across the ulnocarpal joint greater than that seen in diagnostic pronated grip radiographs which increase the longitudinal relationship of the ulna relative to the radius and the load transmitted across the TFCC [12, 13]. As a result, it is not uncommon to encounter acute or chronic tears in baseball players who have neutral or even negative ulnar variance.

Pertinent Anatomy and Classification

Components of the TFCC

Much of our understanding of the anatomy of the TFCC was originally defined by Palmer and colleagues beginning in the early 1980s [1, 14, 15]. The DRUJ is an inherently unstable joint with a shallow radius of curvature, which places a great amount of importance on the surrounding soft tissues. This collection of structures which make up the triangular fibrocartilage complex include the articular disk, volar and dorsal radioulnar ligaments, meniscal homologue, ECU tendon sheath, ulnar capsule, and volar ulnocarpal ligaments [16] (Fig. 12.1). The articular disk is a thin, poorly vascularized, fibrocartilaginous sheet that originates from the distal sigmoid notch of the radius and extends ulnarly, blending at its margins with the thickened, horizontally oriented fibers of the dorsal and palmar radioulnar ligaments. These stout ligaments are each composed of deep and superficial portions, which have distinct insertions and functional implications. The superficial or distal fibers insert into the ulnar styloid, ECU sheath, and ulnar capsule. The variably shaped structure known as the meniscal homologue represents the ulnar extent of these superficial fibers and contains a central opening known as the prestyloid recess which can easily be mistaken for a tear on MRI and arthroscopy. The deep fibers of the radioulnar ligaments insert deep at the ulnar fovea rather than the styloid and have been referred to as the ligamentum subcruentum [17]. These thick, stout fibers play a greater role in the stability of the DRUJ, and failure to recognize and appropriately address their avulsion is a common source of persistent DRUJ instability following attempted TFCC repair [18, 19].

The ECU sheath is a longitudinally oriented, dorsal structure which originates from the dorsal triquetrum and inserts at the base of the ulnar styloid via the dorsal radioulnar ligament [20]. It is one of the most commonly injured structures in association with tears of the articular disk, and its repair is an essential component of successful surgical treatment [21]. The sheath itself is very thick in comparison to the ulnar joint capsule with which it blends, and it is routinely used as a target for suturing the superficial fibers of the articular disk back to during repairs of ulnar-sided tears. Volarly, the superficial fibers of the radioulnar ligaments blend into the longitudinally oriented ulnotriquetral (UT) and ulnolunate (UL) ligaments, which run from their broad origin at the palmar radioulnar ligament and radial aspect of the base of the ulnar styloid, to their insertions at the volar carpus. These ligaments are difficult to differentiate arthroscopically.

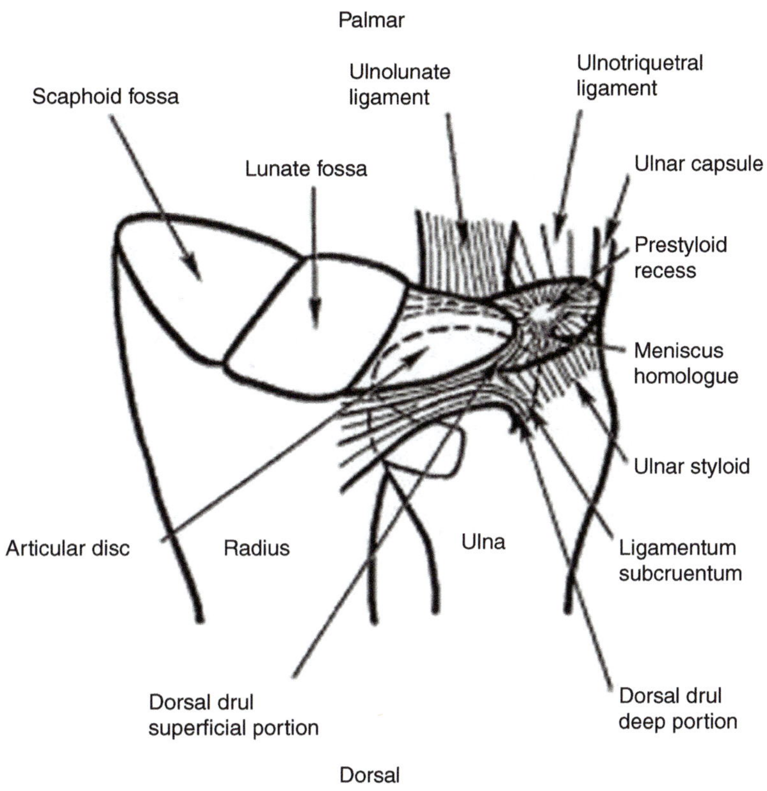

Fig. 12.1 The components of the TFCC. (With permission. From: Ishii et al. [16])

Blood Supply and Innervation

The primary arterial supply of the TFCC is provided by the ulnar artery via its dorsal and palmar radiocarpal branches, with additional blood flow provided by the dorsal and palmar branches of the anterior interosseous artery [22]. Clinically, it is essential to understand the uneven distribution of this blood flow throughout the TFCC. Much like the menisci of the knee, studies of the microvasculature of the TFCC have helped us to understand which portions are amenable to healing following repair. Through their classic India ink cadaver studies, Bednar and colleagues demonstrated that only the peripheral 10–40% of the articular disk is penetrated by vasculature from the peripheral capsule and synovium in a radial fashion [23]. Additionally, they found that no vessels entered the radial portion of the disk from its subchondral attachment to the sigmoid notch (Fig. 12.2). As a result, the central and radial portions of the articular disk are avascular with limited healing potential, while the peripheral portions are well vascularized and amenable to surgical repair.

Functional Implications of the Anatomy

In neutral rotation, the ulnar bears 18–20% of the axial load transmitted across the wrist [14]. Lengthening the ulna by 2.5 mm increases its proportion of total axial load from 18.4% to 41.9%, while shortening by 2.5 mm decreases its proportion to just 4.3% [24]. The concept of ulnar variance describes the longitudinal relationship of the ulnar head relative to the articular surface of the distal radius. During maximal grip, ulnar variance has been demonstrated to increase an average of 1.95 mm, while maximal grip and pronation cause an average increase of 2.5 mm [25, 26]. Ulnar deviation also serves to increase this force. When considering the role of the TFCC as

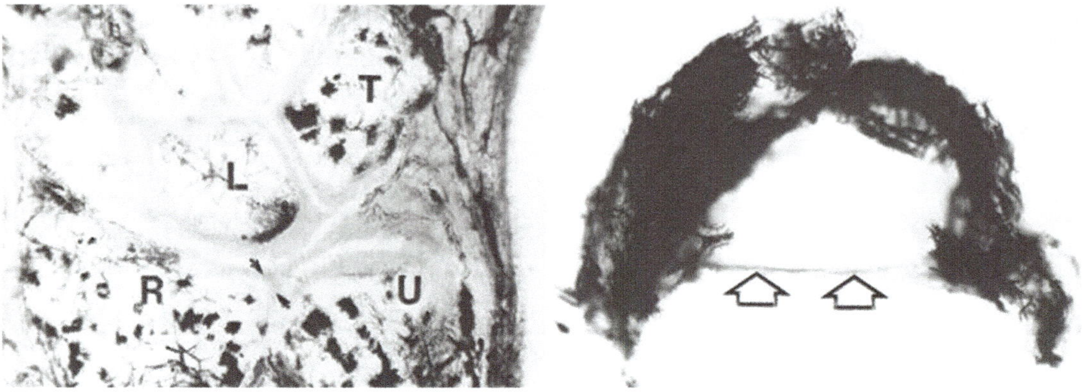

Fig. 12.2 Vascular anatomy of the TFCC. Left: coronal section of the wrist. Vessels from the soft tissues of the joint capsule and synovium can be seen penetrating the triangular fibrocartilage complex. Note that no vessels penetrate the TFCC from its radial attachment (arrows). Right: axial view of en bloc specimen of the TFCC after vascular perfusion and tissue clearing. The inner (horizontal) portion of the TFCC is devoid of vessels. In addition, no vessels could be seen entering the TFCC from its radial attachment (arrows). (With permission. From: Bednar et al. [23])

a shock absorber between the carpus and distal ulna, it is important to understand that ulnar variance is inversely proportionate to the thickness of the TFCC [27]. In other words, the articular disk is thicker and more robust in ulnar negative than in ulnar positive wrists. With this is mind, it is intuitive that repetitive loading across a thinner, less robust TFCC in ulnar positive patients is likely to increase the incidence of articular disk perforation seen in these patients [13]. Maximal grip, pronation, and ulnar deviation are all necessary to the successful execution of the baseball swing. These repetitive motions, as well as the occasional acute pronated axial load created by sliding headfirst or decelerating into the outfield wall, place baseball players at risk for acute and chronic tears of the TFCC.

As previously stated, the TFCC also functions as the primary stabilizer of the DRUJ. Biomechanical studies by Adams and colleagues have shown that the central portion of the articular disk does not significantly contribute to DRUJ stability. They used cadaver models to demonstrate that as long as the peripheral 2 mm of the articular disk is left intact, up to 2/3^{rds} of the total area can be excised without affecting the structural integrity of the TFCC [28]. It is for this reason that central tears of the articular disk can be surgically debrided without creating instability. Conversely, the thickened volar and dorsal radioulnar ligaments are essential to DRUJ stability throughout the range of pronation and supination. Historically, there has been conflicting evidence as to whether the volar or dorsal radioulnar ligaments provide stability in pronation or supination, respectively. The source of this confusion is likely due to the fact that the deep and superficial fibers of the radioulnar ligaments differentially tighten at different positions of the wrist [17]. For the purposes of this discussion, it is most important to understand that the deep fibers of the ligamentum subcruentum, which insert at the ulnar fovea, play the primary role in maintaining DRUJ stability [18].

Classification Systems

In 1989, Palmer classified injuries to the TFCC based their location and etiology as acute type 1 or chronic type 2 tears [15] (Fig. 12.3). This classification is particularly useful for its ability to guide treatment decisions. Type 1A tears involve perforation of the central, avascular portion of the articular disk, and are thus amenable to simple debridement. Type 1B tears represent peripheral avulsion of the ulnar fibers of the articular disk from their insertions at the ulnar styloid and

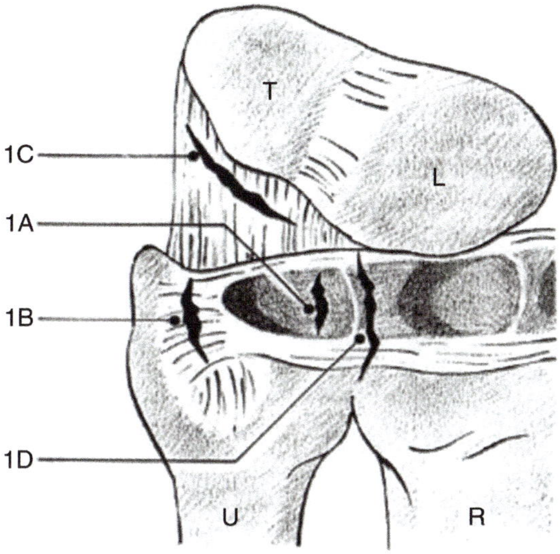

Fig. 12.3 Palmer classification of acute tears by anatomic location. (With permission. From: Böhringer et al. [92])

fovea, and a variety of techniques for their repair have been described [29]. Type 1C tears involve distal avulsions through the ulnocarpal ligaments and include the recently described longitudinal split tear of the ulnotriquetral ligament which has been shown to benefit from repair [20]. Radial-sided type 1D avulsions are generally debrided for their poor vascularity, though some authors advocate transosseous repair, especially in the presence of a radial avulsion fracture. Chronic type 2 tears represent the natural progression of ulnocarpal impaction syndrome from TFCC wear and perforation to involvement of the lunotriquetral ligament and eventual ulnocarpal arthritis. Not all tears of the TFCC fit neatly into this classification, as there is a high incidence of combined lesions and associated injuries reported throughout the literature including partial/complete rupture of the lunotriquetral, scapholunate, and radiocarpal ligaments, as well as fractures of the distal radius and ulnar styloid [19, 30, 31].

More recently, Atzei and colleagues created a new classification which subdivides Palmer's classic 1B tear into six classes [18]. The authors liken the structure of the TFCC to that of an iceberg, with the superficial fibers of the radioulnar ligaments representing the minor, visible portion, while the deep fibers inserting at the ulnar fovea make up the bulk of the structure and provide the majority of DRUJ stability. Failure to recognize injury to these deep, foveal fibers has been cited as a common cause of persistent DRUJ instability following traditional capsular repairs of the peripheral TFCC [19]. Atzei's class zero injury involves an isolated ulnar styloid fracture without TFCC tear and is managed conservatively. Class 1 tears involve only the superficial radioulnar ligament fibers, with or without an associated ulnar styloid fracture. Stability of the DRUJ is maintained, and they advocate treatment with traditional capsular repair. Class 2 and 3 tears both involve injury to the deep fibers and require foveal repair to restore DRUJ stability. Class 4 injuries represent unrepairable tears requiring tendon graft reconstruction of the DRUJ ligaments, and class 5 denotes progression to DRUJ arthritis.

Finally, Melone and colleagues studied their series of 42 cases of open, ulnar-sided repairs performed mostly on athletes, to create their own classification of the pathoanatomy of peripheral TFCC tears [21]. They discovered a consistent pattern of injury beginning with peripheral detachment of the articular disk as the initial insult, followed by extension of the traumatic force to the adjacent ECU sheath, distally to the ulnocarpal ligaments and ultimately the lunotriquetral ligament and midcarpal joint (Fig. 12.4). Each subsequent stage of injury results from greater traumatic force, and each contributes to a spectrum of worsening instability. While all of their cases began with peripheral avulsions, only 33% were classified as isolated tears of the articular disk. This demonstrates the prevalence of injury to surrounding structures, and the importance of recognizing these injuries in order to adequately address posttraumatic instability.

Mechanism of Injury

Acute tears of the TFCC most commonly result from moments of forced wrist extension and axial loading, which can commonly occur during headfirst slides, diving for an outfield catch, or jamming oneself on inside pitch [12]. As previ-

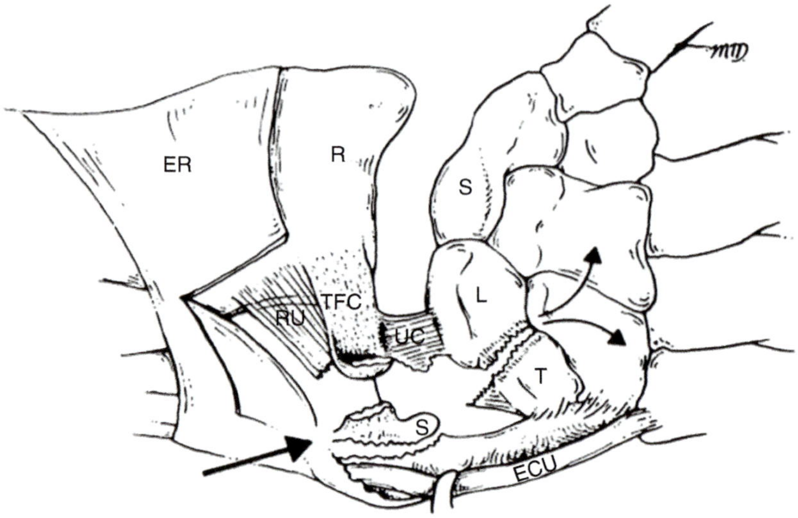

Fig. 12.4 The pathoanatomy of posttraumatic TFCC disruption comprised a spectrum of injury that has been categorized into five stages of increasing severity. The hallmark of stage I, and the common feature of all injuries, was peripheral detachment of the articular disk (TFC) from the ulnar styloid (S). Stage II additionally involved the ECU subsheath. Stage III involved the UC ligaments; stage IV the LT interosseous ligament; and stage V, the triquetral-capitate and triquetral-hamate ligaments. The consistent spectrum noted in this series of cases suggests a continuum of injury beginning at the ulnar styloid and, owing to increasing magnitude of force, extending to the midcarpal joint. (With permission. From: Melone and Nathan [21])

ously mentioned, the combination of grip, ulnar deviation, and forceful pronation required for the baseball swing can also result in acute or chronic tears of the TFCC [11]. During pronation and grip, the head of the ulna is driven both dorsally and distally, creating dynamic ulnar positive variance. This causes compression across the relatively thinner dorsal fibers of the articular disk between the ulna and lunate, leading to both acute perforations as well as dynamic ulnar impaction which can progress to Palmer type 2 degenerative change.

History and Differential Diagnosis

Ulnar-sided wrist pain is commonly referred to as the "black box" of the wrist because of the high concentration of complex structures within this small space which can make definitive diagnosis difficult. When treating a baseball player with ulnar-sided wrist pain whom you suspect may have a tear of the TFCC, it is essential to elicit a thorough history beginning with the timing of onset, mechanism of injury, location of their pain, and positions of the wrist which exacerbate their symptoms. Patients will most frequently complain of ulnar-sided wrist pain, exacerbated by activity with or without a click during forearm rotation. Their pain may also be associated with feelings of instability and weakness of grip affecting both the throw and swing [11]. Players presenting with acute tears may be able to pinpoint the onset of injury after a fall or a single painful swing. They are less likely to recall a specific injury mechanism in the case of chronic tears caused by ulnocarpal impaction, and instead will often complain of the insidious onset of progressive, ulnar-sided pain with loss of grip strength and wrist motion [32].

The differential diagnosis for suspected TFCC tears is broad and includes the plethora of injuries that may occur at the ulnar side of the wrist (Table 12.1) For this reason, a thorough physical exam, focused on ruling out potential distracting or associated injuries is essential to successful diagnosis and treatment.

Table 12.1 Differential diagnosis and associated injuries

ECU tendinosis and subluxation
DRUJ instability
DRUJ osteoarthritis
Ulnar styloid and distal radius fractures
Hook of hamate fracture
Ulnocarpal and radioulnar ligament injury
Ulnocarpal impaction/abutment
Ulnocarpal instability
Lunotriquetral instability
Pisotriquetral osteoarthritis

Directed Physical Exam

Physical exam begins with inspection of the painful and contralateral wrist for swelling and deformity. The piano key sign represents excessive dorsal prominence of the distal ulna in relation to the radius and carpus, and can be an indication of instability. Grip strength as well as range of motion of the wrist in all planes should be assessed and documented in comparison to the contralateral side to assess the effectiveness of conservative and surgical treatment. Lunotriquetral and midcarpal instability should also be assessed for, as their presence can have significant treatment implications [32].

The exam can then be focused by asking the patient to their area of maximal tenderness which is most often localized to the ulnar fovea between the ECU and FCU tendons just distal to the ulnar styloid. Recreation of their pain with deep palpation to this area is known as the fovea sign which is the most reliable exam maneuver for the detection of TFCC tears with sensitivity and specificity reported at 95% and 87% compared to arthroscopy as the gold standard [33]. Another commonly performed provocative maneuver has been described by several names throughout the literature including the ulnocarpal stress test [34], ulnar impaction test [35], and TFCC grind test [36]. It is performed by positioning the patient with the elbow at 90° and the wrist in maximal ulnar deviation in order to axially load the TFCC. The wrist is then passively rotated to the limits of pronation and supination, with recreation of pain as a positive result. Although sensitivity for this test has been reported as high as 90%, it can often elicit pain in the presence of any number of ulnar-sided wrist conditions, resulting in a comparatively low specificity [36].

An additional provocative maneuver known as the press test is performed by asking a seated patient to lift himself/herself out of a chair, bearing full weight through their extended wrists. A positive result recreates their ulnar-sided pain and has been reported to be 100% sensitive for the diagnosis of TFCC tears [37]. The ECU tendon should also be assessed for tendinosis and instability, which can be elicited with the wrist in full supination and extension while asking the patient to abduct their small finger against resistance. The lunotriquetral shuck test should also be performed to assess for ligamentous instability.

Finally, evaluation of DRUJ stability is an essential portion of the physical exam, as instability indicates likely avulsion of the deep fibers of the ligamentum subcruentum [18]. This is performed by placing the patient in a seated position facing the examiner, with their elbow on a flat surface flexed to 90° and the fingers extended. The distal ulna is stabilized while the radius is translated volarly/dorsally with the wrist in neutral, pronation, and supination. Excessive translation compared to the contralateral side indicates instability. This test should routinely be performed before surgery while the patient is anesthetized as the muscular stabilizers of the wrist can often be misleading during examination of the awake patient.

Imaging Including Advanced Methods

Radiographs

Imaging evaluation begins with standard PA/lateral and oblique radiographs in comparison to the contralateral wrist. These plain films allow for the assessment of multiple bony abnormalities including ulnar styloid fracture which can suggest an acute TFCC tear, associated radial avulsion fractures, and DRUJ congruity [11]. Ulnar

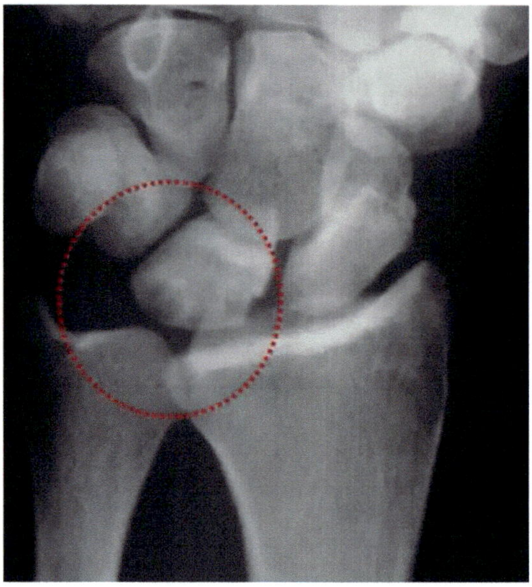

Fig. 12.5 Radiograph demonstrating degenerative change of the proximal ulnar corner of the lunate in the setting of ulnar positive variance indicative of chronic ulnar impaction syndrome

variance is assessed on PA radiograph by positioning the forearm in neutral pronosupination, 90° of shoulder abduction, and 90° of elbow flexion. The longitudinal distance is measured between parallel lines drawn tangential to the articular surfaces of the ulnar head and the lunate fossa of the radius to determine the patient's neutral variance [35, 38]. Pronated grip views should also be obtained to determine the degree of dynamic ulnar positive variance which has been demonstrated as 2.5 mm on average [26]. The proximal ulnar corner of the lunate should also be assessed for subchondral sclerosis and cystic change suggestive of chronic ulnocarpal abutment (Fig. 12.5). Additionally, the presence of a prominent ulnar styloid should be noted, as an arthroscopic wafer resection will be unable to address degenerative symptoms driven by ulnar styloid-carpal impaction.

Magnetic Resonance Imaging

The use of MRI with or without gadolinium arthrography has supplanted X-ray arthrography as the gold standard of advanced imaging for assessment of the TFCC. Numerous studies have reported on the diagnostic accuracy of MRI, with high variability across the literature due to differences in magnetic field strength, use of a dedicated wrist coil, contrast usage, and enhancement techniques. In a 2008 study by Anderson and colleagues, 3-Tesla MRI demonstrated sensitivity, specificity, and accuracy of 94%, 88%, and 91%, respectively, compared to just 85%, 75%, and 83% for 1.5Tesla scans [39]. Faber et al. pooled data from 22 publications and found the average sensitivity and specificity of high-resolution 3T MRI to be 86.1% and 82.1%, with positive and negative predictive values of 85.4% and 82.8%, respectively [40]. Magnetic resonance arthrography (MRA) achieved sensitivity, specificity, negative, and positive predictive values of 81.7%, 87.1%, 86.6%, and 82.4%, respectively. The role of gadolinium remains controversial; however, multiple studies have reported greater diagnostic accuracy of MRA compared to conventional MRI [41–43].

When considering the diagnostic yield of MRI and MRA, it is important to understand that the accuracy of advanced imaging varies with location of the tear [36]. Specifically, both conventional MRI and MRA demonstrate greater accuracy in diagnosing central compared to peripheral tears because of the focal synovitis and granulation tissue which develops over peripheral tears and can make signal interpretation difficult [3, 7, 44–46].

The experience level of the interpreting radiologist has also been shown to affect the accuracy of advanced imaging for diagnosis of TFCC tears. A study by Blazar and colleagues in 2001 compared the interpretations of preoperative MRI scans by attending versus fellow level radiologists and found differences in sensitivity of 86% versus 80%, specificity of 96% versus 80%, and accuracy of 83% versus 61% [44]. These significant differences based on observer experience underscore the limitations and difficulty of interpretation of advanced imaging methods for the diagnosis of TFCC tears. Additionally, MRI studies of asymptomatic patients have demonstrated abnormal TFCC signal in 27–33% of subjects under the age of 50 years old [47, 48]. While the diagnostic utility of advanced imaging continues to improve, diagnostic arthroscopy remains the gold standard. Arthroscopy allows for the assessment of tear size and mechanical stability, with the added benefit of facilitating treatment at the time of diagnosis, and should be considered early in the treatment of elite athletes to avoid delays and errors in diagnosis [11, 29, 49].

Conservative Treatment

In the general population, initial treatment of TFCC tears typically begins with a period of immobilization, activity modification, NSAIDs, and possible corticosteroid injection, with most authors advocating 4–6 months of conservative care before consideration of surgical intervention. However, when treating the competitive baseball player, modifications should be made which focus on early diagnosis and minimizing the time away from competition [8]. For athletes in the midst of a competitive season, activity modification can initially be attempted without complete cessation of game play. Bracing between events and taping during games/workouts may be sufficient. If these measures fail, activity modification to avoid provocative maneuvers, and if necessary, a period of rest and immobilization can be attempted with or without corticosteroid injection [32]. In the absence of DRUJ instability, Baratz and colleagues recommend wrist immobilization in a short arm splint for 5–7 days followed by re-evaluation [12]. However, an unstable DRUJ represents a serious threat to a player's career and should warrant early consideration of arthroscopy in most cases.

Although not specifically studied in athletes, the natural history of nonoperatively treated TFCC tears has been reported by multiple authors. Lee et al. reviewed 72 patients with TFCC tears without DRUJ instability diagnosed by clinical exam and advanced imaging who underwent 4–12 weeks of immobilization in a short arm wrist splint. Complete recovery was reported in 30% of patients at 6-month follow-up and 50% of patients at 1 year [50]. In 2010, Park and Yao reviewed 84 patients with clinical evidence of a TFCC tear who initially underwent 4 weeks of immobilization in a short arm cast or volar wrist splint. In their study, 57% of patients experienced complete symptom resolution after immobilization, while 43% went on to MRI and operative arthroscopy. Interestingly, the use of a volar resting splint versus a short arm cast did not affect the likelihood of progression to surgery [51].

When considering the optimal treatment strategy for the competitive baseball player, it is essential to gain an understanding of their short- and long-term goals, the functional demands of their position, and the timing of their injury in the context of their season. For the casual junior baseball player with a suspected TFCC tear, it is reasonable to attempt 4 or more weeks of rest, immobilization, and NSAIDs as a first line. However, if scholarship potential or professional earnings are at stake, early diagnosis and intervention with arthroscopy should be pursued to avoid prolonged time on the disabled list [4, 11]. If the injury occurs during the playoffs or a similarly critical period of the season, the athlete can be allowed to play through their injury if there is no DRUJ instability and their level of pain and function allows. Corticosteroid injection may be particularly useful in these cases. In such circumstances, players should be counseled that they are unlikely to cause additional damage or injury by playing in the short term, and shared decision-making should be undertaken between the player, physician, and coaching staff to determine if operative intervention should be delayed until the conclusion of the season [12].

Surgical Treatment

A multitude of surgical procedures have been described to address injuries of the TFCC. Most athletes can expect a successful outcome and return to sport, as long as the choice of surgery is guided by an understanding of the location of the tear, its etiology as acute or chronic, and the presence of any associated injuries. Arthroscopic techniques have largely supplanted open surgery in the debridement and repair of acute tears due to the reduced surgical site morbidity and potential for quicker return to function [8, 31, 52]. Although few studies have focused specifically on surgical outcomes in athletes, the wealth of outcomes data reported on the general population can be extrapolated to guide treatment of the competitive baseball player. For the purposes of this section, we will divide our discussion in terms of the aforementioned Palmer classification which has become the most widely utilized throughout the literature [15].

Type 1A

Acute, central tears of the articular disk which do not respond to conservative measures are treated with arthroscopic debridement due to their avascularity which precludes repair [23]. Arthroscopic debridement is performed through a standard arthroscopy set up with an arthroscope placed in the 3–4 portal, and a 2.0–3.0 mm shaver, biter, or other ablative device inserted through the 6-R portal [7, 29, 49]. The tear is then debrided back to stable margins, with removal of any unstable flaps which can become caught between the ulna and carpus during forearm rotation and cause mechanical irritation. It is often necessary to switch the arthroscope to the 6-R and shaver to the 3–4 portal to complete debridement of the most ulnar portion of the tear. Care must be taken to leave at least a 2 mm rim of articular disk without debriding the dorsal and volar radioulnar ligaments in order to preserve DRUJ stability [28]. Difficult-to-visualize central tears can be exposed by applying external compression to the DRUJ, causing the tear to gap open, occasionally allowing for DRUJ synovium to herniate distally through the tear [49].

Numerous studies have demonstrated relief of pain and patient satisfaction following debridement of acute, central tears [29, 49, 52–55]. In 1994, Bednar et al. reported good to excellent results in 90% of patients after debridement [52]. Their results are similar to those reported by Arsalan and colleagues in 2018 who found improved symptoms in 41/44 patients, with 93% of patients stating that they would undergo the same procedure again [55]. Despite these positive results, it is important to recognize the subsets of patients for whom simple debridement is not appropriate. Minami et al. reviewed 16 patients with either acute traumatic or degenerative central tears and found significantly poorer outcomes in the degenerative cohort – especially in those with ulnar positive variance, lunate chondromalacia, and/or LT ligament tears [53]. A recent study by Roh et al. found that the presence of a degenerative tear conferred an odds ratio of 3.4 for a dissatisfactory outcome following simple debridement [54]. Patients with ulnar positive variance were also at increased risk for a poor outcome in their study, though other authors have not shared this finding [55]. In general, athletes with central tears an no evidence of degenerative ulnar impaction can expect good to excellent results with arthroscopic debridement alone. Patients with ulnar positive variance should be counseled on the possibility of future surgery for ulnar shortening if their pain persists, but should be offered the option of acute debridement to speed return to play [29].

Type 1B

Peripheral, ulnar-sided tears of the TFCC represent a spectrum of injury which requires a careful assessment of the affected structures in order to select the appropriate surgical treatment. Superficial capsular tears should first be differentiated from foveal avulsions which are more likely to cause DRUJ instability [18]. This can be difficult to determine with advanced imaging, and thus several arthroscopic techniques have been described to aid in diagnosis. First is the trampoline test which is performed by inserting a probe through the 6-R or 4–5 portal and applying distal to proximal pressure to the articular disk in order to assess its resilience. A soft and compliant central disk typically indicates the presence of a peripheral tear [18, 56]. The foveal insertion of the deep radioulnar ligaments is further assessed by the hook test which is performed by inserting a probe into the site of the tear. If the examiner is able to displace the peripheral TFCC toward the center of the joint, the test is considered positive [30, 57]. The hook test was validated in a cadaver model by Trehan et al. who found 90% sensitivity and specificity for the diagnosis of foveal detachment [58]. Thus, a positive trampoline test with a negative hook test is indicative of a superficial capsular tear, while positive findings for both tests indicate the presence of a complete tear with foveal injury. Once this distinction is made, the surgeon can then decide from the multiple techniques described for repair.

For superficial ulnar-sided tears, the authors prefer the arthroscopic outside-in technique as described by Whipple [49] and Trumble [59]. This technique is performed with the wrist in a standard arthroscopy tower, distracted by 12-15lbs of traction. The radiocarpal joint is distended with 7 cc of sterile saline and a 2.7 mm 30° arthroscope is inserted through the 3,4 portal. After diagnostic arthroscopy is performed with pump irrigation, a shaver is introduced into the 6R portal for debridement of the inflamed synovium overlying the peripheral tear and dorsal wrist capsule. A standard meniscal repair kit is then opened, and a curved needle is inserted percutaneously, just dorsal to the ECU tendon, across the peripheral edge of the TFCC from proximal to distal. A second straight needle is then inserted distal to the TFCC. A 2–0 PDS suture is fed through this cannulated straight needle into the radiocarpal joint and passed through a wire loop inserted into the first curved needle under arthroscopic visualization. The PDS suture is then withdrawn through the curved needle creating a horizontal mattress stich across the tear with both limbs present on the ulnar side of the wrist (Fig. 12.6). This process is repeated up to three times depending on the size of the tear, and the sutures are tensioned to ensure satisfactory reduction of the TFCC. A longitudinal incision is then made over the dorsal ulnar wrist, in-line with the sutures, and blunt dissection is carried down to the dorsal capsule, with particular care paid to identification and protection of the dorsal sensory branch of the ulnar nerve. The sutures are then tied over the dorso-ulnar capsule, the incisions are closed, and a well-padded long arm splint is applied with the forearm in 45° of supination. PDS suture is used because it begins to resorb within weeks of surgery, thus limiting mechanical irritation of the subcutaneous suture knots when the athlete returns to play [60].

The inside-out technique has also been described for the repair of superficial ulnar-sided tears [7, 61]. Rather than a meniscal repair set, it utilizes a single Tuohy needle inserted into the 3,4 portal with an arthroscope placed in the 6-R portal for direct visualization. PDS suture is fed through the cannulated Tuohy needle which is passed twice through the tear and out the ulnar side of the wrist in order to create a horizontal mattress stich which is then tied over the ulnar capsule in a similar fashion to the outside-in technique.

Finally, the all-inside technique was developed and popularized by Yao and colleagues as a way to improve repair strength and avoid the potential disadvantages of the outside-in and inside-out techniques including subcutaneous suture knots and iatrogenic nerve injury [62, 63]. The technique utilizes a FasT-Fix pre-tied suture device analogous to those used for all-inside meniscal repairs. The device is inserted into the standard 3,4 portal and pierced through the articular disk 2 mm radial to the tear. Two -L-lactic acid blocks are deposited outside the ulnar capsule, and the pre-tied PDS suture is tightened creating a vertical mattress repair (Fig. 12.7). The safety and strength of this technique were validated in a cadaver model which demonstrated a higher average load to failure and equal safety profile of the FasT-Fix device compared to PDS suture needle techniques [64].

All three techniques have shown clinical success, with no single method demonstrating clear superiority. In 2007, Estrella et al. reviewed 35 patients with peripheral tears repaired by outside-in or inside-out techniques and found 74% of patients reported good or excellent outcomes with significant reduction in pain. Of the 26% of patients who reported an unsatisfactory result, 45% demonstrated persistent DRUJ instability postoperatively [19]. Corso et al. exclusively utilized the outside-in technique and reported 91% good or excellent results in 45 patients [31]. In

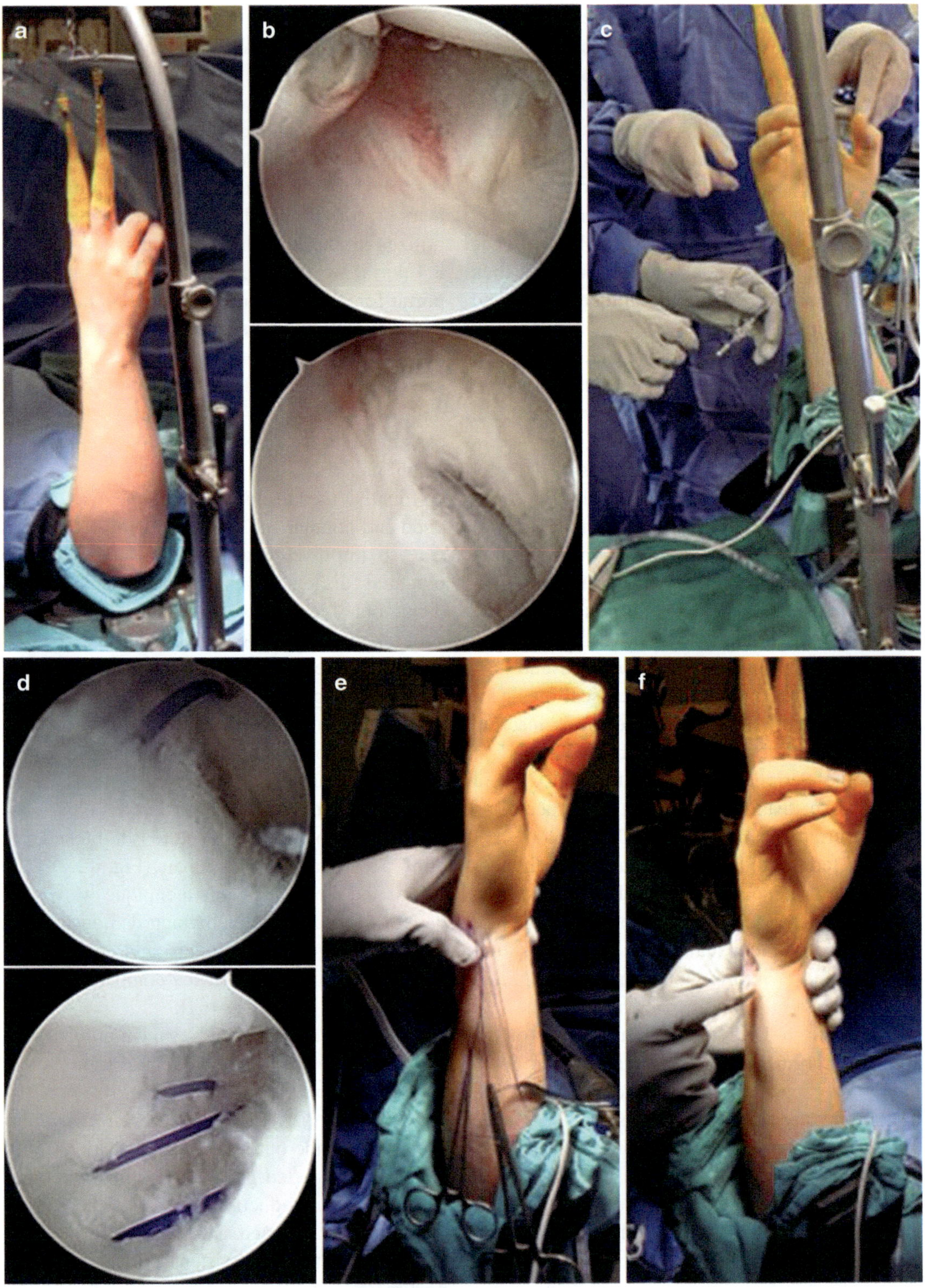
a
b
c
d
e
f

2012, Wysocki et al. reviewed a cohort of 25 patients with superficial, peripheral tears, 11 of whom were high-level competitive athletes. Patients with DRUJ instability were excluded. They found 96% excellent or good results, with 88% of patients reporting that they would undergo the same surgery again. Interestingly, 7 of the 11 elite athletes were able to return to sport at their previous level of play, with 2 gymnasts, 1 volleyball player, and 1 martial artist citing persistent pain with activity for their inability to return [60]. In 2009, McAdams et al. reported on a cohort of 16 high school, NCAA, or professional athletes undergoing repair of a heterogeneous collection of peripheral-sided tears with several associated injuries. They found statistically significant improvements in mean mini-DASH sports module scores and an average return to play of 3.3 months, concluding that arthroscopic repair is successful in treating athletes who require high-level wrist function [7]. The all-inside method has been similarly successful, with studies reporting 83–93% good and excellent results at short to midterm follow-up [57, 63].

Multiple patient factors have been implicated in the success and failure of arthroscopic repair. Among these factors, the role of ulnar positive variance is often over-emphasized as a risk factor for negative outcome [65]. A 2005 case series of 35 patients by Ruch et al. was the first to demonstrate advanced age as an independent risk factor for negative outcome following arthroscopic repair, with patients >50 years old reporting only good or poor results by DASH score [66]. Although this series also demonstrated ulnar positive variance to be associated with worse outcomes compared to ulnar negative variance, this variable should not be viewed in isolation. Equally important factors to consider include the chronicity of the tear, presence of associated DRUJ instability, weight bearing requirements of the wrist, and evidence of ulnar impaction or any other degenerative conditions. In a 2010 follow-up study, Ruch and colleagues compared the results of arthroscopic repair to ulnar shortening osteotomy (USO) in patients with peripheral 1B tears and associated ulnar positive variance. There were no differences in postoperative wrist ROM, DASH, or pain scores between arthroscopic repair and USO, and both groups improved significantly compared to their preoperative baseline [67]. It is critical to understand that this study excluded patients with degenerative tears, as inclusion of these patients in studies reporting on the outcomes of arthroscopic repair alone have demonstrated rates of revision surgery up to 57% [68]. As a result, even in the presence of ulnar positive variance, it is acceptable to attempt arthroscopic repair of acute, traumatic, peripheral ulnar-sided tears in young competitive baseball players without associated DRUJ instability or degenerative changes. Although a subset of these patients may experience persistent ulnar-sided wrist pain following repair [69], they can still benefit from an ulnar shortening procedure in the future [70].

Two additional scenarios which require special consideration and unique treatment options

Fig. 12.6 Outside-in technique for repair of peripheral ulnar-sided tears. (**a**) The wrist is distracted in a standard arthroscopy tower with 12–15 lbs of traction. (**b**) View from the 3,4 portal before and after debridement of the inflamed synovium overlying the tear. (**c**) The curved meniscal needle is inserted percutaneously just dorsal to the ECU tendon across the TFCC from proximal to distal, and the straight meniscal needle is inserted distal to the TFCC. This image shows insertion of the 2–0 PDS suture through the cannulated straight needle into the radiocarpal joint to be retrieved through the curved needle. (**d**) A single horizontal mattress stich is shown spanning the tear (superior), and three sutures are shown under tension demonstrating adequate reduction of the tear. (**e**) Six suture ends are shown exiting the ulnar wrist. (**f**) A small incision is made in line with the exiting sutures at the ulnar wrist, with care taken to identify and protect the dorsal sensory branch of the ulnar nerve. The sutures are tensioned, tied over the ulnar capsule, and cut beneath the skin

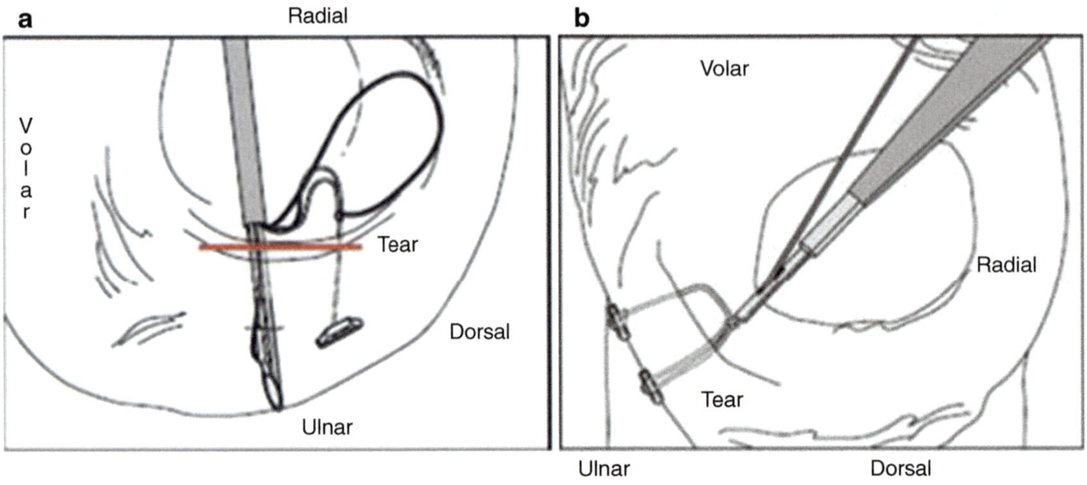

Fig. 12.7 All-inside technique for repair of peripheral ulnar-sided tears. (**a**) Overhead view of the FasT-Fix suture device which deploys 2 PLLA blocks through the capsule on either side of a tear, (**b**) resulting in re-approximation of a peripheral tear when the suture is tightened. (With permission. From: Yao and Lee [63])

include deep foveal avulsions, and nonrepairable tears. These subtypes correspond to class 2, 3, and 4 injuries in the aforementioned Atzei classification of peripheral tears [18]. Foveal avulsion of the deep fibers of the radioulnar ligament contributes to DRUJ instability which represents a risk factor for poor outcome following repair by the capsular techniques described above [19]. Various techniques have been described for foveal repair, either by transosseous bone tunnels or suture anchor fixation, each with high rates of success at restoring DRUJ stability [57, 71]. With regard to nonrepairable tears, reconstruction options have been developed for those thin, friable, often chronic tears with insufficient tissue quality to support an attempt at capsular or osseous repair. The now popular anatomic reconstruction described by Adams and Berger utilizes an autograft tendon weaved through transosseous drill holes to recreate the volar and dorsal radioulnar ligaments [72]. Their initial study reported restoration of DRUJ stability and relief of pain in 12 of 14 patients at 1–4 year follow-up.

Type 1C

Type 1C tears involve injury to the ulnocarpal ligaments with or without associated instability. Their management is controversial and has traditionally involved either nonoperative treatment or simple arthroscopic debridement, though arthroscopic and open repair techniques have been described [29, 59]. A recent area of interest involves the diagnosis and treatment of a subset of these injuries described by Berger and colleagues as longitudinal split tears of the ulnotriquetral (UT) ligament [20]. These intrasubstance tears are hypothesized to occur with radial extension of the wrist, forearm supination, and an axial load which maximally stresses the UT ligament [73]. Patients present with debilitating pain and a positive ulnar fovea sign on physical exam, without associated DRUJ or ulnocarpal instability. MRI may demonstrate signal change within the UT ligament or at its foveal insertion; however, the diagnosis is confirmed arthroscopically. Overlying synovitis is debrided to expose a longitudinally oriented defect within the substance of the UT ligament (Fig. 12.8). An outside-in, PDS suture repair can then be performed in similar fashion to that described for type 1B tears. In their initial 2010 study, Berger and colleagues reviewed their results in 36 patients, at an average age of 30 years old, and found an 89% satisfaction rate with 90% of patients reporting no limitation in activity after repair [20]. They propose a modification to the Palmer 1C classification to

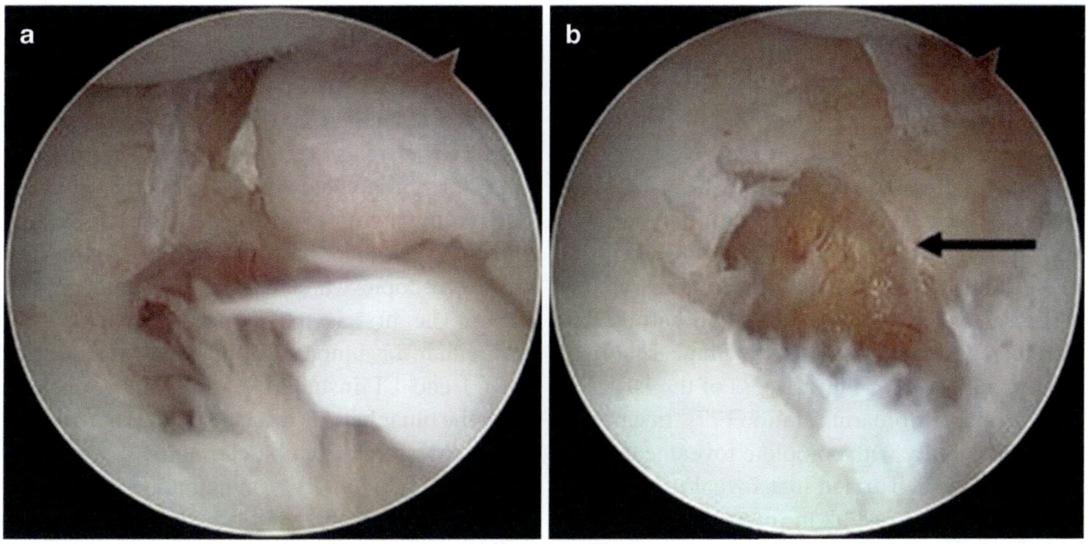

Fig. 12.8 Longitudinal split tear of the ulnotriquetral ligament viewed through the 3–4 portal, (**a**) before and (**b**) after debridement of overlying synovitis. (With permission. From: Tay et al. [20])

include both the traditionally described transverse avulsion injuries of the ulnocarpal ligaments and their underrecognized longitudinal split tear of the UT ligament.

Type 1D

Type 1D tears represent a traumatic avulsion of the articular disk from its origin at the distal aspect of the sigmoid notch. These tears are frequently associated with avulsion fractures of the distal radius, which are amenable to reduction and pinning under arthroscopic visualization. In the absence of an associated fracture, treatment is controversial due to the avascular nature of the radial aspect of the articular disk [23]. Sagerman and Short were the first to describe a technique for arthroscopic repair of these lesions [74]. After debridement of the tear, a burr is inserted through the 6-U or 6-R portal and used to decorticate the sigmoid notch back to bleeding bone in order to facilitate a healing response. Two bone tunnels are then created across the distal radius in an ulnar to radial direction with 0.062 K-wires. Meniscal needles are used to pass a 2–0 PDS suture across the tear in a horizontal mattress fashion, through the bone tunnels, and out the radial side of the wrist where the two suture ends are pulled taught to reduce the tear and tied over the radial capsule. A retrospective study of 19 patients with 1D tears compared simple debridement to transosseous repair as described by Sagerman and found no difference in Mayo wrist scores between groups. They report that compared to repair, isolated debridement is faster, technically easier, allows for quicker rehabilitation, and is associated with lower complications with equivalent functional outcomes [75].

Degenerative Tears

Palmer type 2 TFCC tears represent the spectrum of injuries which result from the degenerative effect of repetitive ulnocarpal impaction. Even in the absence of ulnar positive variance, the dynamic effect of grip on ulnar variance makes baseball players uniquely susceptible to impaction due to the repetitive power grip and pronation required for the swing [25, 26]. Simple debridement of degenerative tears should be avoided, especially in the presence of an associated lunotriquetral ligament injury, because of the high risk of persistent pain and need for revision surgery [53, 76]. Ulnar shortening procedures have been described as the panacea for degenerative, ulnar-sided wrist conditions, with arthroscopic wafer resection and ulnar shortening osteotomy representing the two most commonly performed techniques.

Ulnar shortening osteotomy is primarily performed for cases of ulnar impaction syndrome, with or without evidence of LT or DRUJ instability. Shortening not only decompresses the forces between the ulnar head and carpus, but also increases the tension of the ulnocarpal ligaments and increases the stiffness of the DRUJ in all positions of forearm rotation [77]. In cases of DRUJ instability with complete foveal tears, Seo et al. have demonstrated that foveal repair combined with USO results in improved postoperative stability compared with USO alone [71]. The osteotomy is performed either proximal or distal to the origin of the distal oblique bundle (DOB) of the interosseous ligament which originates 5.4 cm proximal to the ulnar head and inserts into the radioulnar ligaments at the sigmoid notch. The DOB is present in just 40% of patients but can confer significant DRUJ stability when tensioned by ulnar shortening osteotomy [78]. It is for this reason that in cases of instability the osteotomy should be performed 6 cm proximal to the articular surface in order to tension the DOB, while in isolated cases of impaction without instability the osteotomy may be performed more distally. Oblique cuts are made and up to 5 mm of bone is removed. Interfragmentary compression can be used in combination with dynamic compression plating for fixation. Outcomes studies in the general population have demonstrated good to excellent results in greater than 90% of patients with improvements in pain, motion, and function following USO [79–82]. The risks inherent to USO include hardware irritation, malunion, and nonunion, though the rates of these complications have decreased in recent years with improved surgical technique and implant design [83].

The arthroscopic wafer procedure involves partial excision of the distal dome of the ulna through a central tear in the TFCC. The articular disk is debrided, and a mini burr is inserted through the tear and used to remove 2–3 mm of the distal ulna under fluoroscopic visualization to ensure even resection back to 1–2 mm of negative ulnar variance [32]. Similar outcomes have been reported compared to USO, and several studies report lower rates of complications and reoperations for symptomatic hardware removal which is seen following up to 50% of USOs [84]. Despite these results, there are three primary limitations of arthroscopic wafer resection as compared to USO. The first is that it does not tighten the radioulnar or ulnocarpal ligaments to address DRUJ and LT instability. Additionally, because only the ulnar head is resected, it does not address those cases of impaction caused by a prominent ulnar styloid. Finally, a maximum resection of 2–3 mm is recommended, which limits its use to mild/moderate cases of ulnar positivity.

Complications

The types of complications seen following treatment of TFCC tears are dependent primarily upon the surgery performed. The most commonly reported complication following arthroscopic debridement or repair is iatrogenic injury to the dorsal sensory branch of the ulnar nerve (DSBUN). A cadaver study of the inside-out technique determined that the nerve courses just 1.9–2.7 mm from the repair sutures on average, which emphasizes the importance careful dissection during these techniques [85]. Injuries range from transient paresthesia to permanent numbness and have been reported to occur at a rate of 7–17% [8, 19, 57, 60].

Patients undergoing arthroscopic debridement or repair should also be counseled on the potential need for additional surgery following their index procedure. This is most commonly performed for persistent DRUJ instability, with patients subsequently requiring USO or allograft tendon reconstruction [70, 86]. A systematic review by Robertson et al. determined the rate of subsequent conversion to USO for persistent ulnar-sided wrist pain to be between 4 and 13% following debridement and 8% following repair [8]. They also report a 4% rate of postoperative ECU tendonitis, 4% rate of re-tears after repair, and a 2% rate of chronic nonspecific postoperative pain. FCR tendonitis and repeat debridement for recurrent synovitis have also been described [19, 60].

Complications following ulnar shortening osteotomy have been extensively reported, and include nonunion, malunion, hardware irritation, and re-fracture through the osteotomy site following plate removal. In 2018, Owens et al. performed a systematic review of the literature which included 1423 patients across 37 studies and found an average rate of nonunion of 4% and an average rate of delayed union of 5.7% [83]. These rates can be mitigated by limiting periosteal stripping during exposure, diligent reduction and fixation, smoking cessation, and insisting that baseball players refrain from chewing tobacco until they demonstrate radiographic union. Rates of plate removal for symptomatic hardware range widely from 10 to 50%, and likely vary by surgeon preference [87–90]. When desired, plate removal is typically delayed 1 year to mitigate the risk of refracture; however, a 2005 study by Pomerance et al. demonstrated safe removal at 6–9 months postoperatively as long as 2 sets of radiographs taken 4 weeks apart demonstrate union at the osteotomy site [89].

Post Treatment Rehab and Return to Play

The timing and method of immobilization and rehabilitation following arthroscopic debridement and repair are variable throughout the literature. In general, for arthroscopic debridement, a volar slab or similar wrist splint is maintained for 7–10 days postoperatively, followed by ROM and strengthening as dictated by player comfort. Most athletes can expect a return to unrestricted play by 4–5 weeks [11, 29, 49].

Players undergoing arthroscopic repair of peripheral tears are most often immobilized in an above elbow splint or muenster cast for up to 6 weeks in order to prevent forearm rotation. Most authors then advocate progressive ROM and strengthening with a goal for return to play by 3 months [7, 8, 11, 19, 29, 49, 57, 63]. In their series of athletes undergoing arthroscopic repair, McAdams et al. utilized a short cast and instructed their athletes not to perform any resistive pronosupination until cast removal at 6 weeks. They feel that this allows the trustworthy athlete to perform other exercises without the disability conferred by a long arm cast [7]. With regard to baseball players specifically, Harvey and Culp immobilize their repairs in a muenster splint for 4 weeks followed by ROM, with strengthening allowed only once grip strength reaches 80% of the contralateral side (with the understanding that the dominant extremity will be 10% stronger at baseline). They allow return to play when the player is able to hit off a tee and field their position without pain.

A recent systematic review by Robertson et al. examined the rates and timing of return to play following various methods of debridement and repair [8]. They found a 97% average rate of return to sport following arthroscopic debridement, compared to an 88% rate for all methods of ulnar-sided repair. When analyzed by repair method, they found a 72% rate of return for outside-in repairs, 81% for inside-out, and 94% for all-inside. The higher rate seen for all-inside compared to outside-in was the only statistically significant difference between groups. The mean return to sport time for debridement was significantly faster at 7.6 weeks compared to 13.6 weeks for repair.

Following arthroscopic wafer resection, patients are generally immobilized in a short arm splint for 1–2 weeks with early ROM and strengthening beginning thereafter. Return to sport is then guided by patient tolerance [29, 91]. Immobilization and rehabilitation protocols are more varied following ulnar shortening osteotomy. Jarrett et al. report immobilization in a short arm cast for 4–6 weeks while encouraging forearm rotation and gentle grip immediately after surgery [32]. A study by Papetropoulos et al. placed patients in a removable wrist splint postoperatively and encouraged daily ROM after wound healing to prevent stiffness [67]. Regardless of initial immobilization, all cited authors restrict full activity until there is radiographic evidence of union, with return to sport expected around 3 months [11, 29, 32, 67].

References

1. Palmer AK, Werner FW. The triangular fibrocartilage complex of the wrist—Anatomy and function. J Hand Surg. 1981;6(2):153–62.
2. Dailey SW, Palmer AK. The role of arthroscopy in the evaluation and treatment of triangular fibrocartilage complex injuries in athletes. Hand Clin. 2000;16(3):461–76.
3. Papapetropoulos PA, Ruch DS. Repair of arthroscopic triangular fibrocartilage complex tears in athletes. Hand Clin. 2009;25(3):389–94.
4. Rettig AC. Epidemiology of hand and wrist injuries in sports. Clin Sports Med. 1998;17(3):401–6.
5. Pang EQ, Yao J. Ulnar-sided wrist pain in the athlete (TFCC/DRUJ/ECU). Curr Rev Musculoskelet Med. 2017;10(1):53–61.
6. Geissler WB, Burkett JL. Ligamentous sports injuries of the hand and wrist. Sports Med Arthrosc Rev. 2014;22(1):39–44.
7. McAdams TR, Swan J, Yao J. Arthroscopic treatment of triangular fibrocartilage wrist injuries in the athlete. Am J Sports Med. 2009;37(2):291–7.
8. Robertson G, Ang KK, Maffulli N, Simpson CK, Rust PA. Return to sport following surgical management of triangular fibrocartilage tears: a systematic review. Br Med Bull. 2019;130(1):89–103.
9. Avery DM, Rodner CM, Edgar CM. Sports-related wrist and hand injuries: a review. J Orthop Surg Res. 2016;11(1):99.
10. Fares MY, Salhab HA, Khachfe HH, Kane L, Fares Y, Fares J, et al. Upper limb injuries in major league baseball. Phys Ther Sport. 2019;41:49–54.
11. Harvey NM, Culp RW. Baseball commentary "Traumatic TFCC Tear". Hand Clin. 2012;28(3):323–4.
12. Baratz ME. Central TFCC Tears in Baseball Players. Hand Clin. 2012;28(3):339.
13. Harley BJ, Pereria ML, Werner FW, Kinney DA, Sutton LG. Force variations in the distal radius and ulna: effect of ulnar variance and forearm motion. J Hand Surg Am. 2015;40(2):211–6.
14. Palmer AK, Werner FW. Biomechanics of the distal radioulnar joint. Clin Orthop Relat R. 1984;187: 26–35.
15. Palmer AK. Triangular fibrocartilage complex lesions: a classification. J Hand Surg Am. 1989;14(4):594–606.
16. Ishii S, Palmer AK, Werner FW, Short WH, Fortino MD. An anatomic study of the ligamentous structure of the triangular fibrocartilage complex. J Hand Surg Am. 1998;23(6):977–85.
17. Kleinman WB. Stability of the distal radioulna joint: biomechanics, pathophysiology, physical diagnosis, and restoration of function what we have learned in 25 years. J Hand Surg Am. 2007;32(7):1086–106.
18. Atzei A, Luchetti R. Foveal TFCC tear classification and treatment. Hand Clin. 2011;27(3):263–72.
19. Estrella EP, Hung L-K, Ho P-C, Tse WL. Arthroscopic repair of triangular fibrocartilage complex tears. Arthroscopy. 2007;23(7):729–737.e1.
20. Tay S-C, Berger RA, Parker WL. Longitudinal split tears of the ulnotriquetral ligament. Hand Clin. 2010;26(4):495–501.
21. Melone CP, Nathan R. Traumatic disruption of the triangular fibrocartilage complex. Clin Orthop Relat R. 1992;275:65–73.
22. Pathi RGT, Ferlic DC, Clayton ML, McClure DC. Arterial anatomy of the triangular fibrocartilage of the wrist and its surgical significance. J Hand Surg [Am]. 1986;11(2):258–63.
23. Bednar MS. The Microvasculature of the triangulra fibrocartilage complex: it's clinical significance. J Hand Surg [Am]. 1991;16:1101–5.
24. Werner FW, Glisson RR, Murphy DJ, Palmer AK. Force transmission through the distal radioulnar carpal joint: effect of ulnar lengthening and shortening. Handchir Mikrochir Plast Chir. 1986;18(5): 304–8.
25. Friedman SL, Palmer AK, Short WH, Levinsohn EM, Halperin LS. The change in ulnar variance with grip. J Hand Surg [Am]. 1993;18(4):713–6.
26. Tomaino MM. The importance of the pronated grip x-ray view in evaluating ulnar variance. J Hand Surg [Am]. 2000;25(2):352–7.
27. Palmer AK, Glisson RR, Werner FW. Relationship between ulnar variance and triangular fibrocartilage complex thickness. J Hand Surg [Am]. 1984;9(5):681–3.
28. Adams BD. Partial excision of the triangular fibrocartilage complex articular disk: a biomechanical study. J Hand Surg [Am]. 1993;18(2):334–40.
29. Ko JH, Wiedrich TA. Triangular fibrocartilage complex injuries in the elite athlete. Hand Clin. 2012;28(3):307–21.
30. Ruch DS, Yang CC, Smith BP. Results of acute arthroscopically repaired triangular fibrocartilage complex injuries associated with intra-articular distal radius fractures. Arthroscopy. 2003;19(5):511–6.
31. Corso SJ, Savoie FH, Geissler WB, Whipple TL, Jiminez W, Jenkins N. Arthroscopic repair of peripheral avulsions of the triangular fibrocartilage complex of the wrist: a multicenter study. Arthroscopy. 1997;13(1):78–84.
32. Jarrett CD, Baratz ME. The management of ulnocarpal abutment and degenerative triangular fibrocartilage complex tears in the competitive athlete. Hand Clin. 2012;28(3):329–37.
33. Tay SC, Tomita K, Berger RA. The "ulnar fovea sign" for defining ulnar wrist pain: an analysis of sensitivity and specificity. J Hand Surg Am. 2007;32(4):438–44.
34. Nakamura R, Horii E, Imaeda T, Nakao E, Kato H, Watanabe K. The ulnocarpal stress test in the diagnosis of ulnar-sided wrist pain. J Hand Surg Br. 1997;22(6):719–23.
35. Minami A, Kato H. Ulnar shortening for triangular fibrocartilage complex tears associated with ulnar positive variance. J Hand Surg Am. 1998;23(5): 904–8.
36. Schmauss D, Pöhlmann S, Lohmeyer JA, Germann G, Bickert B, Megerle K. Clinical tests and magnetic

resonance imaging have limited diagnostic value for triangular fibrocartilaginous complex lesions. Arch Orthop Trauma Surg. 2016;136(6):873–80.
37. Halbrecht J, Levy IM, Gaudinez R. "Press test" for office diagnosis of triangular fibrocartilage complex tears of the wrist. Ann Plast Surg. 1995;35(1):41–5.
38. Palmer AK, Glisson RR, Werner FW. Ulnar variance determination. J Hand Surg Am. 1982;7(4):376–9.
39. Anderson ML, Skinner JA, Felmlee JP, Berger RA, Amrami KK. Diagnostic comparison of 1.5 tesla and 3.0 tesla preoperative MRI of the wrist in patients with ulnar-sided wrist pain. J Hand Surg Am. 2008;33(7):1153–9.
40. Faber KJ, Iordache S, Grewal R. Magnetic resonance imaging for ulnar wrist pain. J Hand Surg Am. 2010;35(2):303–7.
41. Lee YH, Choi YR, Kim S, Song H-T, Suh J-S. Intrinsic ligament and triangular fibrocartilage complex (TFCC) tears of the wrist: comparison of isovolumetric 3D-THRIVE sequence MR arthrography and conventional MR image at 3 T. Magn Reson Imaging. 2013;31(2):221–6.
42. Lee RKL, Ng AWH, Tong CSL, Griffith JF, Tse WL, Wong C, et al. Intrinsic ligament and triangular fibrocartilage complex tears of the wrist: comparison of MDCT arthrography, conventional 3-T MRI, and MR arthrography. Skelet Radiol. 2013;42(9):1277–85.
43. Zanetti M, Bräm J, Hodler J. Triangular fibrocartilage and intercarpal ligaments of the wrist: Does MR arthrography improve standard MRI? J Magn Reson Imaging. 1997;7(3):590–4.
44. Blazar PE, Chan PSH, Kneeland JB, Leatherwood D, Bozentka DJ, Kowalchick R. The effect of observer experience on magnetic resonance imaging interpretation and localization of triangular fibrocartilage complex lesions. J Hand Surg Am. 2001;26(4):742–8.
45. Oneson SR, Timins ME, Scales LM, Erickson SJ, Chamoy L. MR imaging diagnosis of triangular fibrocartilage pathology with arthroscopic correlation. Am J Roentgenol. 1997;168(6):1513–8.
46. Haims AH, Schweitzer ME, Morrison WB, Deely D, Lange R, Osterman AL, et al. Limitations of MR imaging in the diagnosis of peripheral tears of the triangular fibrocartilage of the wrist. Am J Roentgenol. 2002;178(2):419–22.
47. Iordache SD, Rowan R, Garvin GJ, Osman S, Grewal R, Faber KJ. Prevalence of triangular fibrocartilage complex abnormalities on MRI scans of asymptomatic wrists. J Hand Surg Am. 2012;37(1):98–103.
48. Bendre HH, Oflazoglu K, van Leeuwen WF, Rakhorst H, Ring D, Chen NC. The prevalence of triangular fibrocartilage complex signal abnormalities on magnetic resonance imaging relative to clinical suspicion of pathology. J Hand Surg Am. 2018;43(9): 819–826.e1.
49. Whipple TL, Geissler WB. Arthroscopic management of wrist triangular fibrocartilage complex injuries in the athlete. Orthopedics. 1993;16(9):1061–7.
50. Lee JK, Hwang J-Y, Lee SY, Kwon BC. What is the natural history of the triangular fibrocartilage complex tear without distal radioulnar joint instability? Clin Orthop Relat R. 2019;477(2):442–9.
51. Park MJ, Jagadish A, Yao J. The rate of triangular fibrocartilage injuries requiring surgical intervention. Orthopedics. 2010;33(11):806.
52. Bednar JM, Osterman AL. The role of arthroscopy in the treatment of traumatic triangular fibrocartilage injuries. Hand Clin. 1994;10(4):605–14.
53. Minami A, Ishikawa J, Suenaga N, Kasashima T. Clinical results of treatment of triangular fibrocartilage complex tears by arthroscopic debridement. J Hand Surg Am. 1996;21(3):406–11.
54. Roh YH, Hong SW, Gong HS, Baek GH. Prognostic factors of arthroscopic debridement for central triangular fibrocartilage complex tears in adults younger than 45 years: a retrospective case series analysis. Arthroscopy. 2018;34(11):2994–8.
55. Arsalan-Werner A, Grüter L, Mehling IM, Moll W, Wölfle O, Sauerbier M. Results after arthroscopic treatment of central traumatic lesions of the triangular fibrocartilage complex. Arch Orthop Trauma Surg. 2018;138(5):731–7.
56. Hermansdorfer JD, Kleinman WB. Management of chronic peripheral tears of the triangular fibrocartilage complex. J Hand Surg Am. 1991;16(2):340–6.
57. Atzei A, Luchetti R, Braidotti F. Arthroscopic foveal repair of the triangular fibrocartilage complex. J Wrist Surg. 2015;04(01):022–30.
58. Trehan SK, Wall LB, Calfee RP, Shen TS, Dy CJ, Yannascoli SM, et al. Arthroscopic diagnosis of the triangular fibrocartilage complex foveal tear: a cadaver assessment. J Hand Surg Am. 2018;43(7):680.e1–5.
59. Trumble TE, Gilbert M, Vedder N. Isolated tears of the triangular fibrocartilage: management by early arthroscopic repair. J Hand Surg Am. 1997;22(1):57–65.
60. Wysocki RW, Richard MJ, Crowe MM, Leversedge FJ, Ruch DS. Arthroscopic treatment of peripheral triangular fibrocartilage complex tears with the deep fibers intact. J Hand Surg Am. 2012;37(3):509–16.
61. de Araujo W, Poehling GG, Kuzma GR. New Tuohy needle technique for triangular fibrocartilage complex repair: preliminary studies. Arthroscopy. 1996;12(6):699–703.
62. Yao J, Dantuluri P, Osterman AL. A novel technique of all-inside arthroscopic triangular fibrocartilage complex repair. Arthroscopy. 2007;23(12):1357.e1–4.
63. Yao J, Lee AT. All-arthroscopic repair of Palmer 1B triangular fibrocartilage complex tears using the FasT-Fix device. J Hand Surg Am. 2011;36(5):836–42.
64. Yao J. All-arthroscopic triangular fibrocartilage complex repair: safety and biomechanical comparison with a traditional outside-in technique in cadavers. J Hand Surg Am. 2009;34(4):671–6.
65. Whitlock K, Ruch DS. Editorial commentary: ulnar variance is not the sole determinant of arthroscopic wrist triangular fibrocartilage complex repair outcome: considering the forest from the ulnar-positive tree. Arthroscopy. 2020;36(9):2423–4.
66. Ruch DS, Papadonikolakis A. Arthroscopically assisted repair of peripheral triangular fibrocartilage

complex tears: factors affecting outcome. Arthroscopy. 2005;21(9):1126–30.
67. Papapetropoulos PA, Wartinbee DA, Richard MJ, Leversedge FJ, Ruch DS. Management of peripheral triangular fibrocartilage complex tears in the ulnar positive patient: arthroscopic repair versus ulnar shortening osteotomy. J Hand Surg Am. 2010;35(10):1607–13.
68. Kwon BC, Lee JH, Lee SY. What is the effect of the ulnar plus variance on the outcomes of arthroscopic repair for the peripheral ulnar-side TFCC tear? Arthroscopy. 2020;36(9):2415–22.
69. Wolf MB, Haas A, Dragu A, Leclère FM, Dreyhaupt J, Hahn P, et al. Arthroscopic repair of ulnar-sided triangular fibrocartilage complex (Palmer Type 1B) tears: a comparison between short- and midterm results. J Hand Surg Am. 2012;37(11):2325–30.
70. Wolf MB, Kroeber MW, Reiter A, Thomas SB, Hahn P, Horch RE, et al. Ulnar shortening after TFCC suture repair of Palmer type 1B lesions. Arch Orthop Traum Surg. 2010;130(3):301–6.
71. Seo J-B, Kim J-P, Yi H-S, Park K-H. The outcomes of arthroscopic repair versus debridement for chronic unstable triangular fibrocartilage complex tears in patients undergoing ulnar-shortening osteotomy. J Hand Surg Am. 2016;41(5):615–23.
72. Adams BD, Berger RA. An anatomic reconstruction of the distal radioulnar ligaments for posttraumatic distal radioulnar joint instability. J Hand Surg Am. 2002;27(2):243–51.
73. Moritomo H, Murase T, Arimitsu S, Oka K, Yoshikawa H, Sugamoto K. Change in the length of the ulnocarpal ligaments during radiocarpal motion: possible impact on triangular fibrocartilage complex foveal tears. J Hand Surg Am. 2008;33(8):1278–86.
74. Sagerman SD, Short W. Arthroscopic repair of radial-sided triangular fibrocartilage complex tears. Arthroscopy. 1996;12(3):339–42.
75. Osterman AL. Arthroscopic treatment of radial sided TFCC lesions. International Wrist Investigator's Workshop, ASSH; 2014.
76. Osterman AL, Terrill RG. Arthroscopic treatment of TFCC lesions. Hand Clin. 1991;7(2):277–81.
77. Nishiwaki M, Nakamura T, Nakao Y, Nagura T, Toyama Y. Ulnar shortening effect on distal radioulnar joint stability: a biomechanical study. J Hand Surg Am. 2005;30(4):719–26.
78. Kitamura T, Moritomo H, Arimitsu S, Berglund LJ, Zhao KD, An K-N, et al. The biomechanical effect of the distal interosseous membrane on distal radioulnar joint stability: a preliminary anatomic study. J Hand Surg Am. 2011;36(10):1626–30.
79. Iwasaki N, Ishikawa J, Kato H, Minami M, Minami A. Factors affecting results of ulnar shortening for ulnar impaction syndrome. Clin Orthop Relat Res. 2007;465:215–9.
80. Hulsizer D, Weiss A-PC, Akelman E. Ulna-shortening osteotomy after failed arthroscopic debridement of the triangular fibrocartilage complex. J Hand Surg Am. 1997;22(4):694–8.
81. Baek GH, Chung MS, Lee YH, Gong HS, Lee S, Kim HH. Ulnar shortening osteotomy in idiopathic ulnar impaction syndrome. J Bone Jt Surg. 2005;87(12):2649–54.
82. Moermans A, Degreef I, Smet LD. Ulnar shortening osteotomy for ulnar ideopathic impaction syndrome. Scand J Plast Reconstr Surg Hand Surg. 2009;41(6):310–4.
83. Owens J, Compton J, Day M, Glass N, Lawler E. Nonunion rates among ulnar-shortening osteotomy for ulnar impaction syndrome: a systematic review. J Hand Surg Am. 2018;44(7):612.e1–612.e12.
84. Oh W-T, Kang H-J, Chun Y-M, Koh I-H, An H-M-S, Choi Y-R. Arthroscopic wafer procedure versus ulnar shortening osteotomy as a surgical treatment for idiopathic ulnar impaction syndrome. Arthroscopy. 2018;34(2):421–30.
85. McAdams TR, Hentz VR. Injury to the dorsal sensory branch of the ulnar nerve in the arthroscopic repair of ulnar-sided triangular fibrocartilage tears using an inside-out technique: a cadaver study. J Hand Surg Am. 2002;27(5):840–4.
86. ADAMS BD. Anatomic reconstruction of the distal radioulnar ligaments for DRUJ instability. Tech Hand Up Extrem Surg. 2000;4(3):154–60.
87. Bernstein MA, Nagle DJ, Martinez A, Stogin JM, Wiedrich TA. A comparison of combined arthroscopic triangular fibrocartilage complex debridement and arthroscopic wafer distal ulna resection versus arthroscopic triangular fibrocartilage complex debridement and ulnar shortening osteotomy for ulnocarpal abutment syndrome. Arthroscopy. 2004;20(4):392–401.
88. Ahsan ZS, Song Y, Yao J. Outcomes of ulnar shortening osteotomy fixed with a dynamic compression system. J Hand Surg Am. 2013;38(8):1520–3.
89. Pomerance J. Plate removal after ulnar-shortening osteotomy. J Hand Surg Am. 2005;30(5):949–53.
90. Constantine KJ, Tomaino MM, Herndon JH, Sotereanos DG. Comparison of ulnar shortening osteotomy and the wafer resection procedure as treatment for ulnar impaction syndrome. J Hand Surg Am. 2000;25(1):55–60.
91. Tomaino MM, Shah M. Treatment of ulnar impaction syndrome with the wafer procedure. Am J Orthop (Belle Mead NJ). 2001;30(2):129–33.
92. Böhringer G, Schädel-Höpfner M, Petermann J, Gotzen L. A method for all-inside arthroscopic repair of Palmer 1B triangular fibrocartilage complex tears. Arthroscopy. 2002;18(2):211–3.

Part III

Tendon and Nerve Injuries of the Hand and Wrist

Flexor Tendon and Flexor Pulley Injuries

13

Fraser J. Leversedge

Anatomy: Flexor Tendon and Pulley Apparatus

Zones of Injury

Kleinert and Verdan described five zones of injury that consider the anatomy of injury, the biologic mechanisms of repair, and functional outcomes [1] (Fig. 13.1).

Extrinsic Flexor Tendon Anatomy

The extrinsic flexor muscles originate in the volar forearm and include the flexor digitorum profundus (FDP), flexor digitorum superficialis (FDS), and flexor pollicis longus (FPL). The FDP arises from the anterior-medial aspect of the ulna and interosseous membrane and forms a common tendon origin, although typically the index finger has greater independence. The anterior interosseous nerve (AIN) innervates the FDP muscle bellies to the index and middle fingers and the ulnar nerve innervates the ring and small fingers, although variations to this pattern are not uncommon. The superficial flexor muscle, the FDS, is innervated by the median nerve and originates from the medial epicondyle of the humerus, the sublime tubercle of the proximal medial ulna, and the anterior radius. In the forearm, the FDS is separated from the deeper FDP muscle by the median nerve which exits from this interval between the FDS and flexor

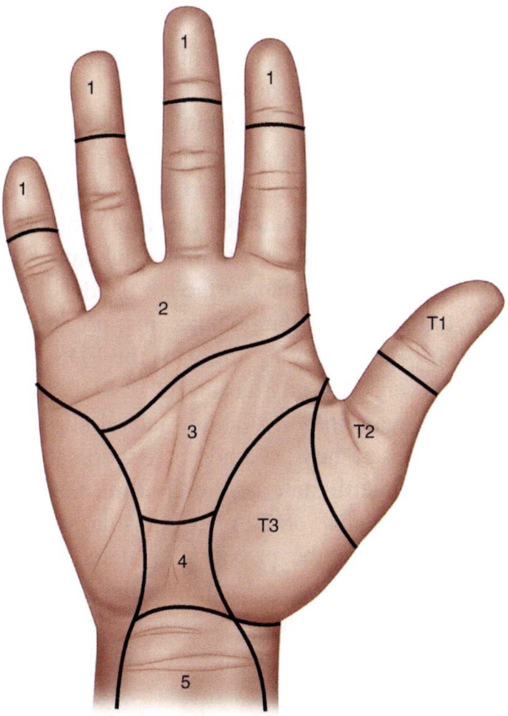

Fig. 13.1 Flexor tendon zones of injury for the fingers and thumb

F. J. Leversedge (✉)
Department of Orthopedic Surgery, University of Colorado, Aurora, CO, USA
e-mail: fraser.leversedge@cuanschutz.edu

G. M. Lourie (ed.), *Hand and Wrist Injuries in Baseball*,
https://doi.org/10.1007/978-3-030-81659-9_13

carpi radialis (FCR) muscles to course distally to the carpal tunnel with the FDS, FDP, and FPL tendons [2].

The FDS and FDP tendons exit the carpal tunnel deep to the superficial palmar arterial arch and are enveloped by a specialized, multi-layered synovial sheath before entering the fibro-osseous digital retinacular system. The common digital neurovascular bundles and the flexor sheath are separated by the vertical retinacular septae of Legeau and Juvara that attach palmarly to the transverse ligament of the palmar aponeurosis and dorsally to the deep intermetacarpal ligament. These eight septae create seven longitudinal compartments: four that contain the flexor tendons, and three that contain the neurovascular bundles and the lumbricals [3].

At the level of the first annular pulley (A1 pulley), the FDS flattens and bifurcates to allow the deeper FDP to pass distally to its insertion at the base of the distal phalanx. The footprint of the FDP insertion is substantial, encompassing nearly the entire palmar surface of the distal phalanx to the neck of the phalanx, just proximal to the tuft [4]. Bifurcating limbs of the FDS rotate laterally and dorsally around the FDP before dividing again into medial and lateral slips. The medial slips of the FDS tendon cross dorsal to the FDP and interdigitate as the chiasma tendinum digitorum manus, or Camper chiasma, over the distal aspect of the proximal phalanx and the proximal interphalangeal joint volar plate [2]. The lateral slips of the FDS tendon continue distally to insert at the palmar base of the middle phalanx (Fig. 13.2).

The FPL originates on the anterior surfaces of the radius and interosseous membrane in the mid-forearm and is innervated by the AIN. The FPL tendon courses through the dorsal and radial aspect of the carpal tunnel, through the interval between the adductor pollicis and the thenar musculature before entering the fibro-osseous digital sheath of the thumb, slightly proximal to the thumb metacarpophalangeal (MCP) joint [2]. The FPL inserts into a broad footprint at the palmar aspect of the distal phalanx.

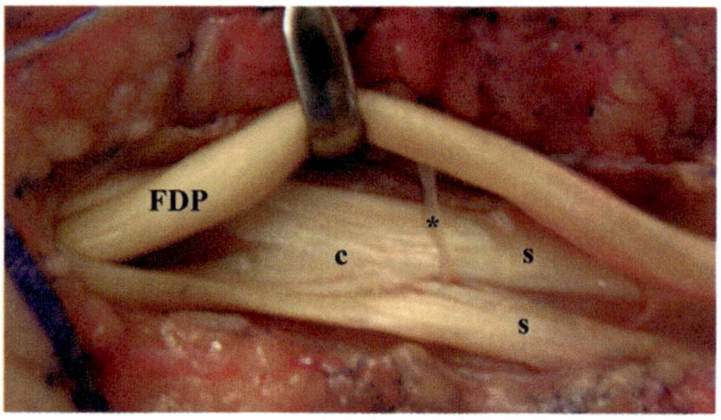

Fig. 13.2 The bifurcating limbs of the FDS tendon rotate laterally and dorsally around the **FDP** tendon and then divide again into medial and lateral slips. The medial slips cross dorsal to the FDP tendon (decussation), rejoining as the chiasma tendinum of Camper (**c**) over the distal aspect of the proximal phalanx and PIP joint volar plate. The lateral slip (**s**) continues distally to insert at the volar base of the middle phalanx. The vincula longum to the profundus tendon (*) is identified as it penetrates the FDS from dorsal to volar. (Reprinted with permission: © Leversedge FJ, Goldfarb CA, Boyer MI. From: Leversedge et al. [2]: 17)

Intrinsic Musculature

The lumbrical muscles originate from the radial aspect of their respective FDP tendon in the hand and course volar to the deep intermetacarpal ligament to contribute to the extensor mechanism of the digit via the oblique fibers of the extensor hood. It is important to consider the anatomic course of the lumbricals as they are palmar to the MCP joint axis of rotation and dorsal to the axis of rotation of the PIP and DIP joints; the lumbricals continue as the oblique fibers of the extensor hood and contribute to the conjoined lateral bands [2, 5–7]. Therefore, the lumbricals assist in flexing the MCP joint and extend the interphalangeal joints. Understanding the relationship between the FDP and the lumbrical musculotendinous units is essential in explaining the phenomenon of paradoxical digital extension following flexor tendon injury and repair.

Flexor Pulley Apparatus

The digital fibro-osseous sheath provides both biomechanical efficiency and a source of nutrition to the flexor tendons. The visceral paratenon envelopes the flexor tendons and the parietal paratenon lines each pulley and the retinacular system [8, 9]. Condensations of the synovial sheath, or pulleys, form at strategic points along the digit to work in conjunction with the transverse carpal ligament and the palmar aponeurosis pulley to maximize efficiency of joint rotation and force transmission.

Classically, five annular (A) and three cruciform (C) pulleys are described for the fingers, as well as the palmar aponeurosis pulley [2, 8–12] (Fig. 13.3). The A1, A3, and A5 pulleys take their origin from volar plates of the MCP, PIP, and DIP joints, respectively, and the A2 and A4 pulleys originate from the proximal and middle phalanges, respectively. The C1, C2, and C3 pulleys are less substantive and are positioned in the A2 and A3, the A3 and A4, and A4 and A5 pulley intervals, respectively. The A2 and A4 pulleys are the most important pulleys biomechanically [13, 14], although several studies have indicated improved clinical outcomes with sacrifice or venting of the critical A4 pulley when its integrity may restrict gliding of the repaired flexor tendon [15, 16]. The anatomical arrangement of the flexor pulleys of the thumb is different from the finger with the A1, oblique, and A2 pulleys described. The A1 pulley is located at the level of the MCP joint, the oblique pulley fibers are oriented in a distal and radial direction at the level of the proximal phalanx, and the A2 pulley originates from the interphalangeal joint volar plate. Biomechanical studies have demonstrated that the A1 and oblique pulleys are most important for resisting FPL bowstringing; biomechanical efficiency is maintained when at least one of these two pulleys is preserved clinically [13].

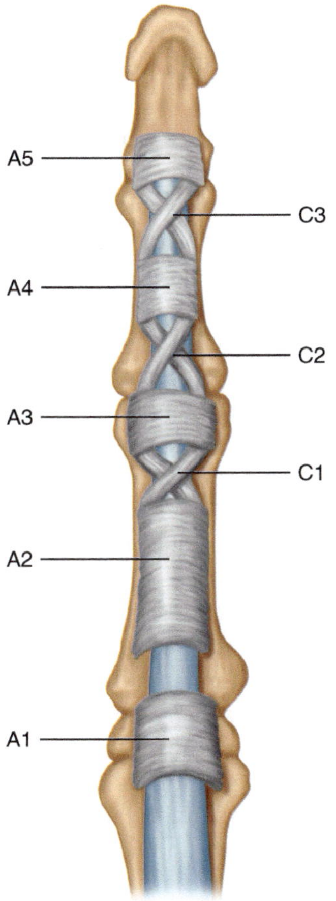

Fig. 13.3 Illustration of the digital flexor pulley system and flexor sheath of the finger

Flexor Tendon Nutrition

The intrasynovial flexor tendons have two sources of nutrition: direct vascular supply and synovial diffusion. The direct vascular system is based on the digital arteries that supply the transverse digital arteries, or "ladder branches," and the vincular system, as well as the intraosseous vessels that percolate the tendinous insertions [17, 18] (Fig. 13.4a, b). Synovial diffusion occurs in the relatively hypovascular zones of the FDS and FDP within the flexor tendon sheath via intratendinous canaliculi [8, 9].

Injury Assessment: Clinical Evaluation

Clinical History

A thorough history is obtained regarding the timing and mechanism of injury. While the timing of open injuries such as a laceration will be obvious, detection of a closed injury to the flexor mechanism may be subtle, leading to a delay in presentation and/or treatment. Pertinent history such as prior extremity injury and pre-existing digital

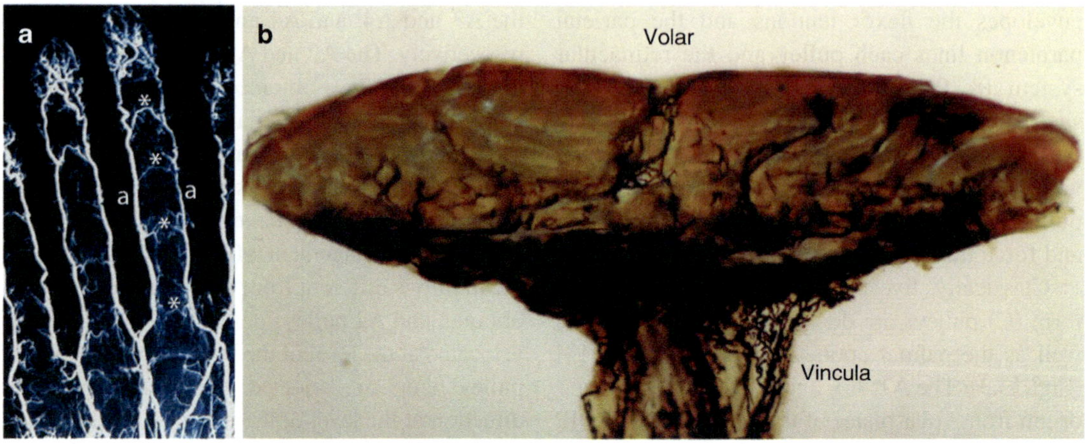

Fig. 13.4 (**a**) Arterial system of the fingers highlighting the digital arteries (a) and the transversely oriented arterial ladder branches (*) that provide perfusion to the flexor tendons via the vincular system. (**b**) Transverse section of the intrasynovial portion of the digital flexor tendon (clarified following India Ink arterial injection) demonstrating the dorsal vincula or mesotenon that arise from the transverse digital arterial "ladder" branches. (Reprinted with permission: © Leversedge FJ, Goldfarb CA, Boyer MI. From: Leversedge et al. [2]: 18)

stiffness is noted, and new symptoms such as alterations in sensibility (sensory nerve injury), digital triggering or pain with tendon excursion (tenosynovitis, partial tendon laceration), perceived reduction in strength or flexion lag (loss of tendon integrity, pulley injury, tenosynovitis), or loss of motion/stiffness are recorded. The player may report an audible or palpable "pop" at the time of a specific loading activity to the hand or digit, commensurate with a soft-tissue avulsion injury, such as a pulley rupture [19]. The mechanism of injury, specific to a particular event or play, or to a particular position-dependent activity, is important to review as this knowledge may shed light on the anatomy of injury. For example, a sudden eccentric loading through the DIP or PIP joints may be accentuated with use of a glove or catching mitt, contact with the ground or fencing, by being struck with the ball, or with incarceration in another player's jersey. Alteration in pitching mechanics and a reduction in accuracy or velocity may be early warning signs of a tendinopathy, intrinsic muscle injury [20], or pulley injury [19] that could progress to a chronic condition in the throwing athlete.

Clinical Examination

A global assessment is critical as concomitant injuries such as fracture or nerve injury may influence treatment recommendations. Inspection of the limb and involved digit(s) confirms an open or closed injury, evaluates for deformity (fracture or dislocation), considers the location of ecchymosis and swelling, and may provide information regarding the neurovascular status of the affected limb. For example, ecchymosis of the digital pulp in the setting of a closed, eccentric extension loading of the distal fingertip is concerning for an FDP avulsion injury and/or fracture. The resting posture of the hand and digits will reflect the influence of the tenodesis effect; observation of tenodesis during inspection and during dynamic testing of the hand and wrist may provide useful information regarding the integrity of the flexor apparatus (Fig. 13.5).

Focal palpation of the injured hand and wrist progresses through a logical anatomical assessment: the location of injury may be highlighted; however, secondary findings such as the location of a retracted proximal tendon stump, sub-

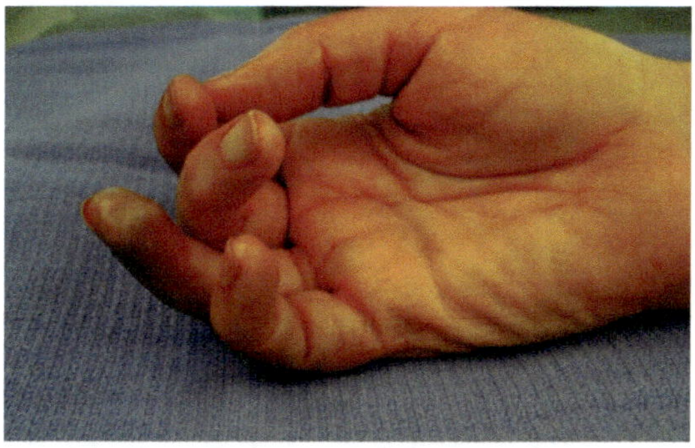

Fig. 13.5 Typical presentation of a closed, FDP avulsion injury demonstrated in the ring finger. Note the mild swelling and ecchymosis of the distal digit with a characteristic loss of DIP joint tenodesis with the hand in a resting position. (Reprinted with permission: © Leversedge FJ, 2004)

tle crepitus or triggering with tendon excursion, or local joint instability may improve diagnostic accuracy. Investigation of possible prodromal symptoms or progressive tendon pathology is helpful for considering diagnostic evaluation, serial examinations and/or timely intervention as indicated. Diagnostic clues may improve prophylactc management of an impending tendon injury such as in the setting of hardware prominence following distal radius volar plating or with irregular bony prominences at the hand or wrist such as a hook of the hamate nonunion sustained by a direct palmar injury during batting.

A neurovascular assessment is essential, particularly in the setting of an open injury. Often, digital or palmar lacerations will involve a neurovascular injury and, therefore, sensory and motor examination is routine as well as digital Allen's testing, where applicable. Although less common, ulnar nerve motor exam is critical prior to surgical intervention for flexor tendon attritional rupture in the setting of a hook of hamate nonunion [21, 22].

The assessment of intrinsic and extrinsic tendon integrity should consider the anatomy of injury, but also anatomic variations that may or may not be present. Evaluation of the FDP tendon involves initial assessment as to presence of the tenodesis effect on the DIP joint during wrist flexion and extension. Discontinuity of the FDP tendon will cause an absence of DIP joint flexion as the wrist is extended (loss of tenodesis), although in rare cases a closed avulsion of the FDP tendon without substantial retraction may exert a flexion force to the distal phalanx via the intact vinculum and / or volar plate of the DIP joint. Active motion of the FDP tendon is assessed with blocking of the middle phalanx as the patient is asked to flex the DIP joint (Fig. 13.6a). Intact but reduced motion may be caused by a partial injury or an impediment to tendon gliding such as flexor tenosynovitis.

Independent FDS tendon evaluation is performed by preventing the indirect influence of the potentially intact FDP tendon on PIP joint motion. During assessment of active FDS function, all the other fingers are held in full extension such that the tenodesis effect of the common FDP origin prevents proximal FDP excursion in the finger being tested, although this may be of limited value in the index finger where a more independent FDP origin has been described (Fig. 13.6b). Absence of the FDS to the small finger is a common anatomic variant and may be unilateral or bilateral [23].

In certain conditions, particularly with open injuries to the hand or with a metacarpal fracture, compromise of digital flexion may be caused by intrinsic muscle dysfunction. The delicate balance between intrinsic and extrinsic function for supporting normal hand function is critical, and alterations in this relationship may cause stiffness or paradoxical digital extension via diversion of the extrinsic flexor forces through the lumbrical muscle and extensor tendon mechanism. A Bunnell intrinsic tightness test is performed by assessing the relative resistance to passive interphalangeal joint flexion with the metacarpophalangeal (MCP) joint in flexion (intrinsics are lax) versus in hyperextension (intrinsics are taut) [24]. Increased resistance to passive interphalangeal joint flexion with the MCP joint in hyperextension (versus flexion) is consistent with intrinsic tightness.

In the thumb, FPL integrity is assessed in similar fashion as for the suspected FDP injury with

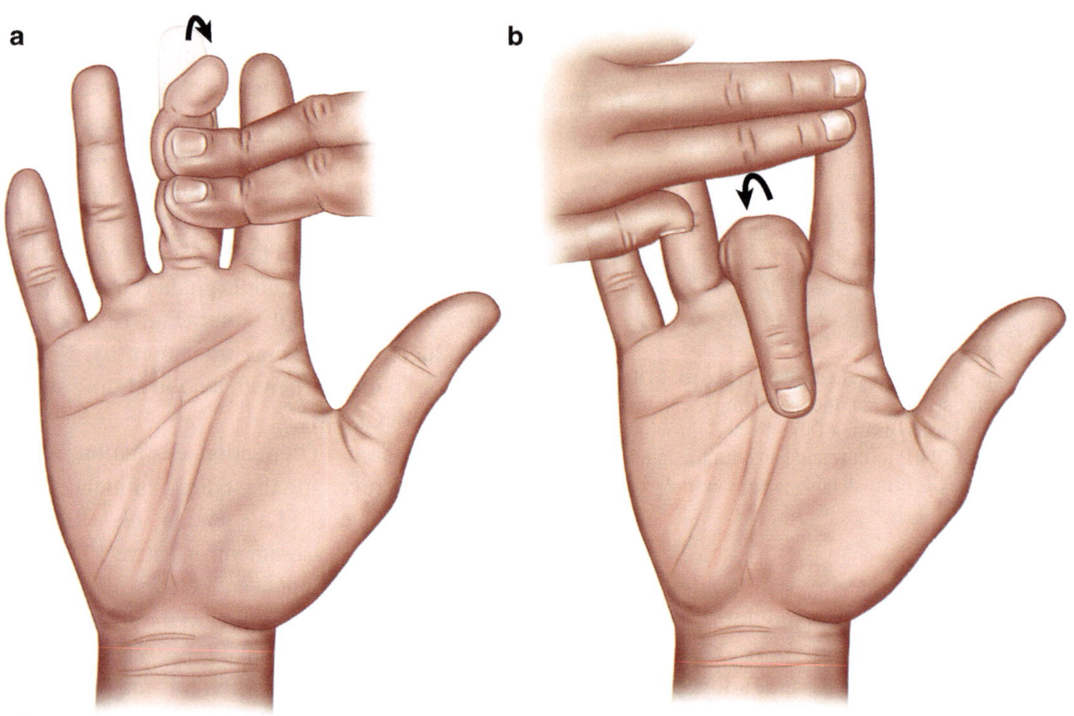

Fig. 13.6 (**a**) Illustration of the clinical examination technique for evaluating active function of the FDP tendon. (**b**) Illustration of the clinical examination technique for evaluating active function of the FDS tendon by limiting the indirect action of the FDP tendon

use of tenodesis and with active tendon function assessment with blocking of the proximal phalanx.

The integrity of the flexor pulley apparatus and fibro-osseous digital sheath may be difficult to assess, particularly in the setting of an acute injury where local swelling may influence digital motion. Increased inflammation associated with injury to the flexor apparatus may cause a reduction in digital extension. A loss of flexor pulley integrity may be difficult to confirm by clinical examination alone; however, focal tenderness typically over the critical A2 or A4 pulleys and a concomitant loss of biomechanical efficiency manifest as a flexion lag should raise the suspicion for a pulley rupture when the mechanism of injury is consistent with forceful loading of the flexor pulley system.

Finally, in the setting of a flexor tendon repair and / or reconstruction, evaluation as to the presence/absence of the bilateral palmaris longus tendons is useful, in the event that a source of tendon graft is necessary [25].

Injury Assessment: Imaging

Radiographs

In general, radiographic assessment includes three views of the injured digit(s) to evaluate for possible tendon avulsion with an associated osseous fragment and/or an associated digital fracture or joint subluxation/dislocation. Careful identification of an avulsion fragment along the flexor sheath, particularly at the volar aspect of the PIP joint, may provide useful information regarding the proximal retraction of a closed tendon avulsion injury.

Ultrasound

Improvements in the quality and resolution of ultrasound, despite this technique being user-dependent, have increased its popularity in the assessment of tendon continuity and the level of retraction of a transected or avulsed tendon [26, 27]. Ultrasound may be useful, also, in evaluating patients with a suspected flexor pulley injury and may provide the advantage over MRI as being a point of care and dynamic study [26–29]. Recently, however, the diagnostic accuracy of ultrasound assessment of certain tendon injuries has been called into question [30].

Magnetic Resonance Imaging

Often, in the setting of a pathologic tendon rupture or tenosynovitis, MRI has been demonstrated to provide useful information prior to surgical exploration and / or tendon reconstruction [29–32]. A dynamic MRI may be considered to evaluate for a symptomatic closed pulley rupture. This may be done by comparing images obtained of a resting hand in full extension with those of the digit actively held in flexion, or images obtained with active flexion against resistance [32]. While the actual pulley injury may not be visible on MR images, T1 sequences may demonstrate bowstringing of the tendon from the phalanx and T2 imaging sequences will characteristically highlight local peritendinous inflammation [28–32].

Injury Classification: Flexor Tendon

- *Tendon Laceration*

Transection or laceration injuries to the flexor tendons are defined by their zone of injury (Fig. 13.1) and as to complete or incomplete lacerations. The anatomic zones of injury permit perioperative planning by the surgeon, both for repair and reconstructive options but also for the coordination of post-repair rehabilitation.

- *Tendon Avulsion*

Avulsion of the FDS from its insertion at the base of the middle phalanx is rare, although it has been described in isolation [33], and mid-substance FDS rupture has been described in combination with a distal FDP avulsion [34]. Avulsion of the FDP from its insertion at the base of the distal phalanx is more common and is known by the descriptive term "jersey finger." The classification system for FDP avulsion injuries emphasizes the variations in both prognosis and treatment choices based on the level of tendon retraction, the remaining sources of nutrition to the avulsed tendon, and the nature of the soft-tissue or bony avulsion fragment. The classification scheme described by Leddy and Packer [35] (Types I, II, and III) was supplemented by Robins and Dobyns through their recognition of a less common, but important Type IIIA injury [36].

Type I

Type I injuries involve a complete avulsion of the FDP tendon and retraction of the tendon (with its bony avulsion fragment, if present) through the flexor sheath and into the palm. The majority of its vincular attachments are striped from the tendon as the tendon is retracted proximally, compromising vascular supply to the tendon.

Type II

Type II injuries involve a complete avulsion of the FDP tendon (with its bony avulsion fragment, if present) and retraction of the proximal stump to the level of the PIP joint. Compared to the Type I injury, there is less disruption of the vincular system. Continuity of the flexor sheath and intrasynovial environment is generally maintained.

Type III

Type III injuries involve avulsion of the FDP tendon from its insertion; however, it retracts no further proximally than the A4 pulley. Proximal retraction of the tendon may be restrained by the vincula and volar plate; however, restriction to proximal retraction of the tendon is typically due to a large bony avulsion fragment that is trapped by the A5 or A4 pulley. In contrast to Type I and II injuries, the vinculae and synovial sheath remain in continuity, improving tendon nutrition.

Type IIIA

The less common Type IIIA/Type IV injury involves a Type III injury, however with avulsion of the FDP tendon from the bony avulsion fragment following incarceration of the bony fragment by the flexor pulley system. The subsequent FDP tendon retraction can, therefore, replicate a Type I or Type II injury. The potential for this injury mechanism highlights the importance of confirming by direct visualization the continuity of the FDP tendon with the bony avulsion fragment at the time of surgical repair. This injury should not be confused with an FDP avulsion injury that occurs incident to a peri-articular fracture of the base of the distal phalanx.

- *Tendon Rupture*

Mid-substance tendon rupture is rare; however, this may be caused by progressive attritional changes associated with local factors such as retained hardware (e.g., distal radius hardware) or bone irregularity (e.g., hook of hamate fracture), or underlying medical condition such as inflammatory tendinopathy or gout.

Management of Flexor Tendon Injuries

Pre-Repair Considerations

Clinical suspicion for a flexor tendon injury on the field of play is important as the absence of pain or open injury could promote continued participation and compromise injury outcomes through the increasing migration of the proximal tendon stump. This escalation of injury should be avoided by protecting the digit from further injury by application of a forearm-based resting hand splint application and immediate restriction of activity that might promote further tendon retraction. For open injuries, appropriate wound care should be instituted (debridement and irrigation, hemostasis, sterile dressing care), with an appropriate antibiotic regimen and tetanus update, as indicated.

Injury Management: Surgical Repair

General Principles

Surgical repair of flexor tendons is done in an operating room setting under a general anesthesia or upper extremity regional block. The surgeon (and player) should be prepared for the potential scenarios of tendon repair and reconstruction, including the need for multiple incisions for tendon retrieval, the potential need for a tendon graft source for pulley reconstruction or primary tendon graft reconstruction, use of a silicone tendon implant, and consideration for salvage procedures in the event that primary repair is not feasible. Associated injuries should be considered during the surgical exposure and determination as to an effective strategy for the sequence of repairs. Preoperative antibiotics are given in timely fashion within 1 h of incision, and tetanus toxoid and/or tetanus immunoglobulin are administered when indicated. Repairs are done using loupe optical magnification.

In general, a mid-axial or Bruner-type incision is used to facilitate exposure of the flexor tendon system. Open injuries or lacerations are incorporated into the exposure, maintaining adequate and viable soft-tissue flaps for subsequent closure. The digital neurovascular bundles are protected and meticulous hemostasis is maintained during dissection.

A strategy for exposing and retrieving the injured flexor tendons should be considered prior to opening the digital flexor sheath in order to preserve the biomechanical integrity of the digital flexor sheath system. Iatrogenic peritendinous adhesion formation will be reduced through the careful handling of the gliding surfaces of the flexor tendons and the fibro-osseous digital sheath [37]. Where possible, the A2 and A4 pulleys are preserved, although venting of these critical pulleys or complete release of the A4 pulley is reasonable depending on the level of injury [13]. Preserving the adjacent pulleys, therefore, will assist in reducing the work of flexion in the event that the integrity of the critical A2 and A4 pulleys are compromised, either through the original injury or by venting during surgical exposure.

Often, the retracted tendon stump may be identified within the sheath by the presence of local hemorrhage. The proximal tendon stump may be "milked" distally within the tendon sheath to facilitate retrieval with the wrist and MCP joints held in flexion. The exposed interior substance of the tendon stump may be grasped using fine-toothed forceps. If the tendon stump is not able to be retrieved in an atraumatic manner, then the retracted proximal tendon stump may be retrieved using a pediatric feeding catheter passed retrograde within the flexor sheath from the initial wound or at the distal tendon sheath to a transverse incision in the palm or within the membranous portion of the flexor sheath distal to the A2 pulley [38] (Fig. 13.7). As the tendon(s) are retrieved and brought distally for repair, the FDS and FDP relationship is restored at the level of the FDS bifurcation.

Acute Injuries

Zone I flexor tendon injuries involving avulsion of the FDP tendon from its insertion or a distal laceration of the FDP tendon with insufficient distal tendon for end-to-end repair are treated by advancement of the proximal stump and reinsertion into the distal phalanx. In general, up to 1 cm of advancement may be permissible to avoid the limitations of a post-repair quadriga effect, although the more independent index FDP may tolerate up to 1.5 cm [39]. Various methods of tendon to bone repair have been described including use of: (1) a pullout suture passed through osseous tunnels in the distal phalanx and tied over a well-padded suture button placed on the nail (Fig. 13.8a, b); (2) a pullout suture construct is created similar to (1); however, the suture is passed around the distal phalanx instead of through the phalanx; (3) a suture tied deep to the skin overlying the extensor tendon insertion after passage from volar to dorsal via trans-osseous tunnels; and (4) one or two suture size-appropriate anchors [40–44] (Fig. 13.9).

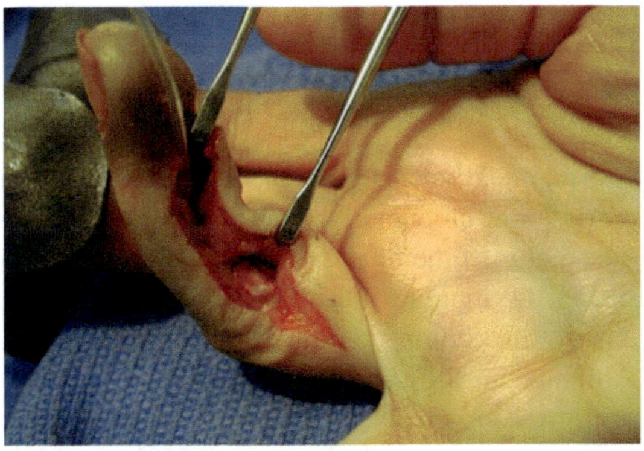

Fig. 13.7 Intraoperative photograph demonstrating the use of a pediatric feeding catheter to retrieve the retracted FDP stump at the PIP joint following a closed avulsion injury (Type II) of the ring finger. (Reprinted with permission: © Leversedge FJ, 2004)

For each of the repair methods, in general, the distal tendon stump is debrided and the volar base of the distal phalanx, distal to the insertion of the volar plate of the DIP joint, is prepared for tendon reattachment by debridement of residual tendon fibers and exposure of the phalangeal cortex, although elevation of a periosteal flap may be used.

If a pullout button repair method is used, the button and suture are removed at approximately 8 weeks postoperatively. It is important to inform the patient as to signs or symptoms of soft-tissue complications while the button is in place as such issues are not uncommon [45], and osseous complications including osteomyelitis can complicate non-pullout suture methods of repair [46]. Suture anchor use should be critically assessed, also, as technique-related studies have demonstrated the risk of intra-articular placement and potential dorsal cortical penetration concerning for nailbed injury and / or infection [47, 48].

Open flexor tendon injuries may involve one or both of the flexor tendons. When both tendons are transected, typically the FDS is repaired first as its inserting limbs are located dorsal to the FDP tendon. Many suture configurations have been described for zone II flexor tendon repair and, while the exact techniques are beyond the scope of this chapter, it is important to consider a modern core suture method which includes the following: (1) at least four suture strands of 4–0 or 3–0 suture, (2) a suture configuration that

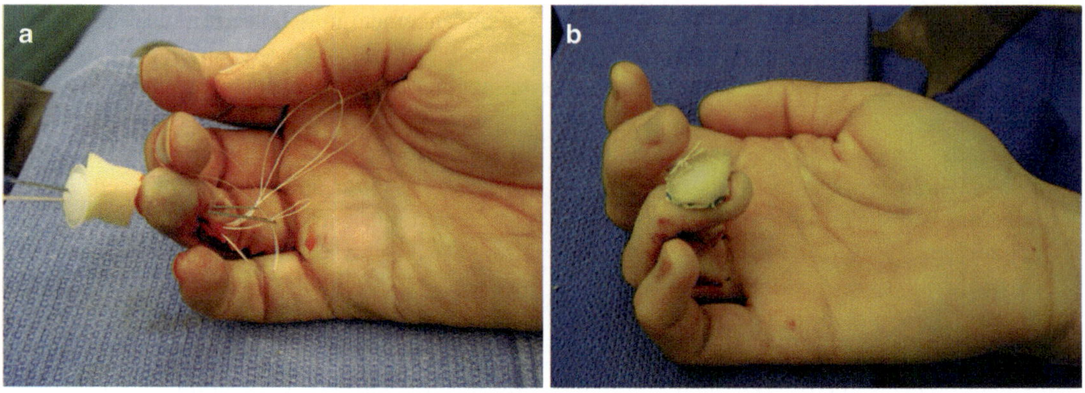

Fig. 13.8 (**a**) Intraoperative photograph demonstrating an FDP tendon repair using a well-padded, tie-over suture button. Sutures are passed through an osseous tunnel using straight Keith needles that have been drilled through the base of the distal phalanx, avoiding injury to the germinal matrix of the fingernail. (Reprinted with permission: © Leversedge FJ, 2004). (**b**) Intraoperative photograph demonstrating an FDP tendon repair with the finger held in flexion as the FDP tendon is reduced to its anatomic insertion and the sutures are secured over the polypropylene button. Note that the digital flexion cascade ideally shows slightly increased tension in the repaired digit. (Reprinted with permission: © Leversedge FJ, 2004)

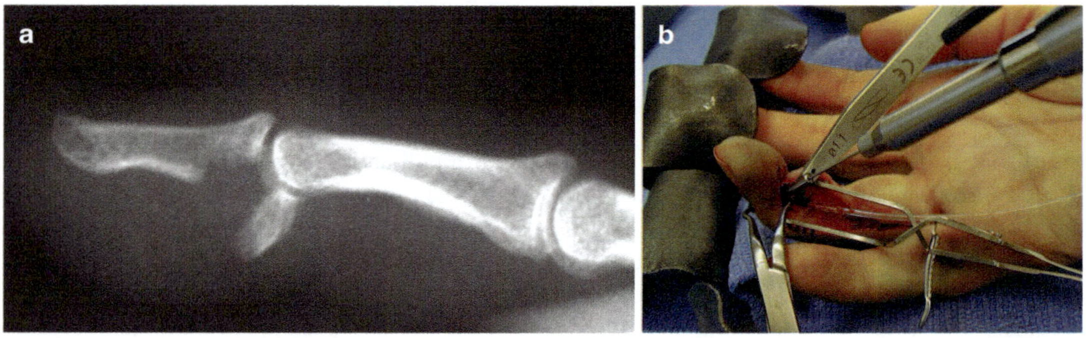

Fig. 13.9 (**a**) Lateral radiograph of the finger demonstrating an avulsion fracture from the volar base of the distal phalanx fracture consistent with a possible Type III or Type IIIa FDP avulsion injury. (Reprinted with permission: © Leversedge FJ, 2004). (**b**) Intraoperative photograph demonstrating open fracture reduction and internal fixation of a displaced volar base fracture of the distal phalanx, consistent with an FDP avulsion injury. (Reprinted with permission: © Leversedge FJ, 2004)

interacts with the tendon substance in an appropriate grasping or locking fashion, and (3) a method that is finished with an epitendinous suture repair that not only reduces the tendon ends, but also increases the ultimate strength of the tendon repair construct. The use of wide-awake local anesthesia, no tourniquet (WALANT) methods for anesthesia have improved intraoperative assessment of the repaired tendon in regard to tendon gliding and avoidance of gap formation during active tendon excursion [49].

Treatment of partial tendon injuries should consider the amount of tendon involvement appreciated at the time of open tendon exploration or a patient's symptoms if there is uncertainty as to the extent of injury during clinical evaluation. Although the difficulty in determining the percentage of tendon involvement in a partial tendon laceration has been demonstrated [50], multiple investigators have concluded that partial lacerations involving less than 60% of the tendon's cross-sectional area should not be repaired. Debridement of the injured tendon may be indicated if the laceration site presents a risk for tendon triggering or entrapment and tendons lacerated greater than 60% should be repaired, typically with a core suture and epitendinous suture repair, as appropriate, to minimize the risk of tendon triggering, entrapment, or rupture [51, 52].

Delayed Repair/Reconstruction

Consideration for tendon reconstruction should account for the level of injury and the functional goals of the individual in the setting of a delayed presentation of flexor tendon injury. The time from injury and the level of tendon retraction will influence whether a primary repair is considered; the length-tension relationship of the musculotendinous unit will be altered by the retracted stump resulting in higher risks of contracture and secondary complications such as the adverse effects of quadrigia. Also, a loss of the favorable gliding environment within the "empty" flexor sheath may require recreation of the potential gliding space through the use of a silicone tendon implant. Second-stage flexor tendon reconstruction is delayed until optimal conditions exist for grafting: (1) a supple and mature wound, free of signs of infection or soft-tissue compromise; (2) maximal recovery of passive digital motion to provide the greatest potential for restoring active motion following tendon reconstruction; and (3) patient compliance with therapy and postoperative care [37].

There are several considerations for reconstructing the flexor tendon-deficient digit. In the finger, patients with an FDP injury but an intact FDS tendon may consider staged flexor tendon grafting; however, procedures that involve excision of the injured FDP tendon (to reduce interference with FDS function) and either DIP joint arthrodesis or DIP joint tenodesis may provide reasonable outcomes [35]. The loss of DIP joint motion, however, may impact adversely the ability of certain position players. Importantly, while these DIP joint stabilization procedures remove the potential for independent FDP function, they are regarded as definitive procedures with consistent results. Typically, the DIP joint is stabilized in neutral or in a slightly flexed position of function. Staged flexor tendon reconstruction, however, typically involves considerable patient investment and commitment with multiple procedures with variable outcomes and, therefore, these factors should be discussed in detail with the patient preoperatively [37]. Similarly, in the thumb, reconstruction of the FPL tendon with intercalary grafting, ring finger FDS tendon transfer, or interphalangeal joint arthrodesis may be considered in light of the patient's underlying condition and expectations for recovery of function.

Injury Management: Post-Repair Rehabilitation

Post-repair rehabilitation protocols should emphasize several principles: (1) player education is essential to minimize the risk of postoperative repair site rupture and to maximize tendon function; (2) communication with the player, training staff, and therapist is imperative regarding the nature of the injury and the specific protocol to be used; (3) the timing for the initiation of post-repair rehabilitation is ideally between 3 and 5 days to reduce work of flexion; (4) the use of a low-force, high-excursion protocol will maximize tendon gliding, but minimize the risk of repair site failure [53, 54].

The timing for the return to unrestricted activity following flexor tendon repair is not well-defined; however, decisions should be guided by a recognition of the accrual of repair site strength with time and the influence of associated injuries. Typically, return to unrestricted activity is permitted between 4 and 6 months from surgical repair, although it is the author's preference to delay the release to unrestricted activity until 6 months post-repair, consistent with the recent recommendations of Ruchelsman et al. [55]. Associated injuries and treatments such as fracture of nerve repair may influence the timing of incremental rehabilitation strategies.

Despite well-intended protective splinting or casting of the injured extremity to facilitate early return to play, the high risk of repair site rupture persists due to the inability to restrict tensile forces created by the contracting muscle-tendon unit. Therefore, return to upper extremity contact sport and activities involving higher loading forces through the hand and wrist are not advised for 4–6 months. Throwing, catching, and batting all place high-tensile loads through the flexor system and should be restricted for 6 months from repair. Buddy-strapping of the injured digit to an adjacent digit will reduce the risk of inadvertent eccentric loading or passive extension of the isolated injured digit, particularly in the setting of peritendinous adhesion formation and the relative tethering of the affected tendon(s). A hand-based or forearm-based thermoplastic splint or cast may provide reasonable protection for the healing flexor tendon for non-contact (upper extremity) training activities that present low fall risk.

The indications for flexor tenolysis, typically considered at 4–6 months post-repair, include a failure to regain adequate active and independent gliding of the repaired tendon(s) and to restore functional activities despite achieving excellent passive digital motion. This demanding procedure requires close cooperation between the surgeon, patient/player, therapist, and training staff to ensure optimal outcomes [37].

Flexor Pulley Injury

Injury Classification

Injury to the flexor pulley system may be caused by a closed or an open injury. Often, the treatment of open injuries is considered in conjunction with flexor tendon injury repair; however, rarely, a longitudinal laceration of the digit may cause isolated injury to the retinacular pulley system, and treatment should be considered based on the preservation and / or reconstruction of the A2 and A4 pulleys, as described below.

Closed pulley injuries are rare in the general population, but these have been described more commonly in rock climbers, associated with the high forces placed on the pulley system with the demands of certain climbing maneuvers on the hands, such as with the hanging and crimping positions [28, 29, 56]. In the hanging position, all of the digital joints are resisting force in a flexed position (MCP, PIP, DIP), whereas in the crimp grip position, the DIP joints are hyperextended maximally, the PIP joints are flexed approximately 90°, and the MCP joints are extended. Previous analysis by Lin et al. [14] demonstrated maximum tear load of the A2 pulley to be approximately 400N although antagonistic forces acting on the A2 pulley may exceed these tolerances during the crimp grip position [28, 29, 56].

Nonsurgical Treatment

Typically, isolated, closed pulley ruptures are treated with nonsurgical management, supported by both biomechanical studies and outcomes evaluations [29]. Initial treatment with anti-inflammatory measures, activity restrictions, and emphasis on tendon gliding and range of motion to prevent stiffness or contracture is encouraged. Protective digital taping at the approximate level of the injured A2 or A4 pulley has been advocated in the recovery period, but also with return to strenuous lifting and grasping activities [57].

A case series involving isolated A4 pulley ruptures in the middle fingers of the throwing hands of four baseball pitchers has been reported [19]. In each of the reported injuries, A4 pulley ruptures were confirmed by MRI or dynamic ultrasound and treatment consisted of rest, anti-inflammatory modalities, and return to play in 6 weeks (1 player), 3 months (2 players), and 6 months (1 player). The injury mechanism was described as "repetitive extension force placed on an acutely flexed finger when throwing a fastball." The authors recommended return to play at between 6 and 12 weeks, "only after painless range of motion and proper rehabilitation of the throwing arm" and avoidance of corticosteroid injection during treatment, due to the potential adverse effects of pulley rupture and delayed tissue healing [19].

Surgical Treatment

Although treatment for isolated flexor pulley injuries is nonsurgical, injuries involving multiple pulley ruptures may require surgical recon-

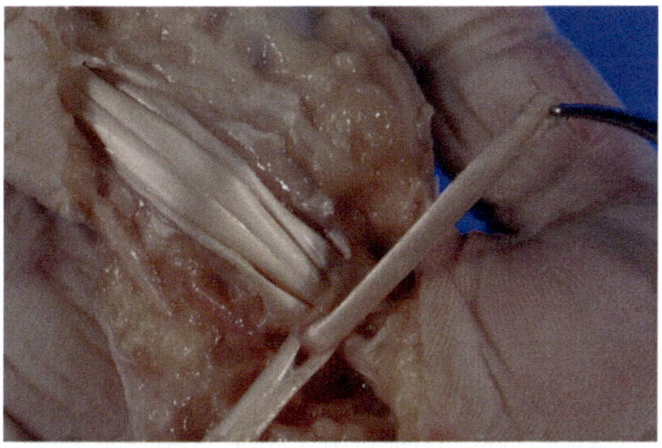

Fig. 13.10 Intraoperative photograph demonstrating an A2 pulley reconstruction using the first of two (side-by-side) palmaris longus tendon grafts, secured with a "belt-loop" configuration. (Reprinted with permission: © Leversedge FJ, 2004)

struction in order to restore biomechanical efficiency of the flexor system. Several reconstruction options exist which emphasize the restoration of the biomechanically important A2 and A4 pulleys [58] (Fig. 13.10). Consideration of ideal graft sources, such as an extrasynovial tendon (palmaris, plantaris) or intrasynovial tendon (excised FDS, single FDS slip, or extensor retinaculum) may take into account ease of harvest and resistance to tendon gliding [59, 60]. The A2 pulley reconstruction typically employs a graft passed volar to the extensor tendon apparatus, whereas during A4 pulley reconstruction the graft is passed dorsal to the terminal extensor tendon.

Post-Repair Rehabilitation

Postoperative protocols emphasize early, protected independent tendon gliding, avoiding resisted activity that could compromise the pulley repair. Tenodesis should be incorporated into early motion exercises to reduce forces applied to the repaired tissues; preoperative patient education regarding anticipated post-repair rehabilitation methods may improve patient understanding and compliance with therapy. Anti-edema modalities are critical for reducing the work of flexion associated with swelling in the first 3–5 days following surgery [61]. Supportive taping or use of a thermoplastic pulley ring is utilized for all activities for 3 months, and with higher loading activities until 6 months postoperatively.

Summary

In 1948, R. Guy Pulvertaft, a British surgeon, noted that regarding flexor tendon injuries: "it is not difficult to suture tendons and prepare the ground for sound union; the real problem is to obtain a freely sliding tendon capable of restoring good function" [62]. His observation almost 75 years ago highlights the challenges of flexor tendon injuries faced even today. Flexor tendon and pulley injuries in the baseball player present similar challenges to those same injuries in other athletes or non-athletes, however with the added complexity of a condition that influences directly one's ability to return to play, often conflicting with an obligate period of tendon healing. Advances in our understanding of the biology of tendon injury and repair and the potential application of adjuvant biologic treatments to accelerate tendon healing hold promise for improved therapies. The diagnosis and treatment, and ultimately the outcomes of flexor tendon injuries remain influenced greatly by a comprehensive understanding of pertinent anatomy, the timely recognition and treatment of the condition, and careful patient, training staff, and therapist education and communication in order to reduce the risk of adverse events during the recovery process and to maximize tendon sliding capable of restoring good function.

References

1. Kleinert HE, Verdan C. Report of the committee on tendon injuries (International Federation of Societies for Surgery of the Hand). J Hand Surg Am. 1983;8:794–8.
2. Leversedge FJ, Goldfarb CA, Boyer MI. A pocketbook manual of hand and upper extremity anatomy – Primus Manus. Philadelphia: Wolters-Kluwer/Lippincott Williams & Wilkins; 2010. p. 57–65.
3. Bilderback KK, Rayan GM. The septa of Legeau and Juvara: an anatomic study. J Hand Surg Am. 2004;29:494–9.

4. Chepla KJ, Goitz RJ, Fowler JR. Anatomy of the flexor digitorum profundus insertion. J Hand Surg Am. 2015;40(2):240–4.
5. Eyler DL, Markee JE. The anatomy and function of the intrinsic musculature of the fingers. J Bone Joint Surg. 1954;36A:1–9.
6. Smith RJ. Intrinsic muscles of the fingers: function, dysfunction, and surgical reconstruction. AAOS Instr Course Lect. 1975:200–20.
7. Eladoumikdachi F, Valkov PL, Thomas J, Netscher DT. Anatomy of the intrinsic hand muscles revisited: part II. Lumbricals. Plast Reconstr Surg. 2002;110:1225–31.
8. Lundborg G, Rank F. Experimental intrinsic healing of flexor tendons based upon synovial fluid nutrition. J Hand Surg Am. 1978;3:21–31.
9. Manske PR, Lesker PA. Flexor tendon nutrition. Hand Clin. 1985;1:13–24.
10. Doyle JR, Blythe WF. Anatomy of the flexor tendon sheath and pulleys of the thumb. J Hand Surg Am. 1977;2:149–51.
11. Manske PR, Lesker PA. Palmar aponeurosis pulley. J Hand Surg Am. 1983;8:259–63.
12. Doyle JR. Anatomy of the flexor tendon sheath and pulley system. J Hand Surg Am. 1988;13:473–84.
13. Idler RS. Anatomy and biomechanics of the digital flexor tendons. Hand Clin. 1985;1:3–11.
14. Lin GT, Amadio PC, An KN, Cooney WP, Chao EY. Biomechanical analysis of finger flexor pulley reconstruction. J Hand Surg Br. 1989;14:278–82.
15. Tang JB. Release of the A4 pulley to facilitate zone II flexor tendon repair. J Hand Surg Am. 2014;39(11):2300–7.
16. Ben IK, Elliot D. "Venting" or partial lateral release of the A2 and A4 pulleys after repair of zone 2 flexor tendon injuries. J Hand Surg Br. 1998;23(5):649–54.
17. Ochiai N, Matsui T, Miyaji N, Merklin RJ, Hunter JM. Vascular anatomy of flexor tendons. I. Vincular systems and blood supply of the profundus tendon in the digital sheath. J Hand Surg. 1979;4:321–30.
18. Leversedge FJ, Ditsios K, Goldfarb CA, Silva MJ, Gelberman RH, Boyer MI. Vascular anatomy of the human flexor digitorum profundus tendon insertion. J Hand Surg Am. 2002;27A:806–12.
19. Lourie GM, Hamby Z, Raasch WG, Chandler JB, Porter JL. Annular flexor pulley injuries in professional baseball pitchers. A case series. Am J Sports Med. 2011;39(2):421–4.
20. Barrera CM, Damodar D, Henry S, Dong F, Jose J. Lumbrical tear in Major League Baseball player throwing 4-seam fastballs. A case report. JBJS Case Connect. 2019;9:e0115.
21. Crosby EB, Linscheid RL. Rupture of the flexor profundus tendon of the ring finger secondary to ancient fracture of the hook of the hamate. Review of the literature and report of two cases. J Bone Joint Surg Am. 1974;56:1076–8.
22. Milek MA, Boulas HJ. Flexor tendon ruptures secondary to hamate hook fractures. J Hand Surg Am. 1990;15(5):740–4.
23. Austin GJ, Leslie BM, Ruby LK. Variations of the flexor digitorum superficialis of the small finger. J Hand Surg Am. 1989;14A:262–7.
24. Boyes JH. Bunnel's surgery of the hand. 4th ed. Philadelphia: JB Lippincott; 1964. p. 256–60.
25. Reimann AF, Daseler EH, Anson BJ, Beaton LE. The palmaris longus muscle and tendon: a study of 1600 extremities. Anat Rec. 1944;89:495.
26. Cohen SB, Chhabra AB, Anderson MW, Pannunzio ME. Use of ultrasound in determining treatment for avulsion of the flexor digitorum profundus (rugger Jersey finger): a case report. Am J Orthop. 2004;33(11):546–9.
27. Alvarez DA, Ballard DH, Carroll T, Frilot C, Simoncini AA. Ultrasound localization of lacerated flexor tendon ends in the hand: a cadaveric study. Skelet Radiol. 2019;48(12):1941–6.
28. King EA, Lien JR. Flexor tendon pulley injuries in rock climbers. Hand Clin. 2017;33(1):141–8.
29. Schoffl VR, Schoffl I. Injuries to the finger flexor pulley system in rock climbers: current concepts. J Hand Surg Am. 2006;31(4):647–54.
30. Renfree KJ, Dahiya N, Kransdorf MJ, Zhang N, Patel KA, Drace PA. Comparative accuracy of 1.5T MRI, 3T MRI, and static ultrasound in diagnosis of small gaps in repaired flexor tendons. A cadaveric study. J Hand Surg Am. 2021;46(4):287–94.
31. Kumar BA, Tolat AR, Threepuraneni G, Jones B. The role of magnetic resonance imaging in late presentation of isolated injuries of the flexor digitorum profundus tendon in the finger. J Hand Surg Br. 2000;25:95–7.
32. Schellhammer F, Vantorre A. Semi-dynamic MRI of climbing-associated injuries of the finger. Skelet Radiol. 2019;48(9):1435–7.
33. Ferrier JA, Atkinson RE. Acute flexor superficialis avulsion. J Hand Surg Am. 1993;18A:514–5.
34. Tan V, Mundanthanam G, Weiland AJ. Traumatic simultaneous rupture of both flexor tendons in a finger of an athlete. Am J Orthop. 2005;34(10):505–7.
35. Leddy JP, Packer JW. Avulsion of the profundus tendon insertion in athletes. J Hand Surg Am. 1977;2: 66–9.
36. Robins PR, Dobyns JH. Avulsion of the insertion of the flexor digitorum profundus tendon associated with fracture of the distal phalanx. A brief review. In: American Academy of Orthopaedic Surgeons Symposium on tendon surgery in the hand. St. Louis: CV Mosby; 1975.
37. Boyer MI, Strickland JW, Engles DR, Sachar K, Leversedge FJ. Flexor tendon repair and rehabilitation: state of the art in 2002. J Bone Joint Surg Am. 2002;84:1684–706.
38. Sourmelis SG, McGrouther DA. Retrieval of the retracted flexor tendon. J Hand Surg Br. 1987;12: 109–11.
39. Malerich MM, Baird RA, McMaster W, et al. Permissible limits of flexor digitorum profundus tendon advancement: an anatomical study. J Hand Surg Am. 1987;12:30.

40. Dovan TT, Ritty T, Ditsios K, Silva MJ, Kusano N, Gelberman RH. Flexor digitorum profundus tendon to bone tunnel repair: a vascularization and histologic study in canines. J Hand Surg Am. 2005;30:246–57.
41. Dovan TT, Gelberman RH, Kusano N, Calcaterra M, Silva MJ. Zone I flexor digitorum profundus repair: an ex-vivo biomechanical analysis of tendon to bone repair in cadavers. J Hand Surg Am. 2005;30:258–66.
42. McCallister WV, Ambrose HC, Katolik LI, Trumble TE. Comparison of pullout button versus suture anchor for zone I flexor tendon repair. J Hand Surg Am. 2006;31:246–51.
43. Matsuzaki H, Zaegel MA, Gelberman RH, Silva MJ. Effect of suture material and bone quality on the mechanical properties of zone I flexor tendon-bone reattachment with bone anchors. J Hand Surg Am. 2008;33:709–17.
44. Chu JY, Chen T, Awad HA, Elfar J, Hammert WC. Comparison of an all-inside suture technique with traditional pull-out suture and suture anchor repair techniques for flexor digitorum profundus attachment to bone. J Hand Surg Am. 2013;38:1084–90.
45. Kang N, Marsh D, Dewar D. The morbidity of the button-over-nail technique for zone 1 flexor tendon repairs. Should we still be using this technique? J Hand Surg Eur Vol. 2008;33:566–70.
46. Leversedge FJ, Laino D. Distal phalanx osteomyelitis complicating zone I flexor tendon repair with a non-pullout suture tied over a dorsal button: a report of two cases. JBJS Case Connect. 2014;4(3):e80–e4.
47. Bond S, Rust P, Boland M. The accommodation of bone anchors within the distal phalanx for repair of flexor digitorum profundus avulsions. J Hand Surg Am. 2019;44(11):986.e1–6.
48. Galano GJ, Jiang KN, Strauch RJ, Rosenwasser MP, Tang P. Inflammatory response with osteolysis related to a bioabsorbable anchor in the finger: a case report. Hand. (N.Y.). 2010;5(3):307–12.
49. Lalonde DH. Latest advances in wide awake hand surgery. Hand Clin. 2019;35(1):1–6.
50. Grewal R, Sotereanos DG, Rao U, Herndon JH, Woo SL. Bundle pattern of the flexor digitorum profundus tendon in zone II of the hand: a quantitative assessment of the size of a laceration. J Hand Surg Am. 1996;21:978–83.
51. Schlenker JD, Lister GD, Kleinert HE. Three complications of untreated partial laceration of flexor tendon – entrapment, rupture, and triggering. J Hand Surg Am. 1981;6:392–8.
52. McGeorge DD, Stilwell JH. Partial flexor tendon injuries: to repair or not. J Hand Surg Br. 1992;17:176–7.
53. Silva MJ, Brodt MD, Boyer MI, Morris TS, Dinopoulos H, Amiel D, Gelberman RH. Effects of increased in vivo excursion on digital range of motion and tendon strength following flexor tendon repair. J Orthop Res. 1999;17:777–83.
54. Boyer MI, Gelberman RH, Burns ME, Dinopoulos H, Hofem R, Silva MJ. Intrasynovial flexor tendon repair: an experimental study comparing low and high levels of in vivo force during rehabilitation in canines. J Bone Joint Surg Am. 2001;83:891–9.
55. Ruchelsman DE, Christoforou D, Wasserman B, Lee SK, Rettig ME. Avulsion injuries of the flexor digitorum profundus tendon. J Am Acad Orthop Surg. 2011;19:152–62.
56. Schweizer A. Biomechanical properties of the crimp grip position in rock climbers. J Biomech. 2001;34:217–23.
57. Schöffl I, Einwag F, Strecker W, Hennig F, Schöffl V. Impact of taping after finger flexor tendon pulley ruptures in rock climbers. J Appl Biomech. 2007;23:52–62.
58. Seiler JG 3rd, Leversedge FJ. Digital flexor sheath: repair and reconstruction of the annular pulleys and membranous sheath. J South Orthop Assoc. 2000;9:81–90.
59. Uchiyama S, Amadio PC, Coert JH, Berglund LJ, An KN. Gliding resistance of extrasynovial and intrasynovial tendons through the A2 pulley. J Bone Joint Surg Am. 1997;79(2):219–24.
60. Seiler JG, Uchiyama S, Ellis F, Amadio PC, Gelberman RH, An KN. Reconstruction of the flexor pulley. The effect of the tension and source of the graft in an in vitro dog model. J Bone Joint Surg Am. 1998;80(5):699–703.
61. Zhao C, Amadio PC, Tanaka T, Yang C, Ettema AM, Zobitz ME, An KN. Short-term assessment of optimal timing for postoperative rehabilitation after flexor digitorum profundus tendon repair in a canine model. J Hand Ther. 2005;18(3):322–9.
62. Pulvertaft RG. Repair of tendon injuries in the hand. Ann R Coll Surg. 1948;3:3.

Extensor Tendon Injuries of the Digits: Mallet Finger, Boutonnière Deformity, and Sagittal Band Disruption

14

Jacob W. Brubacher, E. Bruce Toby, and Jake S. Enos

Extensor Tendon Injuries of the Digits

The focus of this chapter will be on injuries to the extensor mechanism in the digits – focusing on mallet finger, boutonnière deformity, and sagittal band disruption. Hand and wrist injuries are quite common in baseball and can lead to long-term morbidity. A large study performed over 10 years investigating the incidence of hand and wrist injuries in various sports, concluded that of the greater than 8000 injuries studied, roughly 9% of these were attributed to the hand and wrist. Of these, 25% were related to baseball, second to only roller hockey [1]. It is imperative that these injuries are appropriately identified as early splinting and rehabilitation can prevent the need for surgical intervention or long-term deformity.

Mallet Finger Also Known as "Baseball Finger"

The terms "mallet finger" and "baseball finger" are descriptors used to describe a specific injury to the terminal extensor tendon. Mallet injuries are the most common tendon injury in athletes and are common in baseball players [2]. One reason for the high frequency in baseball players is the common mechanism in which a ball strikes the actively extended distal phalanx causing a forced flexion moment at the distal interphalangeal joint (DIP) (Fig. 14.1). This forced flexion moment overpowers the actively engaged terminal extensor tendon that is attached at the dorsal base of the distal phalanx causing a tendinous avulsion or an avulsion associated with a bony fragment [2]. Baseball players are at high risk for this injury due to their frequent catching of a ball traveling at high speed with risk of impaction to the fingertip.

Commonly, the player will present with pain and swelling at the dorsal aspect of the DIP joint where the tendinous or bony avulsion has occurred. The finger may be held with the DIP joint in flexion due to the unopposed pull of the flexor digitorum profundus. On examination, there will be decreased active extension of the DIP joint due to the lack of attachment of the terminal extensor tendon [1, 2]. Passive range of motion is typically normal, and this difference between the active and passive motion defines the amount of extension lag. The skin should also be inspected for bruising and abrasion/laceration, and adjacent digits should be inspected for injury.

These injuries can be divided into soft tissue mallet injuries where the tendon is avulsed from the bone and bony mallet injuries where a piece of bone is avulsed with the tendon remaining

J. W. Brubacher (✉) · E. B. Toby · J. S. Enos
Department of Orthopedic Surgery, The University of Kansas Medical Center, Kansas City, KS, USA
e-mail: jbrubacher@kumc.edu

G. M. Lourie (ed.), *Hand and Wrist Injuries in Baseball*,
https://doi.org/10.1007/978-3-030-81659-9_14

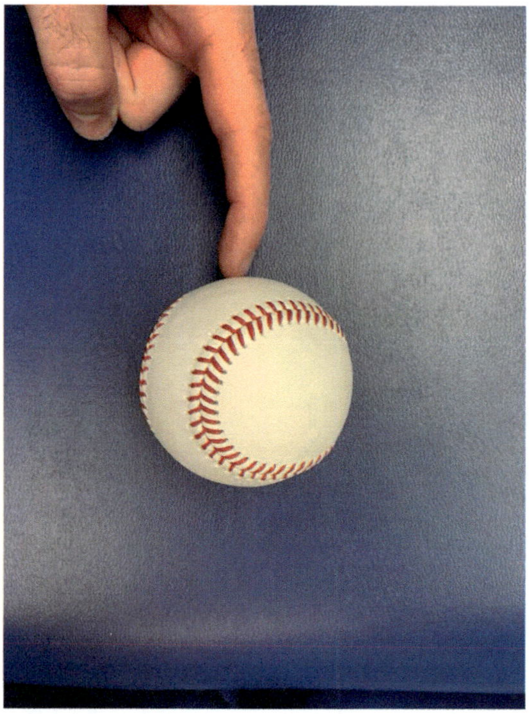

Fig. 14.1 Example of direct impact to distal phalanx as a common mechanism of mallet injury in baseball

attached to this fragment. Plain radiographs should be obtained of all suspected mallet injuries.

PA and lateral radiographs are usually sufficient with particular attention focused on the dorsal and proximal aspect of the distal phalanx [2]. If there is an associated bony fragment, the injury can be further classified based on the characteristics of the dorsal fragment. The lateral radiograph is used to classify the fragment avulsed as either a small fleck fragment, a large fragment (large defined as greater than 1/3 of the articular surface of the distal phalanx), or a large fragment with associated volar subluxation of the distal phalanx at the DIP [2]. The importance of thoroughly evaluating the plain radiographs, in particular the lateral view, is imperative as these findings can change treatment indications and ultimately patient outcome. These radiographs can also be used as a baseline for clinical monitoring throughout the course of recovery.

Treatment is largely dependent upon the abovementioned classification of these injuries. The vast majority of these injuries are closed but it is important to mention that open lacerations do occur. These open injuries should have irrigation and debridement and repair of the extensor mechanism. Surgical repairs of lacerations of the distal extensor are challenging due to the thinness of the terminal tendon. Surgeons can consider suture techniques that include the skin in the tendon repair to increase strength. Transarticular pinning of the DIP is typically necessary to protect the repair postoperatively.

Soft tissue mallet injuries with an intact soft tissue envelope can be treated nonoperatively with DIP extension splinting for 6–8 weeks [3]. Classically, nonoperative extension splinting is prescribed for 6 weeks in bony mallet injuries and 8 weeks in soft tissue mallets. The patient is reexamined at the 6-week mark for assessment of DIP extension strength and range of motion. Extension lag is evaluated and a cutoff of 20° is frequently used to determine whether the patient should continue with DIP extension splinting full time for an additional 2–6 weeks [2, 3]. Full time extension splinting protocol is followed by active range of motion of the DIP, protective DIP taping with Coban for return to sport, and nighttime extension splinting for an additional 4 weeks.

Studies investigating splint style and subsequent outcome concluded that style and cost of splint did not have an impact on patient outcome. Patient compliance was most closely related to good outcome [3]. An important consideration for DIP extension splinting is ensuring the DIP joint is adequately immobilized in extension and that the proximal interphalangeal joint (PIP) is left free for active motion [2]. Additionally, the splint should not be placed too tightly as to restrict microvascular flow or with the DIP joint in a position of hyperextension as this can lead to skin necrosis.

It is difficult for many position players to return to play with rigid DIP extension splinting. Pitchers on the dominant side will be quite limited by the restricted flexion of the DIP joint and unlikely to be able to compete. A glove hand injury can be significantly more rigidly immobilized and play is likely possible. Our preferred method is utilizing the SAM type metal/foam composite splint cut to comfortably cover the middle and distal phalanx (Fig. 14.2). This splint can easily be modulated in terms of rigidity by creating a concavity – increasing the concavity increases the rigidity. Position players may require more malleable splints in their glove hands to allow for required dexterity. For position players, the throwing hand is most hindered by immobilizing the index and long finger. The degree of immobilization that is tolerated while maintaining high performance will need to be individualized. The ring and small finger play more of a role in power grip and therefore will affect batting performance. Treatment here must be individualized to allow for performance.

Although indications for nonoperative treatment of mallet fingers are generally straightforward, surgical indications are more difficult to find consensus. Even with subluxation of the volar fragment, nonoperative treatment has

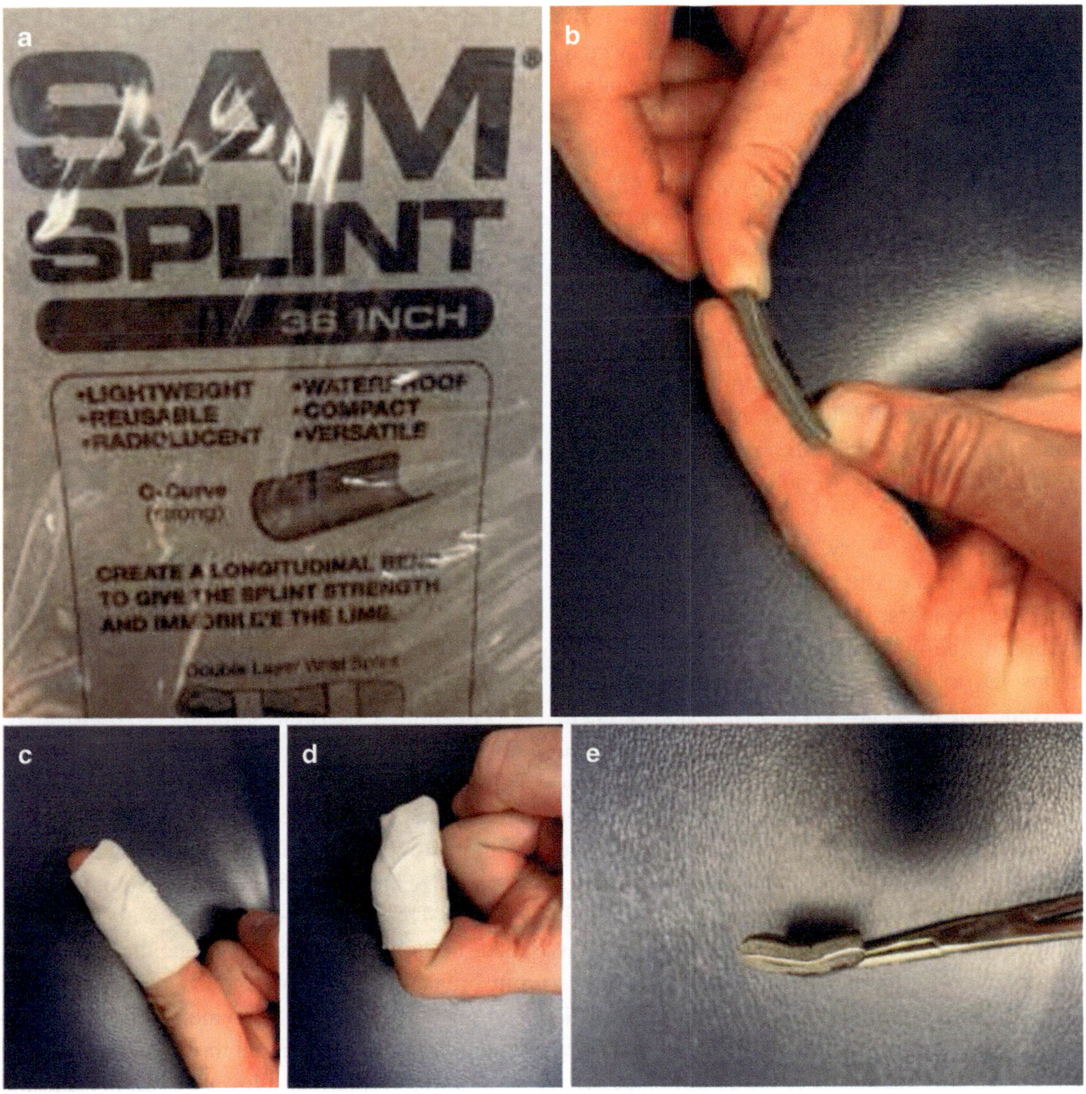

Fig. 14.2 (**a**) Example of SAM splint material in packaging. (**b**) Fitting a piece of SAM splint to middle and distal phalanx for immobilization. (**c**) Affixing the SAM splint to the digit. (**d**) Allowing continued range of motion of the PIP joint. (**e**) Introducing concavity to increase rigidity of SAM splint

shown acceptable results due to significant remodeling capability in this joint [4]. However, in high-level baseball players the restoration of anatomy and return to previous level of function play a central role in considering operative intervention.

If surgery for a large bony mallet injury is performed, a Kirschner wire (K-wire) is used to secure the volar fragment in a reduced position and acts as an internal splint. A variety of methods have been utilized for reduction of the dorsal bony fragment without clear consensus on superior results. Extension block pinning is a well-known and reliable method [5]. A pin is placed at a 45° angle into the head of the middle phalanx with the DIP flexed. A second pin is placed distal to proximal into the distal phalanx and then used to fix the joint in full extension. The 45° pin blocks the dorsal fragment in a near anatomical position. Other methods include using screws, suture anchors, or suture button fixation of the dorsal fracture fragment [2, 3]. At the conclusion of fixation, joint congruity at the DIP joint should be achieved utilizing a lateral plain radiograph. The DIP joint immobilization is typically maintained for 6 weeks while the fracture fragment is given an opportunity to achieve osseous union and joint stability.

As with any injury, a thorough discussion should take place with players educating them on the risks, benefits, and typical outcomes of the proposed treatment plan. The player should be counseled that even with excellent compliance and outcome they can expect a 10° extensor lag at the DIP joint. Additionally, a "bump" over the DIP joint is typical and can have associated tenderness for weeks to months [2]. Off-season or early season, one can consider more aggressive treatment with full-time splinting and possible removal from play until treatment is completed. Delayed intervention may be considered as nonoperative protocols have had successful results when initiated months after the injury date [6]. This may allow players to delay their treatment until after the conclusion of the season. Decision to delay treatment must be considered carefully in the context of player position, location of the injured finger, bony or soft tissue injury, PIP hyperextension, and player expectations and preferences.

The player should be counseled that without treatment, or with incompletely followed treatment recommendations, the finger may be permanently held in a flexed position at the DIP. This is a consequence of lack of terminal extensor continuity which may cause dysfunction at the PIP joint. This resultant hyperextension at the PIP joint and flexion at the DIP is termed a "swan neck" deformity and is caused by dorsal migration of the lateral bands. This deformity can lead to significant disability as PIP function is critical for hand function. This deformity may require splinting or surgical intervention if function is significantly altered. Chronic mallet fingers may be treated with a central slip tenotomy or the salvage procedure of an arthrodesis [7].

Mallet injuries have wide range in the timing and ability to return to play. If a player is able to compete with a DIP extension splint they may be able to return to play immediately. This will depend greatly on hand dominance, specific finger injured, and the player's position. If the player's position, in combination with the specific digit injured, makes them unable to compete, then a treatment and rehabilitation assignment is necessary. Consideration may also be given to season length and timing of injury because, as mentioned above, chronic injuries up to 3 months from injury may do well with a nonoperative treatment protocol [8].

Full-time extension splinting is quite challenging for the actively competing player. Percutaneous pinning of the DIP joint can be an option for mallet finger care in baseball players. It may allow play sooner, with greater ease wearing a glove and protects the player from noncompliance. This strategy does come with increased risks of complications, including infection and pin breakage. Since pin breakage is a potential complication, oblique placement of the transarticular pin with penetration through both cortices is advisable. This will allow easy removal in the case of a broken pin. These buried pins are typically maintained for 6–8 weeks.

Central Slip Injury and Boutonnière Deformity

Boutonnière deformity describes an extensor mechanism imbalance of one or multiple of the second through fifth digits. This is characterized by a flexion posture at the PIP joint with an associated hyperextension deformity at the DIP joint. In contrast to the mallet deformity discussed above, boutonnière deformity is a relatively rare occurrence in baseball players [9]. To understand the acquired deformity, it is pertinent to first understand the extensor mechanism and how tendon disruption leads to altered biomechanics and subsequent digital deformity.

At the level of the PIP joint, the site of pathology leading to boutonnière deformity, the extensor mechanism is rather complex with both intrinsic and extrinsic contributions working in concert to perform fluid, controlled digital extension. The extrinsic extensor tendons enter the digits dorsally and are stabilized at the metacarpophalangeal joint (MCP) by the sagittal bands. These tendons continue distally and trifurcate over the proximal phalanx. The central portion, with contributions from the interossei and lumbricals, forms the central slip. The central slip inserts on the dorsal aspect of the base of middle phalanx of each of the fingers to act as the primary extensor of the PIP joint [10]. The insertion lies just proximal to the dorsally based triangular ligament which acts as a support and dorsal restraint to the adjacent lateral bands. When the triangular ligament becomes attenuated, these lateral bands are no longer dorsally constrained and undergo volar migration which is a key component of the boutonnière deformity.

As outlined, these structures act in concert to ensure continued extensor mechanism balance. In classic boutonnière deformity the initial insult is that of a traumatic injury to the central slip, typically of the avulsion type [10]. This injury is frequently caused by a hyperflexion moment at the PIP joint at which point the central slip insertional force is overcome by forced flexion and is torn off the middle phalanx [9, 10] (Fig. 14.3). Additionally, volar PIP dislocations are frequently associated with central slip injuries. Less

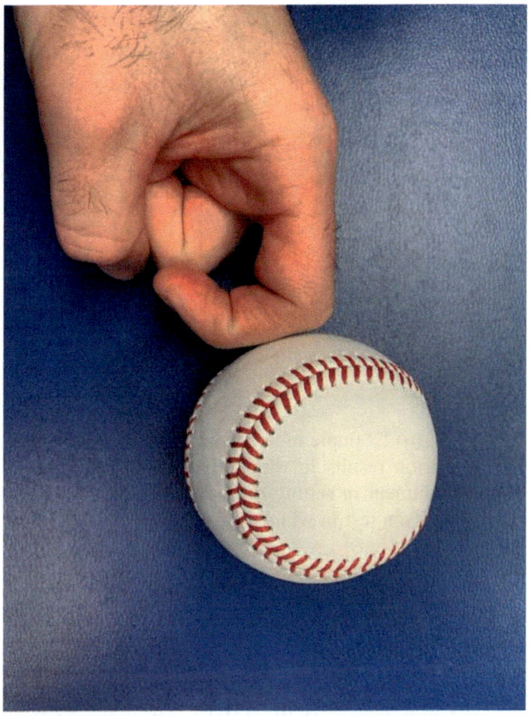

Fig. 14.3 Impaction injury placing PIP in a position of hyperflexion that could lead to central slip injury

frequently, these injuries can be caused by a penetrating injury or laceration over the dorsal base of the middle phalanx and the tendinous central slip insertion is lacerated. With respect to baseball players, this injury most commonly occurs when a ball "jams" a finger or when sliding into a base and the digit is forced into a hyperflexion position.

Given the lower incidence of injury, and the frequently innocuous injury mechanism, training staff must maintain a high index of suspicion for these injuries when athletes present with a chief complaint of a "jammed finger." Players presenting with a chronic injury may present with the classic deformity – flexion contracture at the PIP joint with associated hyperextension deformity at the DIP joint. The more difficult diagnosis is in the acute setting of pain and swelling. Early diagnosis and treatment of a central slip injury can prevent complications and more involved intervention at a later time.

One physical exam maneuver that can be used to assess the integrity of the central slip is the

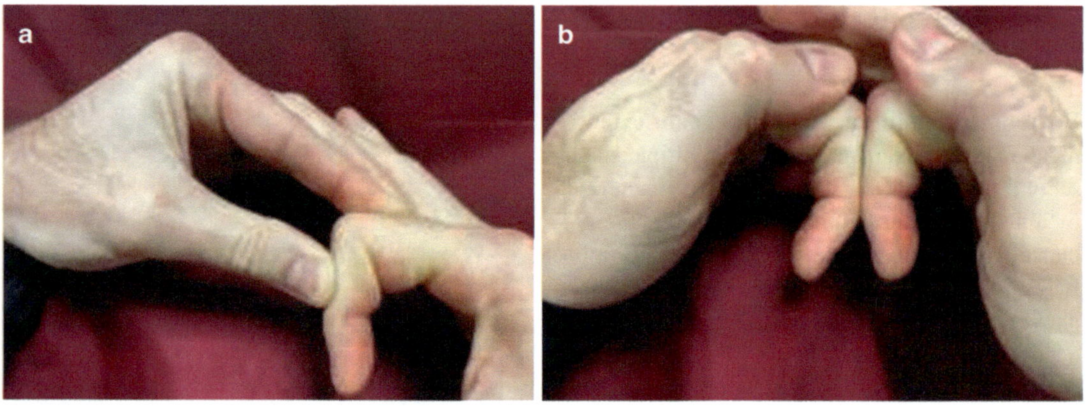

Fig. 14.4 (**a**) Example of abnormal Elson test – resisted PIP extension results in rigid DIP secondary to lateral band recruitment in setting of disrupted central slip. (**b**) Modified Elson test in which two digits are flexed to 90° at the PIP joint and the dorsal aspects are abutted. The patient is instructed to extend the PIP bilaterally and, as demonstrated, the digit on the left has a rigid DIP joint in comparison to the normal, flaccid DIP on the right

Elson test (Fig. 14.4). This test is performed by placing the PIP joint in a position of 90° of flexion and asking the patient to extend the finger against resistance. If the DIP joint remains flaccid, this indicates that the central slip is intact and exerting force on the middle phalanx. In contrast, if the DIP is rigid and extended, this indicates the lateral bands are being recruited to extend the finger. Rigid DIP hyperextension on Elson test confirms central slip incompetence [1, 9]. In the acute setting, the provider can consider a digital nerve block to help with the test without pain confounding the exam.

Orthogonal radiographs of the involved digit should be obtained on initial presentation. These should be assessed for osseous abnormality, specifically at the dorsal proximal middle phalanx in the form of avulsed bone fragment or volar subluxation of the middle phalanx on the proximal phalanx. A true boutonnière must be distinguished from a pseudoboutonniere which is a flexion contracture of the PIP with an intact central slip. These also present after a jamming injury with swelling and pain. However, there is no hyperextension of the DIP and the Elson test is negative. A pseudoboutonniere is typically treated by progressive splinting and occasionally volar plate release.

In the setting of an acute closed central slip injury, management is similar to that of mallet injury in that splinting is typically first-line treatment. The PIP joint is placed in a position of full extension to allow the central slip to heal. The DIP joint is left free to allow motion which maintains the lateral bands in a dorsal position and prevents volar migration and formation of the boutonnière deformity. This splinting is done full time for a period of 6 weeks followed by a period of nighttime splinting for an additional 6 weeks [10]. If compliance with bracing is a concern, pinning of the PIP in extension can be considered. If this intervention is desired, a buried, oblique K-wire traversing the PIP joint would be the recommended treatment. We typically utilize a 0.045 K-wire that exits both the cortex of the proximal and middle phalanx. In case of pin breakage, the pin should be able to be removed both proximally and distally. The pinned PIP joint would be protected with an orthoplast clamshell brace during limited training activities. This treatment comes with increased risks of complications but does improve compliance and alleviates skin concerns with full-time splint wear.

Patients with large osseous avulsion fragments, open injuries, or PIP fracture-dislocation are typically recommended for operative management. Surgical interventions include, but are not limited to, acute central slip repair, open reduction and internal fixation of avulsion fragments, and suture anchor repair. Frequently, a

K-wire is placed obliquely across the PIP joint postoperatively as a form of internal splinting for a period of 4–6 weeks with subsequent removal. A myriad of surgical repair and reconstruction techniques have been described and generally report high levels of success [11, 12]. Surgical repairs or reconstructions carry risk of stiffness, particularly limited flexion, which can be problematic to baseball players. Many patients in the postoperative period will maintain a small degree of extensor lag at the PIP; however, this is infrequently clinically apparent or functionally limiting.

In comparison to the acute setting of central slip disruption, chronic boutonnière deformity presents a different challenge to that of the treating physician. A widely accepted classification system, the Burton classification, is used to characterize the degree of chronicity and help guide treatment. Stage I is a boutonnière deformity that is defined by ability to passively correct the flexion contracture at the PIP joint. Stage II involves extensor mechanism contracture that does not allow the joint to passively correct out of flexion deformity; however, it does not involve the PIP joint itself. Stage III includes a noncorrectable contracture; however, it also includes contracture of the volar plate and collateral ligaments with intra-articular fibrosis. Stage IV includes these findings of stage III with the addition of PIP joint degenerative change, that is, arthritis [13].

Stage I and II injuries can be trialed with nonoperative therapy in the form of serial casting to attempt correction of PIP flexion contracture. If this is unsuccessful, which unfortunately is frequently the case, reconstructive intervention with tendon rebalancing techniques can be considered. This is performed in combination with joint contracture release [1]. An involved preoperative discussion with the patient is of utmost importance in this scenario, especially those patients that are high-level baseball players. Many of these rebalancing techniques may sacrifice flexor function in an attempt to regain extensor function. With these athletes requirement to grip the ball and/or bat, a thorough discussion of expected outcomes should occur as to prevent dissatisfaction in the postoperative period. One such procedure that does not sacrifice flexor function is that of the Fowler tenotomy, also known as Dolphin tenotomy, which involves a distally based extensor tenotomy [1]. This tenotomy reduces the hyperextension force at the DIP joint and through partial retraction gains tension for the extensor mechanism at the PIP joint.

Staged reconstructions are also performed which are more involved but attempt to address deformity in a stepwise manner. Performing the operation utilizing local anesthesia allows interval functional assessment until the surgeon is satisfied with the result. One such staged reconstruction was described by Curtis et al. and begins with performing an extensor and transverse retinacular ligament tenolysis [14]. If desired extension is not obtained, stage II is performed which includes sectioning of the transverse retinacular ligament. Stage III includes the abovementioned Fowler tenotomy and is performed when an extensor lag persists despite sectioning the transverse retinacular ligament. Finally, in stage IV, the central tendon is advanced on the middle phalanx and repaired [14].

Return to play for players with active treatment of a central slip injury is challenging. Player position, digit involved, and hand dominance all factor into a joint decision between player and physician with respect to return to play. Competitive play with a PIP splinted or pinned in full extension would be unusual. Full-time splinting or pinning would be continued for 6 weeks, after which players would begin a return-to-play protocol based on position. Splint may be continued at night for an additional 4–6 weeks and buddy taping for comfort and protection during play can be considered.

Sagittal Band Injury

Sagittal band injury, also known as "boxer's knuckle" secondary to its classic presentation in athletes participating in this sport, is a zone V extensor tendon injury. The injury typically presents after a direct blow to the dorsal aspect of the MCP joint [9]. These injuries can also be sustained with forced radial or ulnar deviation of the

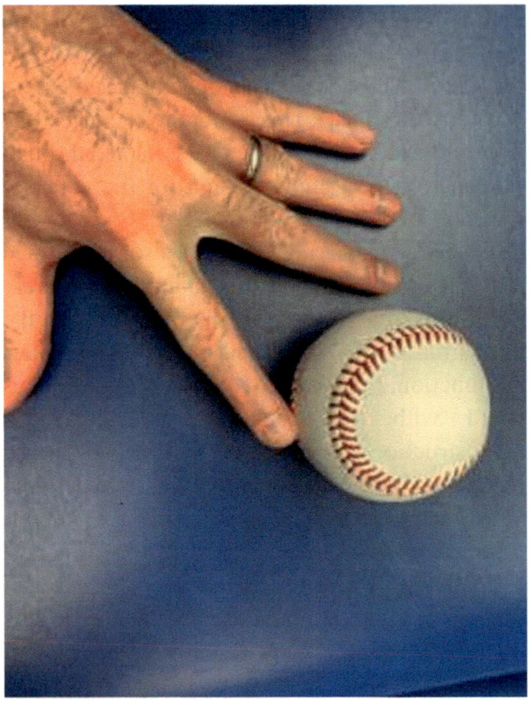

Fig. 14.5 First and second digits placed into radial deviation at the MCP joint that could lead to disruption of the stabilizing sagittal bands

digit causing tears of the supporting sagittal bands and collateral ligaments of the MCP joint (Fig. 14.5). Injury to the extensor mechanism is most common in zone V over the MCP joint, and it is postulated that this is secondary to the prominence of the metacarpal head [3]. The incidence in baseball is less well defined, and it is certainly less frequent than one might expect in professional fighting. However, it certainly has a presence in baseball and the training staff should be versed in classification and treatment algorithms. Sagittal band injuries seen in athletes are different than sagittal band ruptures seen in the elderly or rheumatoid patients. Athletes will more commonly have partial sagittal band injuries without frank extensor dislocation. Additionally, with a traumatic mechanism both radial and ulnar sagittal bands can be injured and damage to the capsule and joint surface is common.

The sagittal bands are ligamentous structures located at the ulnar and radial aspect of each MCP joint with attachments dorsally to the extensor hood and palmarly to the volar plate with a course between these structures. The sagittal bands serve to stabilize the extrinsic extensor tendons over the dorsal aspect of the MCP joint to prevent subluxation or dislocation during range of motion. Classically, the long finger is most commonly affected given that the third metacarpal head is most prominent with a closed fist and thus a direct blow is likely to affect this joint first.

In baseball, one can postulate that a common mechanism involves direct blow from the ball itself either while batting or fielding. As expected, following blunt trauma to the MCP joint, players will present with complaints of pain and swelling about the MCP joint and will likely report a specific trauma. The most common acute presentation is pain; however, players may describe a characteristic "snapping" or "clicking" when flexing and extending at the MCP joint. This sensation is attributed to and explained anatomically by the disruption of the sagittal band. These bands stabilize the extensor tendon over the central dorsal aspect of the MCP joint and when ruptured allow either radial or ulnar subluxation or dislocation of the tendon. The tendon moves toward the opposite direction of the ruptured band which can lead to the snapping sensation reported by patients.

Rayan and Murray classified these injuries into three categories. Type I injuries include sagittal band injuries without instability of the extensor tendon, type II are injuries with associated subluxation of the extensor mechanism, and type III are injuries with associated frank dislocation [14]. Patients with type II and III injuries may report a snapping or clicking. Patients with type III injuries may report an inability to extend the finger due to frank dislocation of the tendon to the intermetacarpal space with subsequent loss of extensor mechanical advantage (Table 14.1) Frank dislocation of the extrinsic tendon occurs most frequently with radial sagittal band injuries but is overall rare in athletes.

Diagnosis of these injuries is largely reliant upon clinical history and examination. It is our recommendation to obtain plain radiographs to rule out associated fracture which may alter treatment recommendations. If there is clinical

Table 14.1 Rayan and Murray classification widely accepted for the classification of sagittal band disruption

Rayan and Murray classification of sagittal band disruption [15]	
Type I	No subluxation or dislocation of extensor tendon
Type II	Subluxation but not dislocation of extensor tendon
Type III	Frank dislocation of extensor tendon

uncertainty, consideration can be given to obtaining advanced imaging in the form of ultrasonography or MRI. Ultrasound or dynamic MRI can be useful in obtaining MCP images with the joint in a position of flexion and extension to evaluate the degree of subluxation or dislocation present [9].

Treatment of these injuries largely depends on the chronicity as well as the clinical findings, that is, stability of the EDC. Like many injuries of the extensor mechanism, a division is made into those patients presenting with an acute injury and those that are chronic. Injuries presenting within 1 month of occurrence are generally considered to be acute and potentially up to 6 weeks post-injury. Patients presenting after 6 weeks from their time of injury are considered to have a chronic injury.

Patients presenting with an acute injury can be trialed with a period of nonoperative management with generally good results [16]. In patients with type I injuries, no subluxation of the EDC tendon, management can consist of buddy taping the affected digit to an adjacent digit for a period of 4–6 weeks with subsequent taping during sport [1]. For patients with type II and III, Catalano et al. advocate the use of a yoke or relative motion splint (Fig. 14.6). This splint places the injured MCP in a position of 25–35° of additional extension relative to adjacent MCP joints. They report good results with an 8-week splinting course with one of 11 patients requiring subsequent operative intervention [17].

Operative intervention should be considered given the inconsistent results of nonoperative management in those patients with type II and III injuries. Potential for failure of splinting makes return to play increasingly uncertain. Operative intervention may provide a more reliable time-frame for return to sport. Operative care for boxer's knuckle involves exploration and repair of the sagittal band which is often partially torn involving primarily the superficial fibers of the sagittal band. Joint exploration may also be considered as capsular and articular injuries are frequently seen. The majority of these injuries in baseball players do not include tendon instability and direct repair of the sagittal band is sufficient. In the rare chronic injury, release of the intact, contracted band may be necessary to realign the tendon. If the tissue quality is poor and the repair not reliable, a slip of the extensor tendon can be looped around the affected side collateral ligament for stabilization of the extensor mechanism dorsally.

With respect to return to play, recommendations are made on a situation-by-situation basis with symptom severity and degree of injury factoring into the treating physician's decision. Patients with minimal discomfort and type I injuries without subluxation or dislocation of their extensor tendon may participate to tolerance. Buddy taping may be helpful for comfort and protection. Patients cleared for return to play may consider different strategies for fielding and batting. Players may employ buddy loops for batting but prefer to go without while fielding. Kinesiology taping can be helpful for some players and may be worn throughout the competition (Fig. 14.7).

Those players presenting with type II or III injuries are more frequently operative candidates given uncertain success with attempted nonoperative management. Postoperatively, players are typically recommended to abstain from play for approximately 8 weeks and are recommended for additional splinting or taping until the 12-week mark. In regard to postoperative rehabilitation, Merritt has proposed a program of relative motion splinting that starts patients moving as soon as 3 to 5 days postoperatively in an effort to accelerate return to play [18, 19]. Patients are allowed to actively range immediately in the relative motion splint, and thus players could return to training or play rather quickly. As mentioned previously, affected hand and digit as well as ability to compete at high level while wearing the splint will factor in to return to play time.

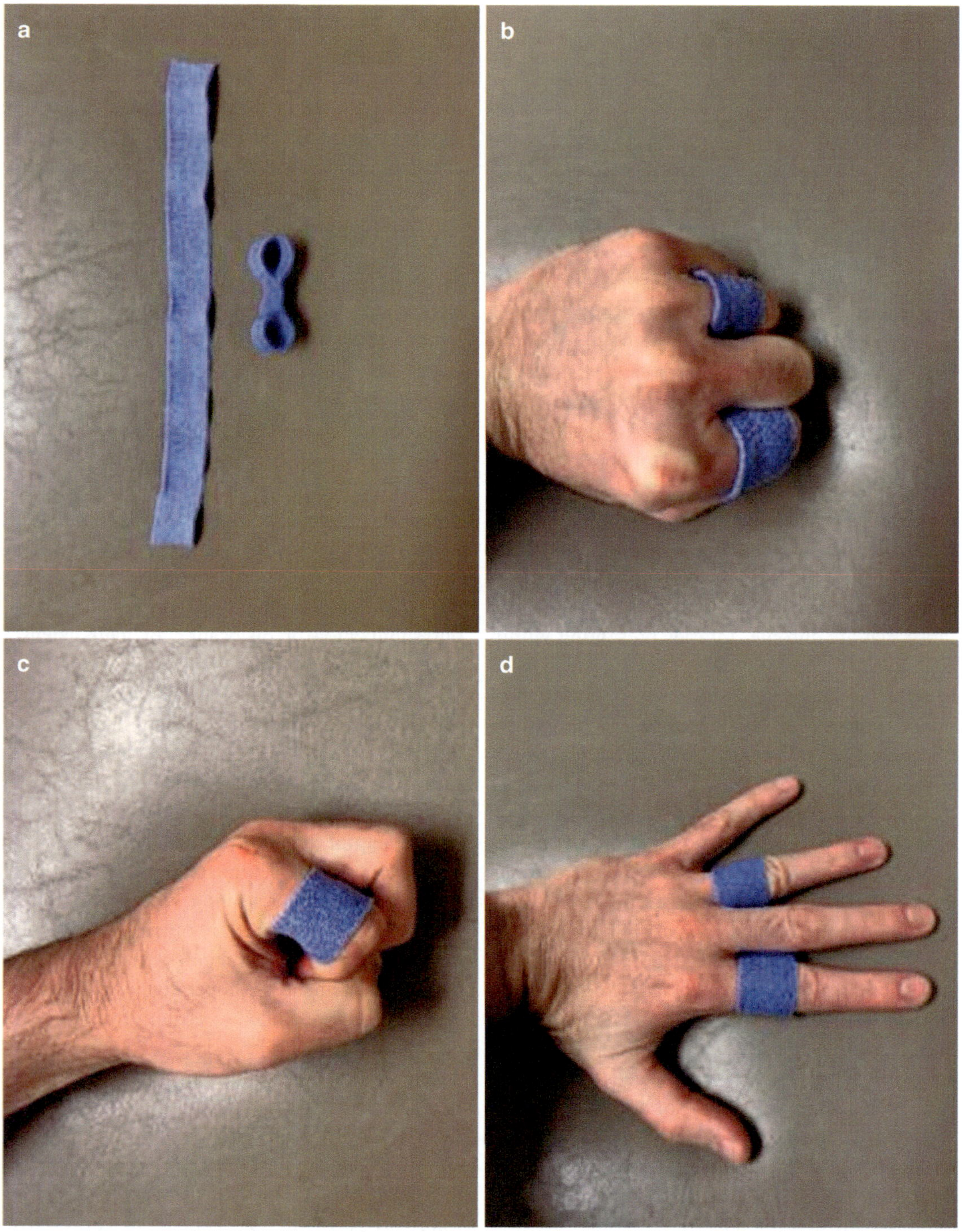

Fig. 14.6 (**a**) Materials used to create relative motion splint. (**b**) Left hand in relative motion splint. Long finger MCP held extended in relation to adjacent digits. (**c**) Lateral projection of third MCP in relative additional extension. (**d**) Extension view

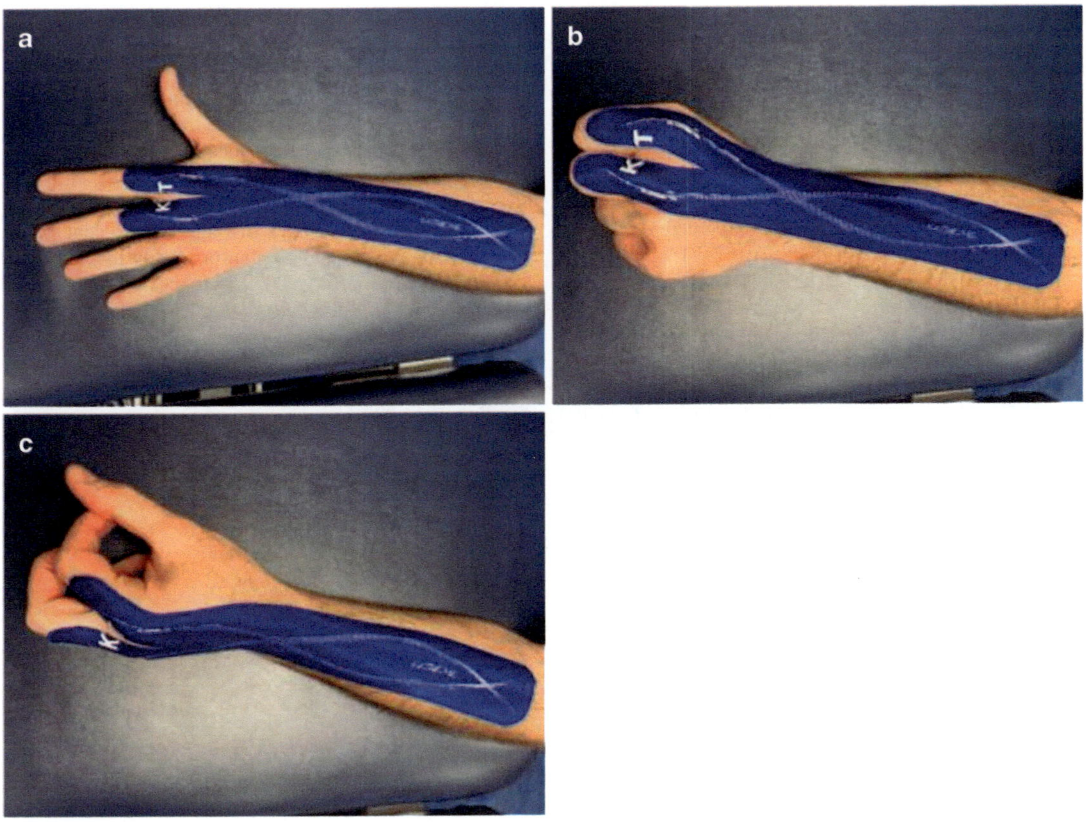

Fig. 14.7 Kinesiology taping technique demonstrated in MCP extension (**a**), flexion (**b**), and lateral projection (**c**)

References

1. Rettig AC. Epidemiology of hand and wrist injuries in sports. Clin Sports Med. 1998;17(3):401–6. https://doi.org/10.1016/s0278-5919(05)70092-2.
2. Aronowitz ER, Leddy JP. Closed tendon injuries of the hand and wrist in athletes. Clin Sports Med. 1998;17(3):449–67. https://doi.org/10.1016/s0278-5919(05)70096-x.
3. Matzon JL, Bozentka DJ. Extensor tendon injuries. J Hand Surg Am. 2010;35(5):854–61. https://doi.org/10.1016/j.jhsa.2010.03.002.
4. Kalainov DM, Hoepfner PE, Hartigan BJ, Carroll C 4th, Genuario J. Nonsurgical treatment of closed mallet finger fractures. J Hand Surg Am. 2005;30(3):580–6. https://doi.org/10.1016/j.jhsa.2005.02.010. PMID: 15925171.
5. Meershoek AJ, Keizer J, Houwert RM, van Heijl M, van der Velde D, Wittich P. Excellent functional recovery after Kirschner-wire extension blocking technique for displaced closed bony mallet finger injuries; results of 36 cases. Acta Orthop Belg. 2019;85(2):240–6. PMID: 31315016.
6. Bachoura A, Ferikes AJ, Lubahn JD. A review of mallet finger and jersey finger injuries in the athlete. Curr Rev Musculoskelet Med. 2017;10(1):1–9. https://doi.org/10.1007/s12178-017-9395-6. PMID: 28188545; PMCID: PMC5344866.
7. Smit JM, Beets MR, Zeebregts CJ, Rood A, Welters CF. Treatment options for mallet finger: a review. Plast Reconstr Surg. 2010;126(5):1624–9. https://doi.org/10.1097/PRS.0b013e3181ef8ec8. PMID: 21042117.
8. Shin SS. Baseball commentary–tendon ruptures: mallet, FDP. Hand Clin. 2012;28(3):431–2. https://doi.org/10.1016/j.hcl.2012.05.041.
9. Grandizio LC, Klena JC. Sagittal band, boutonniere, and pulley injuries in the athlete. Curr Rev Musculoskelet Med. 2017;10(1):17–22. https://doi.org/10.1007/s12178-017-9379-6.
10. Marino JT, Lourie GM. Boutonnière and pulley rupture in elite athletes. Hand Clin. 2012;28(3):437–xii. https://doi.org/10.1016/j.hcl.2012.05.044.
11. Ahmad F, Pickford M. Reconstruction of the extensor central slip using a distally based flexor digitorum superficialis slip. J Hand Surg Am. 2009;34(5):930–2. https://doi.org/10.1016/j.jhsa.2009.01.025.

12. Gama C. Results of the Matev operation for correction of Boutonnière deformity. Plast Reconstr Surg. 1979;64(3):319–24. https://doi.org/10.1097/00006534-197909000-00006.
13. Green D, Wolfe S. In: Green D, Wolfe S, editors. Green's operative hand surgery. 6th ed. Philadelphia: Elsevier/Churchill Livingstone; 2011.
14. Curtis RM, Reid RL, Provost JM. A staged technique for the repair of the traumatic boutonniere deformity. J Hand Surg Am. 1983;8(2):167–71. https://doi.org/10.1016/s0363-5023(83)80009-4.
15. Rayan GM, Murray D. Classification and treatment of closed sagittal band injuries. J Hand Surg Am. 1994;19(4):590–4. https://doi.org/10.1016/0363-5023(94)90261-5.
16. Wu K, Masschelein G, Suh N. Treatment of sagittal band injuries and extensor tendon subluxation: a systematic review. Hand (NY). 2020:1558944719895622. https://doi.org/10.1177/1558944719895622. Epub ahead of print. PMID: 31965857.
17. Catalano LW 3rd, Gupta S, Ragland R 3rd, Glickel SZ, Johnson C, Barron OA. Closed treatment of nonrheumatoid extensor tendon dislocations at the metacarpophalangeal joint. J Hand Surg Am. 2006;31(2):242–5. https://doi.org/10.1016/j.jhsa.2005.10.009.
18. Merritt WH, Wong AL, Lalonde DH. Recent developments are changing extensor tendon management. Plast Reconstr Surg. 2020;145(3):617e–28e. https://doi.org/10.1097/PRS.0000000000006556.
19. Merritt WH. Relative motion splint: active motion after extensor tendon injury and repair. J Hand Surg Am. 2014;39(6):1187–94. https://doi.org/10.1016/j.jhsa.2014.03.015.

Wrist Extensor Pathologies in the Baseball Athlete

15

Thomas J. Graham and Michael J. Moses

Introduction

Consistently balancing hand-forearm unit power and control is the prerequisite for elite-level athletic performance in stick-and-ball sports. The role of the radial wrist extensors and the extensor carpi ulnaris (ECU) is important for spatial positioning, as well as explosive power through the hitting zone.

One of the most rewarding experiences of my quarter-century of caring for professional athletes has been the occasions when our organization's Medical Staff, our Athletic Trainers, and I recognize an unsolved problem, better elucidate its pathophysiology and anatomy, then mutually work toward treatment solutions that return our athletes to their performing status through structured rehabilitation. This has happened on a couple occasions, but none more vividly than our advancement of knowledge about pathologies of the ECU tendon and its investments.

Often considered the "black box" of hand surgery, we have made great strides in understanding pathologies of the ulnar wrist in the baseball athlete. We have tried to be students of how the batting stroke, and other baseball-specific actions, stress this anatomy-packed region. Our proficiency in diagnosis and treatment of TFCC problems, piso-triquetral pathology, midcarpal abutment, and extensor carpi ulnaris (ECU) issues has grown dramatically over the last few years. It is on the latter, pathologies of the ECU and its investments, that we would like to focus our attention for the purpose of this communication.

Incidence in Sports and Baseball

Wrist injuries are common in athletes, with ECU tendon subluxation being unique to those sports in which there is loading of the wrist when the ECU is stressed in wrist flexion, supination, and ulnar deviation. Wrist injuries generally account for nearly 9% of all sports-related injuries. Most commonly, ECU injuries are seen in stick-and-ball sports (tennis, baseball, golf, etc.) or in those sports where the wrist can remain in this vulnerable position during play (rugby). Baseball may predispose athletes to ECU injury due to the wrist position while batting when a strong isometric contraction occurs in conjunction with a sudden laterally based force of the swing as the wrist is in a supinated, flexed, and ulnar-deviated position.

T. J. Graham (✉)
Ohio Hand at Kettering Health, Dayton, OH, USA

Department of Orthopedic Surgery, NYU Langone Health, New York, NY, USA
e-mail: thomas.graham@ketteringhealth.org

M. J. Moses
Department of Orthopedic Surgery, NYU Langone Health, New York, NY, USA
e-mail: Michael.Moses@nyulangone.org

G. M. Lourie (ed.), *Hand and Wrist Injuries in Baseball*,
https://doi.org/10.1007/978-3-030-81659-9_15

One anecdotal observation over my career is that ECU pathologies were considered infrequent, judging by casual references in the literature. I believe that diagnostic sophistication (both clinical and radiographic), coupled with advancement in the knowledge of its unique anatomy and presentation in the athletic environment has proven that pathologies of the ECU and its investments are geing to be seen by those Surgeons engaged in the care of elite athletes.

Pathologies of the Extensor Carpi Ulnaris and Its Investments

In order to understand the pathologies associated with the ECU tendon, knowledge of the functional anatomy is critical as it can dictate while treating elite athletes. Without getting trapped in minute detail of this complex region, there is a collection of facts that all Athletic Trainers and Consultants should appreciate about the ECU and its investments:

As we know, the ECU tendon lies in the sixth dorsal extensor compartment of the wrist in the ulnar groove or sulcus, a concavity of variable depth at the ulna's distal extreme. The osteology of the sulcus is extremely variable; we have encountered nearly flat floors and conversely, the depth could exceed 50% of the diameter of the ECU tendon. Consideration of this bony anatomy will be important in conduct of surgical reconstruction.

The muscle originates on the lateral epicondyle of the humerus and the posterior ulna, as it courses toward its insertion site at the dorsal base of the fifth metacarpal. The trajectory of the ECU tendon from its origin to its insertion forms an obtuse angle in the sixth compartment. The "angle of attack" contributes to function of the tendon, as the ECU is a wrist ulnar deviator in forearm pronation and a wrist extensor in forearm supination. Furthermore, this unique angle predisposes the tendon to positional changes during contraction; like everything in nature, the muscle tendon unit would "prefer" to have a straight line of pull. This created the stress on the soft-tissue investments of the ECU during supination, flexion, and ulnar deviation of the wrist associated with the batting stroke.

The soft-tissue investments considered the "subsheath" constituting the roof of the ulnar sulcus, subjacent to the extensor retinaculum, contribute materially to ECU stability and function. The subsheath was initially described by Spinner and Kaplan who noted that the subsheath's prime function was to stabilize the ECU during forearm rotation in order to prevent ECU subluxation [1]. The senior author (TJG) delineated the ECU "system" and has separated the soft-tissue investments into four separate quadrants and also further elucidated the anatomy of the ulnar ("*labrum*") and radial ("*limbus*") attachments of the subsheath [2] (Fig. 15.1).

This system approach to understanding the ECU investments has also assisted in the classification and ultimate treatment of these injuries. The dorsal/superior quadrant features the transverse fibers of the subsheath and the overlying (but not confluent) extensor retinaculum. The radial quadrant is constituted by the radial limbus, a thinner attachment of the subsheath on its "tension side." The all-important ulnar quadrant presents the buttress of the labrum, reinforced by the *linea jugata*. Finally, the volar quadrant is the osseous floor of the sulcus (Fig. 15.2).

Largely originating from the volar antebrachial fascia with some footprint from the pisiform, the overlying extensor retinaculum does not

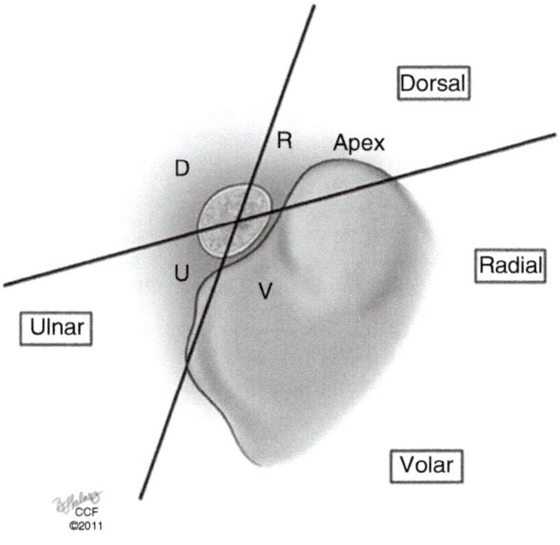

Fig. 15.1 The four quadrants of anatomic consideration for the ECU tendon and its investments

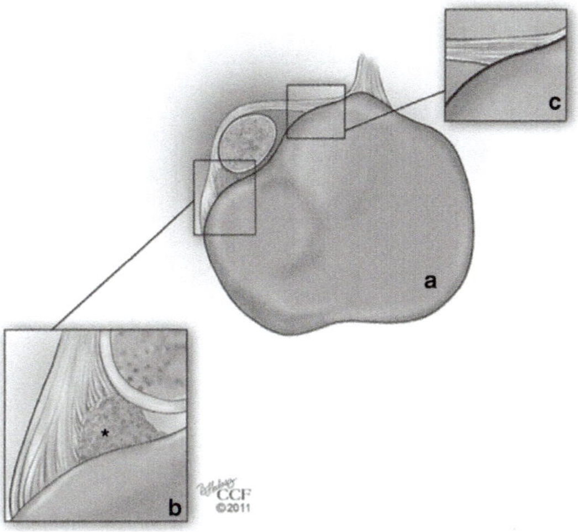

Fig. 15.2 The anatomy of the ECU subsheath is depicted. (A) The level of the subsheath. (B) A magnified view of the ulnar-sided *Labrum* of the subsheath showing the buttress formed by the stout attachment of the subsheath and its reinforcement by the fibers of the *linea jugata* (*). (C) A magnification of the radial-sided *labrum*

contain any direct osseous insertions on the dorsal surface, although there is confluence with interseptal tissue of the fourth and fifth extensor compartments. The retinaculum adds essentially no, and minimal dynamic, stability to the ECU tendon.

Therefore, it is the fibro-osseous subsheath that is approximately 2 cm in length, which prevents subluxation of the ECU tendon from its anatomic location in the sixth dorsal compartment. Injury to the subsheath is the *sine qua non* that contributes to ECU tendon hypermobility/subluxation, while taking into account the osseous elements and the secondary influence of the extensor retinaculum, the germinal lesion that the surgeon must consider is some expression of embarrassment of the subsheath.

There are two classification systems used to communicate about these injuries. These largely differentiate the pattern and extent of subsheath failure and/or osseous pathology [3–5].

However, it is the opinion of these authors that a more simplified and clinically relevant approach should be the intellectual guide to addressing embarrassment ECU investments. Acknowledging that fractures about the ulnar sulcus should be considered in any management scenario, the three basic pathologies that our community will encounter are as follows: (1) intrasubstance ruptures or failures of the transverse fibers of the subsheath, (2) "delamination" of the labrum resulting in the loss of the ulnar buttress, and (3) a combination of intrasubstance attenuation/failure and delamination of the labrum from the ulnar all of the sulcus (Fig. 15.3).

Mechanism of Injury

The typical mode of injury for ECU subluxation occurs when a rapid rotational force occurs as the wrist is in a supinated, flexed, and ulnar-deviated position during the batting stroke. In our experience, the player/patient usually relates that the onset was associated with a check-swing or awkward stroke; rarely do hitters sustain injuries when they "square up" the pitch. The two phases where the hitter's recollection (and now our voluminous video archives) educate us are at the extents of the "hitting zone." When entering the zone, an awkward adjustment to a pitch or check-off, or exiting the hitting zone and attempts to decelerate the bat seem to both create the conditions for eccentric contractions and the ulnar "vector of force" that stresses the radial limbus (in tension) and ulnar buttress that can result in subsheath failure.

History/Differential Dx

Unlike rendering care in the general population, those of us who are privileged to care for the elite athlete benefit from a level and volume of information that is extraordinary. Specifically, we not only have the player's recollection (perhaps some of the most body-aware humans), but we also have multiple trained observers (Athletic Trainers and Hitting Coaches) and adjunct technologies – most stadiums have six or more camera vantage points recording every at bat.

Players may or may not describe a discrete episode of when they felt a sudden onset of ulnar-sided wrist pain and subsequent subluxation of

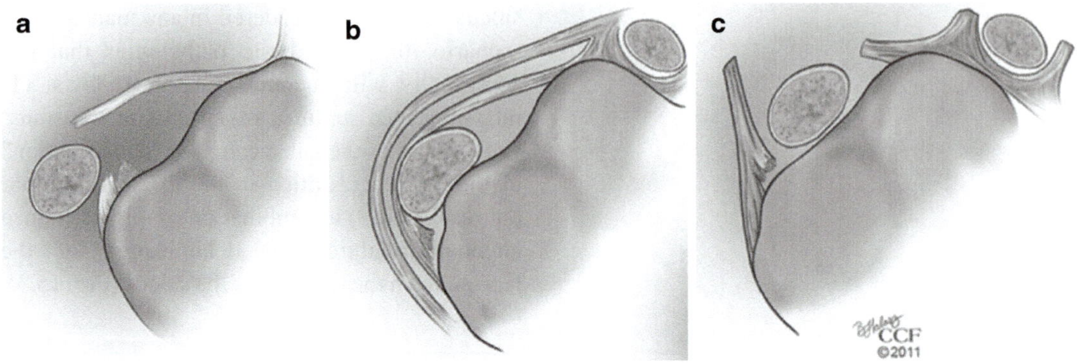

Fig. 15.3 Modes of failure of the investments of the ECU tendon. (**a**) Intrasubstance ruptures or failures of the transverse fibers of the subsheath. (**b**) "Delamination" of the labrum resulting in the loss of the ulnar buttress. (**c**) A combination of intrasubstance attenuation/failure and delamination of the labrum from the ulnar aspect of the sulcus

the tendon; it is true that the volume of swings can lead to a more chronic attritional injury to the investments or basically an overuse attenuation. However, in the majority of cases, the athlete describes a single event that resulted in discomfort, weakness, and was potentially associated with a snapping-type sensation on the ulnar side of the wrist with forearm rotation.

Although we have concentrated our discussion thus far on pathologies that result in mechanical instability, we do want to highlight the spectrum of problems of the ECU and its investments that the consultant will encounter. The four culprits are as follows:

- Inflammatory: Tenosynovitis surrounding the ECU tendon is not uncommon and presents with unusually apparent bogginess surrounding the tendon – made more noticeable because of the relatively subcutaneous position and the proclivity for more florid presentations to show enlarged tumescence in the regions proximal and distal to the subsheath ("dumbbell" presentation). Infrequently, an audible "squeak" can even be detected like we encounter in some other tendinopathies like DeQuervain's.
- Instability: Classic findings like bowstringing and subluxation/dislocation of the ECU tendon, as described; when present, we usually characterize as consistent vs. intermittent subluxation – with or without bowstringing to resistance.
- Tendinopathy: Intrinsic damage or tendinosis of the ECU. This can only be truly diagnosed by cross-sectional imaging.
- Other Mechanical Failure: We have seen overt rupture (usually in the setting of the long-inflamed and multiply injected tendon) and rarely have seen either musculotendinous failure (seldom) or avulsion from the fifth metacarpal insertion (frankly, never without penetrating injury).

The differential diagnosis for ECU tendon subluxation includes those diagnoses typically considered for ulnar-sided wrist pathology: TFCC tears, ulnocarpal abutment syndrome, DRUJ-related pathology, and lunatotriquetral sprain. Rarely would an irritability of the dorsal sensory branch of the ulnar nerve confuse the sophisticated examiner, but we did describe midcarpal impingement in the batter – the slamming together of the hamate and triquetrum that occurs through the hitting zone with ulnar-deviation – that may be one of the "hidden diagnoses" that saw us, but we did not see until we fully recognized its prevalence [6].

Directed Physical Exam

The physical exam is perhaps one of the most telling aspects of the patient and should include the player bringing a bat to the exam to demonstrate or recapitulate the symptoms and so the phase of the hitting stroke in which it is most bothersome can be identified. Mechanical displacement upon provocative testing has obvious implications related to failure of the anatomic constraints we have introduced above and is the hallmark of more advanced pathology.

Simply observing the prominence of the ECU while examining the patient's wrist in ulnar deviation while resisting with a radial deviation force is valuable; this "bowstringing" can be subtle and should be compared to the contralateral side. Patients with gross tendon instability can often demonstrate this in the office, even without a bat or club in their hand. By "rolling" their wrist, they can trap the tendon outside the sulcus, only to relocate it at the end of the maneuver with some modest radial deviation and flexion.

Perhaps not as sophisticated or dramatic, we described the simple act of translating the tendon ulnarward directly at the level of the subsheath with the examiner's thumb, a "strumming" maneuver that allows an appreciation of the palpable displacement of the tendon and comparison to the contralateral side for distinction.

The "ECU Synergy Test" has recently emerged as a physical exam maneuver to diagnose ECU pathology and differentiate it from intra-articular diagnoses [7]. The patient rests their supinated forearm of the affected side on a table and the examiner grasps the patient's thumb and long finger while the patient radially deviates the thumb radially against. The presence of pain upon palpation of the ECU during this maneuver suggests pathology in the ECU rather than intra-articular pathology.

In some confusing cases, those in which both an intra- and extra-articular pathology have been demonstrated on MRI or those in which I am already contemplating injection, I will perform a "differential injection exam." By instilling lidocaine in either the ECU sheath of wrist joint, I can determine the relative contribution to the overall symptom complex, but can then project what a successful cortisone injection can likely provide to the athlete. This also almost eliminates the injudicious use of cortisone which is usually lauded by the athlete who may already harbor trepidation to "shots."

Imaging Including Advanced Methods

Imaging is a helpful adjunct or corroboration to the exam in the diagnosis of ECU tendon pathology and that of its investments. Radiographs will typically be negative for any ECU pathology, but these may be helpful in differentiating the diagnosis from other ulnar osseous pathology or carpal instability. Look for ulnar styloid nonunions or irregularities that may be sources of attritional injury. A "soft call" about the morphology of the sulcus can be made if there is no parallel linear density seen on the PA view, potentially indicating a shallow groove.

Magnetic resonance imaging (MRI) has remained our "go-to" diagnostic imaging modality in approaching suspected ECU-related pathology both for what it tells us about the tendon and its investments as for what it may (or may not) reveal about the surrounding tissues.

Our quick checklist for what we are looking in assessing the non-contrast MRI includes the following: (a) surrounding fluid, inflammatory tissue, especially as to whether it is contained within the subsheath or has "escaped" to the level of the retinaculum; (b) intrinsic quality of the tendon, judge both by the degree of striation or central intra-substance inhomogeneity on the coronal or the intercalary inhomogeneity seen on the sagittal views; (c) positioning of the tendon (within the sulcus, outside the sulcus or "perched"; a variation of this indicator that can be seen on the coronal is the "teardrop" shaped tendon that may indicate that it has started to translate ulnarward because of a labral delamination (Fig. 15.4).

Just a caution, in some patients, a longitudinal raphe in the ECU does not represent pathology, so the radiologist's read of a "split tear," may not be indicative of pathology – it really should be accom-

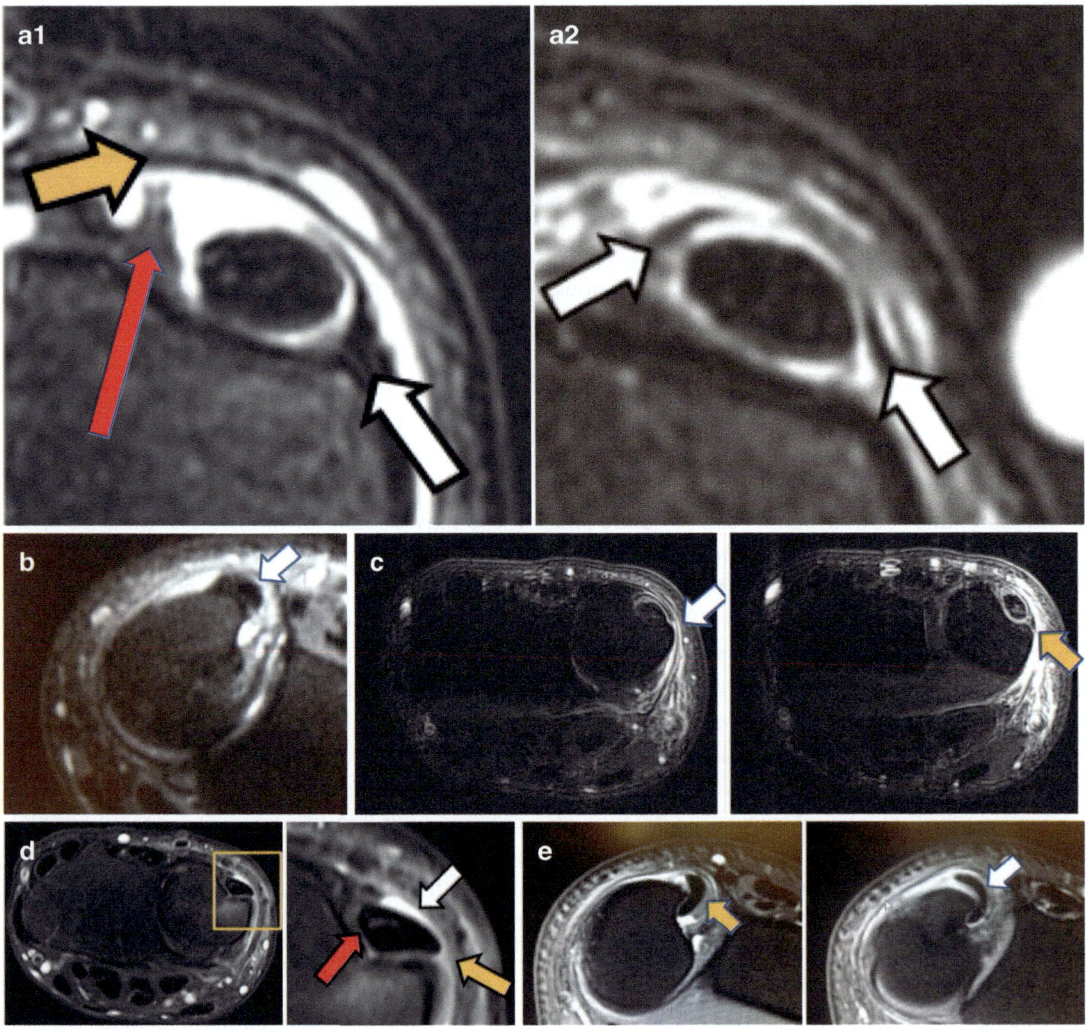

Fig. 15.4 The modern MRI can discern the fine anatomy of the ECU region. (**a1**) In this view of a failure of the midsubstance of the subsheath, the edema fluid nicely highlights the pathology; the stout labrum is nicely seen (white arrow), the red arrow points to the failed *limbus*, and the yellow arrow indicated the *intact* extensor retinaculum, which nicely limits the edema fluid, highlighting the rent in the subsheath. (**a2**) A slice just proximal to the level of subsheath failure shows the radial and ulnar limbs of the subsheath with intact attachments to the ulnar sulcus (white arrows). The modern MRI can discern the fine anatomy of the ECU region. This is a collection of some radiographic findings that may accompany pathologies of the ECU and its investments. (**b**) The surrounding edema indicates the likelihood of a significant acute injury that has left the relatively round tendon (probably indicating a first time injury) "perched" on the ulnar wall of the sulcus; the intact extensor retinaculum still contains the edema, as would be suspected. (**c**) Although the considerable amount of edema would indicate a sever injury to the ECU investments, the tendon is presently located, but the intrinsic damage to the central aspect of the ECU and the labrum (arrows) heralds a serious injury. (**d**) This figure and its magnified view show what we have termed the "teardrop" or "comma" morphology that the ECU adopts when delamination of the labrum permits slight subluxation, but still contains the tendon; there is minor intrinsic change (red arrow), some edema (white arrow), and the ulnarmost extent of the tendon is being deformed by the delaminated labrum. (**e**) A vivid example of a chronic loss of the influence of the ECU investments; not only is the ECU deformed and "draped" over the ulnar wall of the sulcus, but there is fibrosis or tenosynovitis (yellow arrow), again, the extensor retinaculum remains intact, even in these chronic cases (white arrows)

panied by intrinsic changes in the tissue and surrounding fluid/tenosynovitis to verify that finding. Finally, beware the intercalary transverse segment of inhomogeneity at the level of the subsheath; it is worrisome enough when it looks "bright" (on T2) and thickened; it is extremely concerning when it starts to look striated and attenuated (think taffy), indicating significant mechanical compromise.

The advent of in-office ultrasound and our increasing sophistication in its interpretation increased, may rise up to challenge MRI – a trend in which we are most interested in following because of expediency and economy [8].

Right now, we believe that the diagnosis of tendinosis is best made with an MRI, performed without contrast. Although I prefer not to recommend contrast studies, especially in athletes, the value of contrast MRI in assessing ECU pathology was contributed in 2011 by Jeantroux and colleagues, who advocated for gadolinium contrast and dynamic pronation-supination sequences [9]. It is interesting to note, however, that even with MRI as a diagnostic modality, ECU tendon displacement of up to 50% of the tendon width can occur in asymptomatic patients and therefore comparative studies of the contralateral side are usually performed.

With the three hallmarks of ECU pathology firmly in mind, we can develop our admittedly arbitrary, but useful classification system so we can converse with patients, trainers and fellow colleagues. I suggest this simple approach.

Simplified Approach to Classification

Classification: We use the term "Classification" lightly here because we are not proposing the introduction of yet another nomenclature system into the lexicon. Instead, we use to organize the consultant's thinking and facilitate communication throughout the organization and with the patient/player. There is no expectation that it will "stick," but it can be a useful architecture on which to hang the physical and radiographic findings throughout the process and we shall use these distinctions throughout this chapter.

Mild: Swelling in sheath, no bowstringing, no intrinsic abnormality (MRI).

Moderate: Moderate mechanical instability elicited on provocative exam of ECU, possible early intrinsic change (MRI), none or inconsistent subluxation with pronosupination/hitting motion.

Severe: Bowstringing or consistent displacement of the tendon from the sulcus, intrinsic (focal vs. longitudinal) tendon embarrassment seen on the MRI.

Strategies for Treating Pathologies of the ECU and Investments

Nonoperative Treatment

We would never want the relative amount of "real estate" dedicated to operative treatment of pathologies of the ECU and its investments to mislead the reader that our community of baseball consultants should be anything less than conservative and judicious in their approach to treatment. In other venues, we have already revealed our bias against deciding about surgical treatment of acute ECU problems on initial presentation or even snap decisions when a chronic problem presents. The reason behind this is simple and has been played out in my practice dozens of times over my two-plus decades involved in the care of the elite athlete's wrist and hand. Since my thesis has been one of initial nonoperative treatment, we have seen athletes trend toward three different outcomes:

- Complete or near-complete resolution of symptoms, with no lingering discomfort or mechanical manifestations
- Persistence of mechanical symptoms without significant discomfort or impairment of effective play at the elite level
- Continued discomfort and mechanical manifestations that prevent effective and safe play

Appertaining to the "conservative" philosophy and classification we have articulated, my protocol includes the following "phases."

Immobilization Phase: Long-arm splint can be considered, but short-arm splint is usually effective. Wrist can be placed in neutral to slight flexion and radial deviation. Any cardio/leg work permitted per level of comfort.

- *Mild:* 5–7-day initial period of immobilization
- *Moderate:* 7–10-day initial period of immobilization
- *Severe:* 10–14-day initial period of immobilization

[If in removable splint, may ice or perform modalities like iontophoresis. May be out for hygiene if taped around distal aspect of tendon. [I credit George Poulis, the veteran Athletic Trainer who spent many years with the Toronto Blue Jays and is now with the Atlanta Braves and Lonnie Soloff, the Cleveland Indians Senior Director of Medical Services with developing and testing this with me over many years] (Fig. 15.5).

Motion Recovery Phase: After initial immobilization period, assess level of comfort. If pain and swelling persist with gentle motion, consider injection.

Start A/AAROM program to level of comfort along these guidelines:

- For 2–3 days, out 3–5 X/day for motion program (ECU Taped)
- For next 2–3 days, out 6–8 X/day for motion program (ECU Taped)
- For next 2–3 days, out 10–12 X/day for motion program (ECU Taped)
- For next 2–3 days, out 13–15 X/day for motion program (ECU Taped)

[If motion exceeds 75%, may consider start of strengthening program. If at any time during rehabilitation/return-to-play period symptoms dictate (discomfort, swelling, motion limittaion), injection could be considered; typically place in immobilization for 3–5 days post-injection, then resume motion recovery protocol]

Strength Recovery Phase: With ECU taped or splinted (Arnold Palmer-type splint), may commence strength recovery phase as directed by player experience and in collaboration with medical/training staff. When strength exceeds 75%, may start sports-specific preparation.

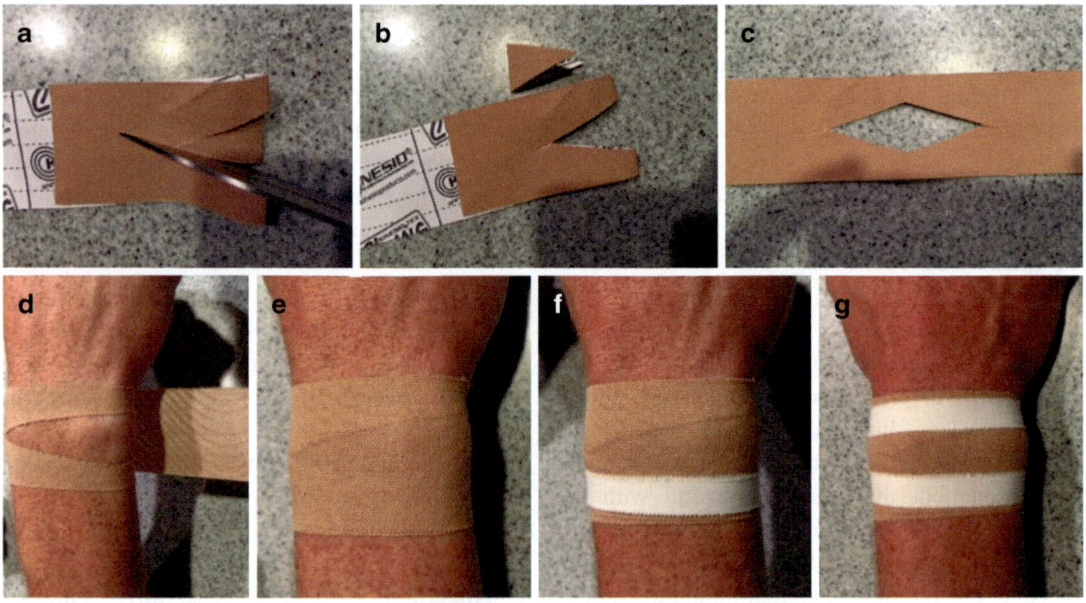

Fig. 15.5 The sequence of preparing and applying the taping method developed by Poulis, Soloff, and Graham for use in the professional baseball player (follow (**a**) through (**g**) consecutively)

Sports-Specific Preparation Phase (Baseball): Obviously, this phase is largely conducted under the purview of the team's medical/training/coaching staff. In our experience, progression through the following stages has allowed appropriate monitoring and focus for this injury:

- Dry swinging with light or fungo bat
- Tee work
- Soft toss
- Cage BP @ 50–75–100%
- Field BP @ 50–75–100%
- Rehab assignment per individual team and player

Return-to-Play

Individual decisions on return-to-play are the complete purview of the player's team. In our experience, the following guidelines can be useful in developing milestones and targets for resumption of elite-level play at the MLB level. Typically, even players in whom symptoms have not completely resolved can return in-season to safe and effective play – in that subset, end-of-season reconstruction (see subsequent sections) remains compatible with completion of the entire rehabilitation protocol so that participation in training camp can be accomplished.

- *Mild:* 25% of players typically return between 2 and 3 weeks, 50% between 3 and 4 weeks, and the remaining 25% after 4 weeks.
- *Moderate:* 25% of players typically return between 3 and 4 weeks, 50% between 4 and6 weeks, and the remaining 25% after 6 weeks.
- *Severe:* 25% of players typically return between 4 and 6 weeks, 50% between 6 and 8 weeks, and the remaining 25% after 8 weeks.

[*NB*. There is a subset of players who have newly developed tendon subluxation after embarrassment of the ECU investments and remain relatively asymptomatic. These players can typically return to elite-level play with taping safely and effectively, requiring symptom monitoring only.]

Surgical Treatment of ECU-Related Pathology: The "Modified Combined" Repair

The reasons we are comfortable recommending nonoperative treatment for problems of the ECU and its investments are that the same form of reconstructive surgery that we perform for acute cases is the same as we perform for remote cases. Stated alternatively, primary repair of the sheath, subsheath, or *linea jugata* is extremely unlikely, so some form of reconstruction and augmentation with a retinacular flap is usually likely for cases of ECU problems, especially tendon subluxation.

Almost every form of reconstruction described features a radially based retinacular flap that is either advanced over the ECU and secured on the ulnar aspect of the sulcus or creates a sling enveloping the tendon and also creating a barrier underneath the tendon, excluding it from the sulcus, which most authors advocate deepening to prevent subluxation [10–14]. There have even been authors who have advocated simple release and bone resection from the ulnar sulcus – I fear that this may not be applicable in a majority of elite athletes and would "burn a bridge" for later definitive reconstruction [15].

I have several reasons why this was always somewhat illogical to me, and why I have been performing a "modified combined" procedure for well over 15 years now consisting of three basic components: (1) labral repair/reinforcement, (2) advancement of an ulnar-based flap of extensor retinaculum, and (3) "contouring" (not necessarily deepening) the ulnar sulcus.

First, I have already provided extreme focus on the unique architecture of the ulnar leaf of the subsheath. The stoutest portion, that which is longitudinally reinforced by the *linea jugata*, is almost always present and robust enough to accept sutures. I believe that this is the primary barrier to ulnarward subluxation of the ECU tendon under contractile force.

Second, I have described the anatomy and favorable mechanics of the extensor retinaculum, particularly, its resilience to mechanical failure. Personally, I have never seen a *primary* failure of this tissue in an athlete (salvage after previous surgery will be discussed subsequently). This is completely compatible with the biomechanical studies quoted [16]. Therefore, I decidedly recommend against sectioning the lone tissue that is essentially intact right over the most important area where reinforcement is needed. Furthermore, the strong septae, especially that between compartments 4 and 5, provides an excellent anchor when securing the radially advanced tissue.

Finally, I certainly understand the intellectual appeal of simply deepening the ulnar sulcus to "capture" the ECU tendon and theoretically prevent recurrent subluxation after surgery. However, on too many occasions, I have seen three problems result: (1) if the ulnar buttress of the labrum and secure retinaculum is not re-established in the presence of a deepened sulcus, the tendon actually has a greater proclivity to subluxate and "perch" on the ulnar lip of the deepened groove; this causes even more intrinsic tendon damage than originally was being experienced with the index pathology. (2) Weakening of the bone in the ulnar sulcus region where additional manipulation (like placement of suture anchors) has been performed to advance a radially based flap – anything from soft-tissue failure to rim fracture ensures and the entire reconstruction fails catastrophically. (3) Exposure of the tendon to a roughened cancellous bone surface (not to mention the bleeding that may have been stirred up when the osseous work was being performed) introduces a potentially problematic variable that creates fibrosis (at minimum) and attritional damage (at maximum).

Technique of the "Modified-Combined" Reconstruction

The accompanying cases (Figs. 15.6 and 15.7) tell a much more vivid story than I can project in words, but I shall summarize the key components in a checklist or "inventory" here:

- Carefully elevate an ulnar-based flap of retinaculum with its proximal extent where the transverse fibers can first be discerned and its distal extent just at or slightly distal to the ulnar styloid. Importantly, I take the flap to include the healthy portion of the 4,5 septum

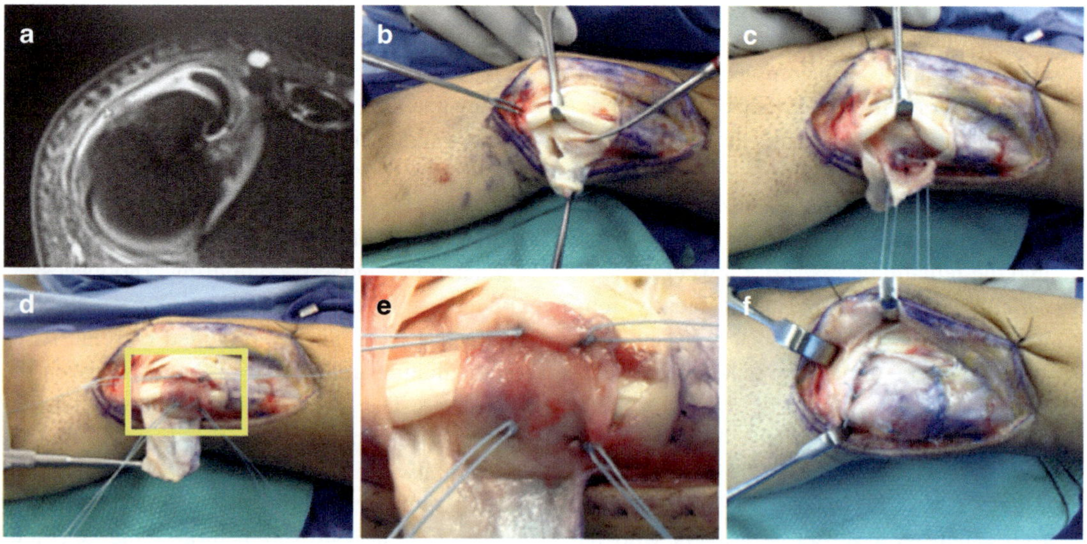

Fig. 15.6 Case of a combined intrasubstance failure and delamination of the ECU subsheath. (**a**) This coronal slice shows a very deformed or "perched" ECU tendon. (**b**) Initial exposure by reflection of the extensor retinaculum from its radial attachment demonstrated the intrasubstance subsheath failure, and the freer elevator highlights the "delamination" of the labrum. (**c**) Recontouring (flattening) of the ulnar wall of the sulcus and reconstruction of the *labrum* with suture anchors establishes the ulnar buttress. (**d, e**) Because of the combination of intrasubstance failure and delamination, the subsheath reconstruction required both *labrum* and limbus reconstruction. (**f**) Reinforcement with the advancement/repair of the extensor retinaculum

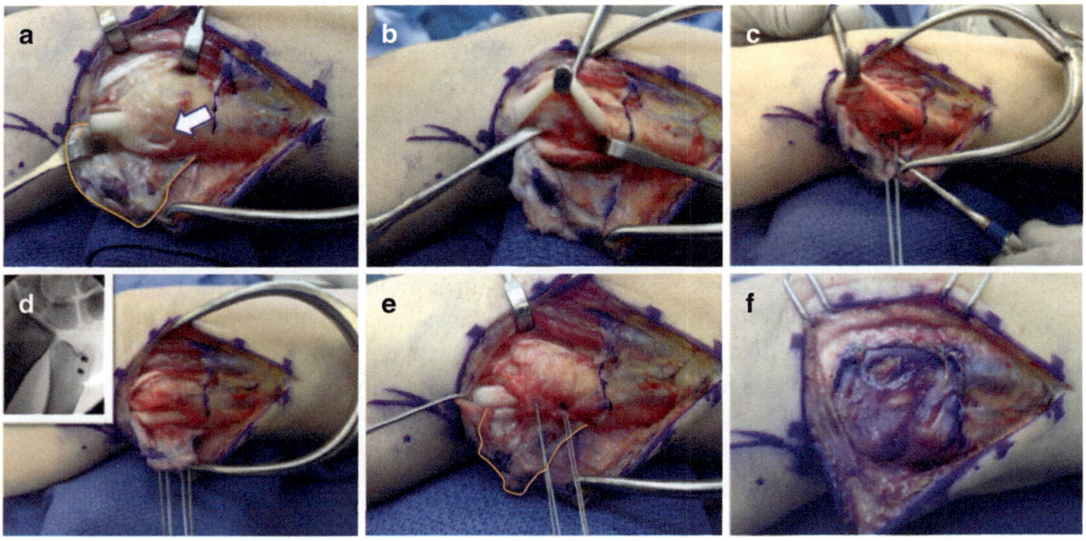

Fig. 15.7 (**a**) A small rent in the subsheath was appreciated upon reflection of the extensor retinaculum as an ulnar-based flap (outlined yellow). (**b**) The longitudinal failure was exploited to expose the ECU, and further delamination of the *labrum* was encountered. (**c**) After recontouring of the ulnar wall of the sulcus – leaving an intact anatomic surface for tendon gliding – suture anchors were placed. (**d**) The ulnar buttress was reestablished by *labrum* reconstruction; the inset shows the level of anchor placement. (**e**) The same sutures were used to both reconstruct the *labrum* and repair the subsheath. (**f**) The extensor retinaculum was advanced and repaired

(and of course, the 5,6 septum). This retinacular layer exposes the subsheath, which should not be disturbed at this time.

- Inspect the subsheath to determine its status; typically, only the thicker region as it approaches the ulnar-sided labral attachment will be intact and useful for repair. Be sure to appreciate how the subsheath has been "delaminated" from the ulnar wall of the sulcus.
- Appreciate the status of the ECU tendon, itself, especially in comparison to the *extensor digiti quinti proprius* (EDQP) tendon that you have now exposed. Record photographically and/or in your operative note the intrinsic status of the tendon.
- "Recontour" the ulnar wall of the sulcus. This is in contradistinction to simply deepening the concavity of the sulcus, which also creates a roughened surface against which the ECU would abrade. This creates a flatter, exposed region to which a combination of the labrum and the advanced retinaculum can be secured with a suture anchor.
- Advance the ulnar-based retinacular flap radially. The amount of tensioning is dependent on individual anatomy, but the stout 4,5 septum allows flexibility to secure the flap to soft tissue or even to the radius through suture anchors. In a minority of cases, I have excluded the EDQP from its native location, electing instead to advance the flap underneath the tendon; I leave a generous amount of retinaculum distally, so this has never created a problem.
- In cases where the EDQP has been relocated anatomically, I suture the proximal and distal edges of the advanced flap to local tissue.

Post-Treatment Rehabilitation

Typical Rehabilitation Plan After Modified-Combined Repair

- First 2 weeks: maintain operative dressing (MI use a "long" short-arm splint to about the maximum girth of the forearm)
  - Work on digital motion *ad lib*
  - Limited pronation/supination is permitted by splint to level of comfort

- At 2 weeks: remove sutures, begin *motion recovery phase*
  - Fashion custom "long short-arm" splint
  - May begin active/active-assisted (A/AAROM) program
  - For wrist flexion (F)/extension (E): accelerate in this plane
    - Start with 20E/20F for 3–4 days
    - Then 30E-30F for 3–4 days
    - Then 40E-40F for 3–4 days
    - Then 50E-50F for 3–4 days
    - Then 60E-60F for 3–4 days
  - For pronation (P)/supination (S), follow similar plan
    - Start with 20P/20S for 3–4 days
    - Then 30P-30S for 3–4 days
    - Then 40P-40S for 3–4 days
    - Then 50P-50S for 3–4 days
    - Then 60P-60S for 3–4 days
- Next milestone is *strength recovery phase*, typically begun when motion exceeds 75% of normal/contralateral (collaboration with team)
- Next milestone *sports-specific recovery phase*, typically begun when strength exceeds 75% of normal/contralateral (collaboration with team)
  - Wrist taping may be considered for comfort and support in practice and competition

Complications/Adverse Events

Aside from the surgical complication profile we all accept when performing open procedures, I should like to simply underscore two pertinent issues. First, the judicious initial surgical handling of the dorsal sensory branch of the ulnar nerve is important. The branch should cross the axial midline roughly at the midpoint between the ulnar styloid and the fifth metacarpal base, but this is variable. In almost all cases, I locate it and make sure it is both protected and in anatomic continuity at the terminus of the case.

The second complication is one I have seen about a dozen times in over two decades of care of elite athletes – rupture of the ECU tendon. The etiology could have been attrition, weakening from chronic inflammation or the use of performance-enhancing substances, or some iatrogenic manipulation (injection or surgical) (Fig. 15.8). We would like to state here that we believe assigning the rupture of the ECU, or any tendon, to inappropriate use of corticosteroid injections is often inaccurate. "Blaming" the physician for rupturing the tendon after judicious performance of a limited number of injections (and not taking into account the primary pathology and other patient-related factors) is unfair and disregards a more complex mosaic of etiologies for tendon failure.

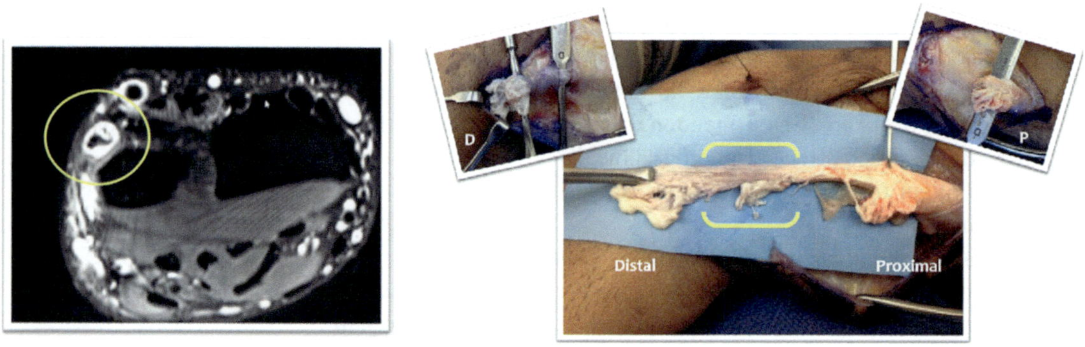

Fig. 15.8 The MRI demonstrates the unusual finding of a florid tenosynovitis contained within the confines of what appears to be an intact ECU subsheath (encircled yellow). In the collage of intraoperative photos, the central figure shows the destruction of the ECU tendon, while photos labeled (D) and (P) show the tendon through "windows" made in the ECU investments

Regardless, we should close this part of the chapter by relating that many of these turned to play at the highest levels. In most, if not all, we have formally resected the tendon ends and "pseudotendon" that seems to bother players when it forms fibrotic tethers to the investments that "pull" with contraction [17]. The ability of these athletes to compensate is remarkable; although there must be weakness, by definition, when you lose the influence of an important muscle, this is overcome by swing changes and other rehabilitation/strengthening techniques [18].

Loss of the ECU does not necessarily translate into a career-ending event, but counseling and flexibility in approaching the craft of hitting will be required to regain playing status. At the time of this writing, we remain advocates for "letting it fly" and not considering any form of ECU reconstruction in the elite athlete. In this case, we believe the simpler approach (vs. an intercalary tendon graft and complex rehabilitation) is more elegant in its simplicity.

Finally, catastrophic failure of the subsheath reconstruction may also occur. I have articulated my bias against sectioning the extensor retinaculum at the ulnar margin and creating a "sling" that envelops the ECU like a pulley – that is the usually the one intact tissue that may be employed for a variety of reinforcement or even subsheath substitution. I cannot argue that some other reconstructions which encircle the tendon in a retinacular sling may prevent ulnar translation, but these are certainly not recapitulating normal anatomy and keeping the ECU in its sulcus.

Seeing the catastrophic failure of the radially based retinacular flap approach lead us to develop a salvage procedure with which we have had success in returning players back to Major League competition (Fig. 15.9).

In this salvage approach, a free tendon graft (*palmaris longus*, if available) is utilized to create both a buttress to ulnar subluxation of the tendon and also an investment of the tendon that provides volar and dorsal protection, while allowing longitudinal excursion. Slight variation of the technique can be elected intra-operatively depending on the surgeon's determination of the "environment in which he or she desires the tendon to reside; protection from possible attrition on the osseous ulna can be affected by enveloping the ECU in tendon graft *versus* securing it in a more intimate position with the sulcus" (Fig. 15.10).

The rehabilitation times are usually lengthened by 10–25% in these salvage situations, but the repair is very sturdy, and can be trusted through the rehabilitation phases once healed.

Early RTP

Projected return to play is approximately 3 months, but if the reconstruction is performed at the end of the season, a slightly protracted rehabilitation can be favored before the start of Spring Training the following season. In our experience, 25% of athletes return between weeks 10 and 12, 50% return between 12 and 14 weeks, and the remaining quarter resume play after week 14.

Pathologies About the Radial Wrist Extensors

Almost forgotten in discussions of wrist extensor pathologies is that of the extensor carpi radialis longus and brevis. In our experience, there are two relevant pathologies that we have seen in the sporting population: intersection syndrome and insertional problems expressed as the carpal boss.

Intersection Syndrome

Of course, most tendinopathies are rather straightforward space:volume inequities – too much anatomy in too little space. The capacity equation creates a downward spiral of friction begets swelling begets more friction and so on.

It is somewhat fascinating that the nexus of the first and second dorsal compartments creates a unique inflammatory nidus. Its presentation, with the distinctive tumescence about the dorsoradial location and the palpable bogginess, differentiates it from DeQuervain's, as does its symptom exacerbation with resisted wrist extension.

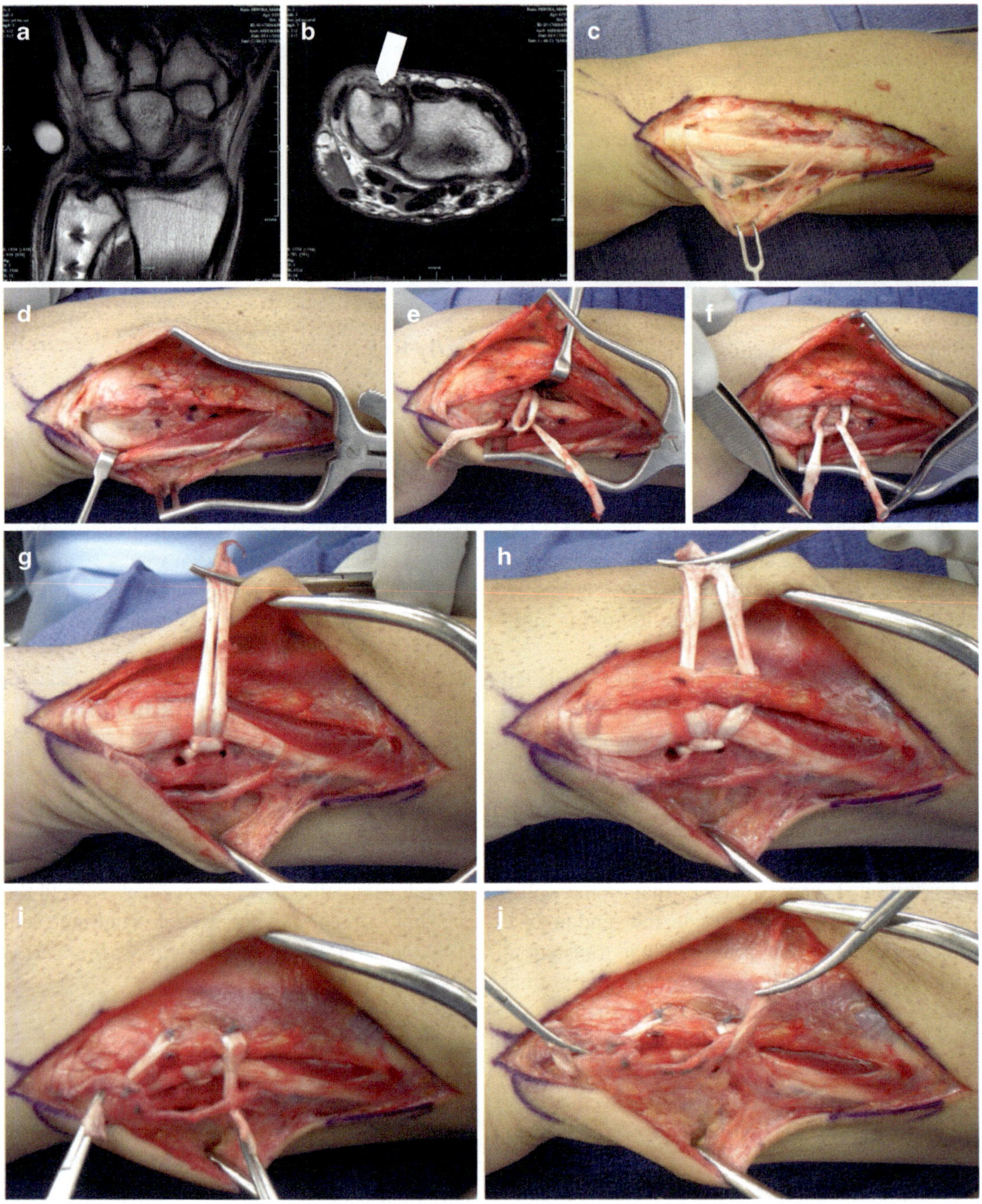

Fig. 15.9 Failure of a "retinacular sling" reconstruction in a professional baseball player. (**a**, **b**) The MRI is revealing of a flattened ECU tendon, demonstrating some longitudinal intrinsic changes, that has completely "escaped" the ulnar sulcus; suture anchors are appreciated. (**c**) Upon exposure, the complete failure of the retinacular sling is encountered (sutures visible), and the ECU is exposed due to lack of any repairable subsheath tissue. (**d**) Adequate debridement of postsurgical scarring and nonviable tissue. (**e**, **f**) After drilling of the ulna, the palmaris graft is passed in a fashion to capture the tendon; it can be weaved to also provide a bed for the ECU if it has been manipulated previous and is unsuitable for tendon gliding. (**g**) In this case, it was more advantageous to capture the ECU tendon with the primary loop, thus relocating in the sulcus that still had a smooth anatomic bed. (**h**) The graft is then passed through the stout interseptal elements of the remaining retinaculum. (**i**, **j**) The graft is used to coapt the remaining retinaculum and reinforce the stabilizing repair

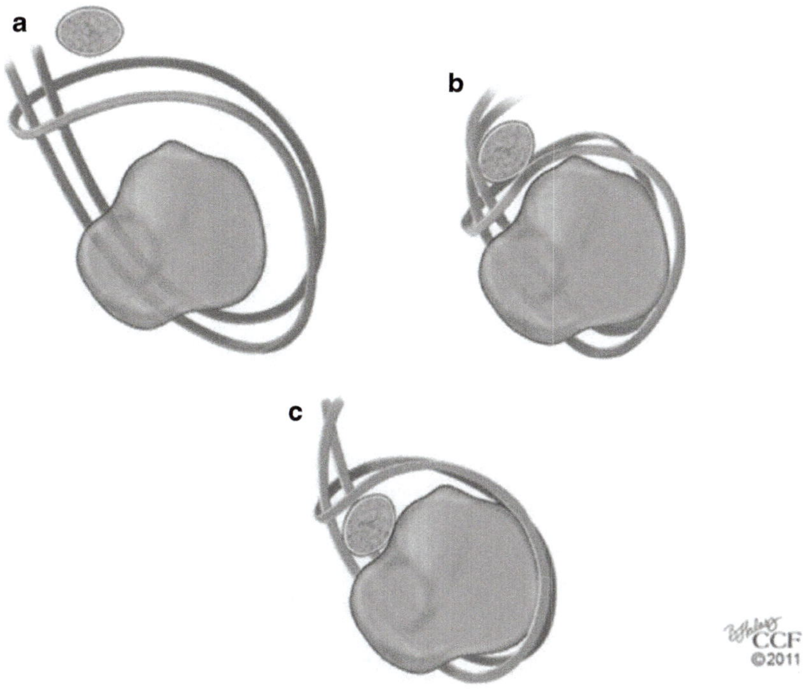

Fig. 15.10 Different techniques to both capture the ECU tendon when its anatomic investments have been destroyed by the pathology or prior attempts at reconstruction. (**a, b**) This technique of encircling the ECU with the tendon graft can be used in any circumstances but has particular merit when the bed has been manipulated by prior attempts to deepen the sulcus and the surface is unfavorable for tendon gliding. (**c**) When the ulnar buttress reconstruction is of utmost important and the floor of the sulcus is favorable, this technique stabilizes the tendon nicely

Intersection syndrome is not typically a diagnostic dilemma and advanced imaging is rarely necessary (however in-office ultrasound may be a welcome supplement to physical examination). There really is almost no other anatomy that can contribute both the patient-reported symptoms and physical signs; embarrassment of the dorsal sensory branch of the radial nerve (Wartnerberg's syndrome) can contribute the symptoms, but normally is physically unimpressive. However, it is not uncharacteristic to have a modicum of DSBRN irritation with intersection syndrome.

Immobilization and injection are the hallmarks of therapy, but occasionally the problem is more florid, requiring release.

Carpal Boss

Whether this entity should be included in a manuscript about extensor pathology is debatable. What is not, however, is the fact that baseball athletes often have morphological changes and discomfort about the carpometacarpal joints of the II and III rays.

The so-called stable unit (CMCs of the index and long rays) is more solidly related to the carpus because of both osseous and soft-tissue anatomy. The tremendous number of repetitions creates enough micromotion over time that even fairly young players can start to manifest the characteristic "beaking" of both the metacarpal base and carpal partner with which it is coapted (Fig. 15.11).

Besides avoiding the embarrassment of mistaking the bony prominence as a ganglion cyst, there is usually no diagnostic dilemma. If the palpation of the excrescence is not enough, a semi-supinated oblique X-ray should show the "kissing lesion." The reason to add it to this chapter is the fact that insertional tendinopathy of the radial wrist extensors can accompany the boss. A subluxation of the ECRB over the boss has been reported [19].

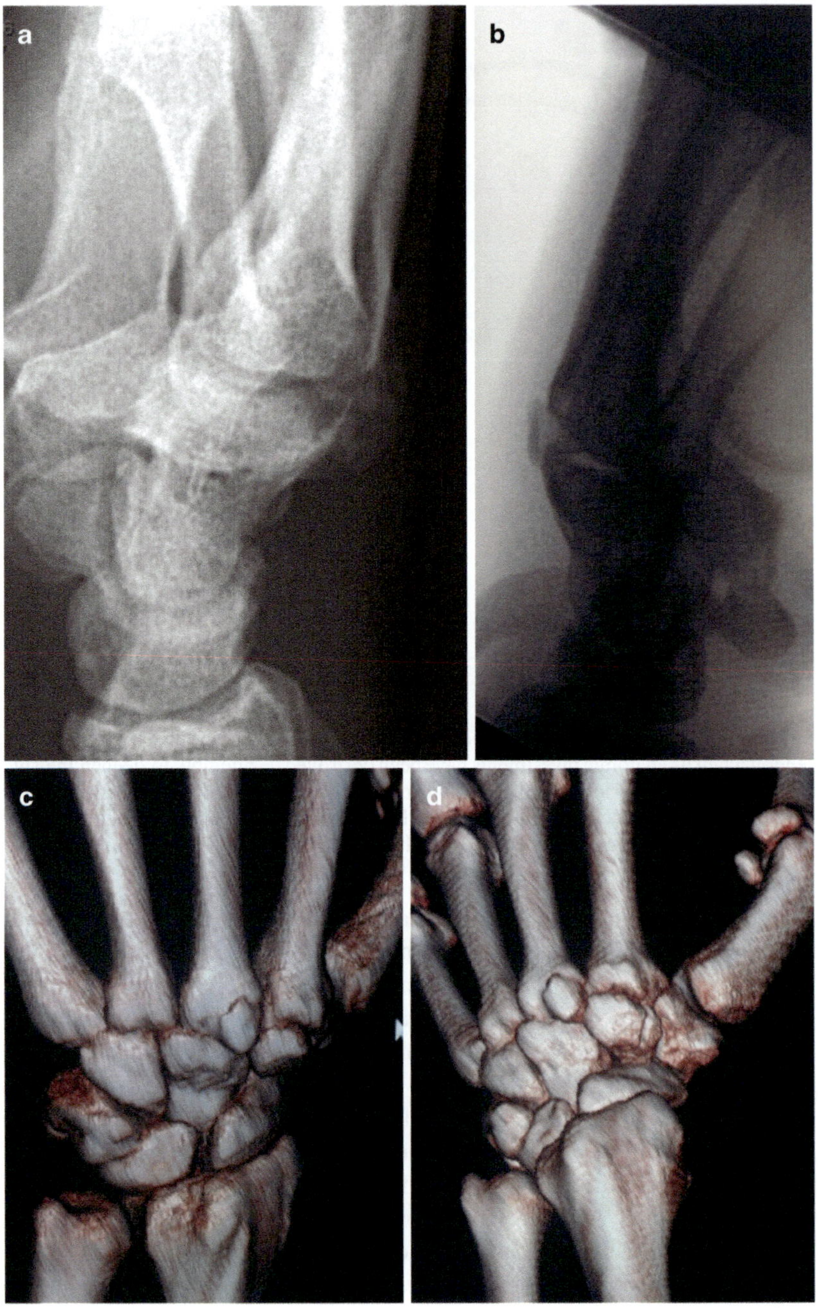

Fig. 15.11 The morphology of the boss or related pathologies, whether a bony excrescence (**a**) or possibly an expression of calcific tendinopathy (**b**), can best be appreciated on a semi-supinated oblique film. (**c**, **d**) Although rarely required, cross-sectional imaging, here a CT scan with three-dimensional reconstruction, can be interesting and informative

In our experience, treatment of the carpal boss is challenging and our default is almost always conservative. Besides icing and anti-inflammatories, injection can be helpful, but be aware that the CMC is a difficult joint to enter in the best of circumstances, let alone when narrowed and "protected" by overlying osteophytosis.

If surgery is the last remaining options, decades of experience have told us that even when one believes that they have excavated the boss adequately, it seems like the bump persists to a greater degree than predicted. Of course, protection of the tendon insertions is paramount. Recommendations vary regarding the percentage of joint resection that is safe, so as not to introduce instability, but there is inherent stability even when the dorsal margin is sacrificed. Fusion is rarely required, but it could be considered a rather aggressive primary or salvage option.

Admittedly, our patients have had ambivalent feelings about the appearance, but have been satisfied with the pain relief; other authors report uniform good results, but we just want to honestly communicate our admonition to consider nonoperative treatment, if possible [20].

Conclusion

Those of us who get the privilege of working with elite athletes maintain a slightly different epidemiological perspective and surgical "playbook." Pathologic entities that are thought rare in the general population will present with unusual frequency in a selected small population, like stick-and-ball athletes. Pathologies of the ECU tendon and its investments represent one of the most important pathologies that the subset of hand surgeons "in this game" must know and with which they need to be comfortable.

Surgery is not always required, and we have outlined the nonsurgical approach to which most athletes deserve initial exposure. However, if the problems like mechanical dysfunction and chronic inflammation are recalcitrant, then I hope the descriptions of the surgical approaches and reconstructions are valuable.

Do not forget that elite athletes can also present with "normal" problems about the radial wrist – DeQuervain's, intersection syndrome, and carpal bossing. Although there may be some additional time-sensitivity, treating these in the manner that has been successful in your general practice is never the wrong answer.

We should all be humbled if we get to enjoy the unique "laboratory" in which to test the validity of our surgical approaches and rehabilitation plans. Working with a supremely healthy, extremely motivated group of patients, who have at their disposal essentially all potential resources is an optimal environment for a surgeon. That is why it is so valuable to share information like this, as it will assist all of us to introduce new techniques and technologies into our entire practice and enhance our specialty.

References

1. Spinner M, Kaplan EB. Extensor carpi ulnaris. Its relationship to the stability of the distal radio-ulnar joint. Clin Orthop. 1970;68:124–9.
2. Graham TJ. Pathologies of the extensor carpi ulnaris (ECU) tendon and its investments in the athlete. Hand Clin. 2012;28:345–356, ix.
3. Goldfarb CA, Puri SK, Carlson MG. Diagnosis, treatment, and return to play for four common sports injuries of the hand and wrist. J Am Acad Orthop Surg. 2016;24:853–62.
4. Inoue G, Tamura Y. Recurrent dislocation of the extensor carpi ulnaris tendon. Br J Sports Med. 1998;32:172–4.
5. Allende C, Le Viet D. Extensor carpi ulnaris problems at the wrist – classification, surgical treatment and results. J Hand Surg Br. 2005;30:265–72.
6. Spangler J, Bamberger H, Graham T. Midcarpal impingement: a cause of ulnar-sided wrist pain in batters. 2013.
7. Ruland RT, Hogan CJ. The ECU synergy test: an aid to diagnose ECU tendonitis. J Hand Surg. 2008;33:1777–82.
8. MacLennan AJ, Nemechek NM, Waitayawinyu T, Trumble TE. Diagnosis and anatomic reconstruction of extensor carpi ulnaris subluxation. J Hand Surg. 2008;33:59–64.
9. Jeantroux J, et al. Athletic injuries of the extensor carpi ulnaris subsheath: MRI findings and utility of gadolinium-enhanced fat-saturated T1-weighted sequences with wrist pronation and supination. Eur Radiol. 2011;21:160–6.
10. Vulpius J. Habitual dislocation of the extensor carpi ulnaris tendon. Acta Orthop Scand. 1964;34: 105–8.
11. Eckhardt WA, Palmer AK. Recurrent dislocation of extensor carpi ulnaris tendon. J Hand Surg. 1981;6:629–31.
12. Burkhart SS, Wood MB, Linscheid RL. Posttraumatic recurrent subluxation of the extensor carpi ulnaris tendon. J Hand Surg. 1982;7:1–3.
13. Rayan GM. Recurrent dislocation of the extensor carpi ulnaris in athletes. Am J Sports Med. 1983;11: 183–4.
14. Rowland SA. Acute traumatic subluxation of the extensor carpi ulnaris tendon at the wrist. J Hand Surg. 1986;11:809–11.
15. Oka Y, Handa A. Recurrent dislocation of the ECU tendon in a golf player: release of the extensor reti-

naculum and partial resection of the ulno-dorsal ridge of the ulnar head. Hand Surg. 2001;6:227–30.
16. Iwamoto A, Morris RP, Andersen C, Patterson RM, Viegas SF. An anatomic and biomechanic study of the wrist extensor retinaculum septa and tendon compartments. J Hand Surg. 2006;31:896–903.
17. Kiyono Y, Nakatsuchi Y, Saitoh S. Ulnar-styloid nonunion and partial rupture of extensor carpi ulnaris tendon: two case reports and review of the literature. J Orthop Trauma. 2002;16:674–7.
18. Wang C, Gill TJ, Zarins B, Herndon JH. Extensor carpi ulnaris tendon rupture in an ice hockey player: a case report. Am J Sports Med. 2003;31:459–61.
19. Park MJ, Namdari S, Weiss A-P. The carpal boss: review of diagnosis and treatment. J Hand Surg. 2008;33:446–9.
20. Fusi S, Watson HK, Cuono CB. The carpal boss. A 20-year review of operative management. J Hand Surg Br. 1995;20:405–8.

Nerve Injuries of the Wrist

16

Dimitrios V. Papadopoulos,
Loukia K. Papatheodorou,
and Dean G. Sotereanos

Carpal Tunnel Syndrome

Introduction

Carpal tunnel syndrome, a compressive neuropathy of the median nerve within the carpal tunnel, is the most common compressive neuropathy affecting 0.1–10% of the general population [1]. It is also the most common focal compression neuropathy in athletes, having been reported in various athletic populations such as in cyclists, body builders, tennis players, baseball players, hockey players, and swimmers [2–4].

Anatomy

The carpal tunnel is an osteoligamentous space located on the volar aspect of the wrist. The floor of this space is made from the proximal carpal row, the roof is formed from the transverse carpal ligament, while its radial boundaries are the scaphoid tubercle and the trapezium, and its ulnar boundaries are the hook of the hamate and the pisiform. In the distal forearm, the median nerve is located deep to the palmaris longus between the flexor carpi radialis and flexor digitorum superficialis, and enters the hand passing deep transverse carpal ligament. The motor fibers of the median nerve innervate the abductor pollicis brevis, the two radial lumbricals, the superficial head of the flexor pollicis brevis, and the opponens pollicis, while its sensory fibers innervate the volar aspect of the thumb, index, and middle finger, and the radial half of the ring finger. A high division of the median nerve resulting in a bifid median nerve can be noted in 1–3.3% of the cases [5]. There are also four main variations regarding the branching of the motor branch of the median nerve. The extraligamentous branching is the most common form, identified in 46% of the cases, while the subligamentous form is the second most common form accounting for 31%, and the transligamentous the third most common form taking 23% of the cases [6, 7].

Etiology

Compression of the median nerve can be caused by space-occupying lesions such as hand tumors or can be due to repetitive motion in patients with normal anatomy [8]. In the latter case, carpal tunnel syndrome is called idiopathic and a common finding in these patients is pathologic and inflamed tenosynovium. In many cases, symptoms of carpal tunnel syndrome are pre-

D. V. Papadopoulos
University of Pittsburgh School of Medicine – UPMC, Pittsburgh, PA, USA

L. K. Papatheodorou · D. G. Sotereanos (✉)
Department of Orthopaedic Surgery, University of Pittsburgh School of Medicine – UPMC, Pittsburgh, PA, USA

G. M. Lourie (ed.), *Hand and Wrist Injuries in Baseball*,
https://doi.org/10.1007/978-3-030-81659-9_16

cipitated by periods of excessive work or activities that require repetitive motions. Baseball players are exposed to forceful repetitive wrist dorsi-palmarflexion coupled with prolonged wrist posture, or they can sustain blunt impacts during activities such as throwing/catching the ball or holding the baseball bat. Sustained local compression of the median nerve can result in carpal tunnel syndrome. Cyclists develop carpal tunnel syndrome since these athletes experience long-standing loading and vibration from the handlebars onto their wrists. Other risk factors for carpal tunnel syndrome include inflammatory arthropathies, pregnancy, amyloidosis, traumatic disorders of the wrist, and endocrine disorders (diabetes mellitus and hypothyroidism) [9]. Carpal tunnel syndrome must be differentiated from other compressive neuropathies of the median nerve along its course in the arm, and from cervical radiculopathy. Moreover, although diabetic neuropathy may present with similar symptoms, many patients with diabetic neuropathy have concomitant carpal tunnel syndrome.

History

Numbness and tingling in the thumb, index, and middle fingers are the most common symptoms, although many patients note that their entire hand feels numb. Although pain usually does not prevent patients from falling asleep, very commonly patients complain of awakenings after a number of hours during sleep [10]. Often patients describe that in order to return to sleep they feel the urge to move and shake their hands to alleviate symptoms. Morning stiffness and hand clumsiness are also some other atypical symptoms.

Numbness, pain, or discomfort can be incited by certain activities in which the wrist is held in a flexed position for a long period of time (e.g., holding a steering wheel, or holding a bicycle handle bar), or by activities that require repetitive flexion of the wrist (e.g., throwing a ball in baseball players). Although symptoms are mainly located in the wrist, discomfort and pain may radiate proximal up to the shoulder or neck. Moreover, patients often complain of clumsiness with certain tasks such as unscrewing a jar top, or can experience difficulty in holding objects such as a glass or a cup.

Physical Examination

In severe, long-standing cases, inspection can reveal atrophy of the thenar eminence since thenar muscles are innervated by the median nerve. Percussion on the skin over the median nerve just proximal to the carpal tunnel can elicit a positive Tinel sign, with the patient complaining of an electric or tingling sensation radiating down to the ring, middle, index, and thumb fingers. Neurologic examination should include muscle strength testing and sensory examination. On muscle strength testing, thumb abduction strength may be decreased compared to the contralateral side, due to weakness of the abductor pollicis brevis muscle. Sensory examination includes the two-point discrimination test and Semmes-Weinstein monofilament test. Patients with carpal tunnel syndrome often present with diminished two-point discrimination ability over the fingers' pulps. The Semmes-Weinstein monofilament test is considered the most sensitive test for the early detection of sensory dysfunction and evaluates a single nerve fiber that innervates group of receptors over a defined area. There are also some provocative tests that are helpful for the diagnosis of carpal tunnel syndrome. The Phalen wrist flexion test is considered by many to be more sensitive and diagnostic than the Tinel sign. It is considered positive when passive wrist flexion with the elbow maintained in extension elicits numbness along the median nerve distribution. The time between the onset of wrist flexion and development of symptoms, and the location of paresthesias should be recorded. Onset of symptoms within 60 s is considered supportive of the diagnosis of carpal tunnel syndrome. The wrist compression test (Durkan's test) is considered positive when carpal tunnel syndromes are provoked within 30 s following pressure over the median nerve proximal to the wrist [11].

Diagnostics

Although electrodiagnostic studies including nerve conduction studies and electromyography are not required to establish the diagnosis, these studies can be helpful in localization of the nerve compression in the arm and can evaluate the residual neural and motor function [12, 13]. A distal motor latency greater than 3.5–4.0 ms is considered the best indicator of carpal tunnel syndrome. The surgical outcomes are usually worse for patients with severe electrodiagnostic findings or, on the other hand, with normal findings compared to patients with moderate findings.

Ultrasound as a diagnostic modality in carpal tunnel syndrome has been proposed in the recent years as an alternative confirmatory study to nerve conduction studies. To have proper and consistent measurements of the cross-sectional area of the median nerve, the ultrasound probe should be positioned perpendicular to the long axis of the forearm and the nerve should be measured at the carpal tunnel inlet just proximal to the level of the pisiform. The outline of the median nerve is defined as the margins within the hyperechoic nerve sheath. Ultrasound has been shown to have 89% and 90% sensitivity and specificity, respectively, for the diagnosis of carpal tunnel in patients whose cross-sectional area of the median nerve is measured $\geq$10 mm^2 [14].

Treatment

Since symptoms of carpal tunnel syndrome are usually precipitated by sustained wrist flexion (usual sleep posture), sustained extension, or by repetitive wrist motions and vibrations, the first line of treatment include night splint that maintains the wrist in a neutral position, NSAIDs, and activities modification. Activities modification may include simple measures such as adjustment of keyboard height or decreasing the frequency of the provoking athletic activities [15]. The diagnosis of carpal tunnel syndrome is further supported if symptoms improve with this simple measure.

Steroid injection in the carpal tunnel may improve symptoms by decreasing the inflammatory response around the flexor tendons and can be the second step in the treatment of carpal tunnel syndrome if the previous measures fail. Injection of the carpal tunnel is usually performed with a 25-gauge 1.5-inch needle which is placed at the level of the palmar wrist crease just ulnar to the palmaris longus tendon. In cases of absent the palmaris longus, the needle is placed along the line of the radial border of the ring finger down to the wrist crease. Patients that report a transient relief of symptoms after injection are more possible to have a favorable surgical outcome following release of the carpal tunnel. Although the reported success rate for temporary improvement of symptoms is 80%, only 20% of patients report symptom relief at 1 year.

Surgical treatment is indicated in athletes with ongoing symptoms despite an adequate trial of conservative measures. However, in more severe cases, surgical treatment may be recommended from the beginning [16]. The main goal of surgical release of the carpal tunnel is the complete transection of the transverse carpal ligament. Surgical release can be performed through either open (extended open, limited, or mini-open) or endoscopic approach. Each surgical approach has its own advantages and disadvantages. The open carpal tunnel release approach remains the gold standard and the most commonly used technique.

A small longitudinal incision (2–4 cm) is created distal to the wrist crease in line with the third webspace for the mini-open technique (Fig. 16.1). Following incision of the palmar fascia longitudinally, the transverse carpal ligament is exposed and divided under direct visualization. This incision avoids injury to the palmar cutaneous branch of the median nerve. The endoscopic carpal tunnel release can be performed though either a single incision (at the level of the proximal wrist flexion crease) or through two incisions (one proximal to the wrist crease and one midpalmar).

Open and endoscopic carpal tunnel release can both result in excellent functional outcomes. Neither technique has been shown to be superior

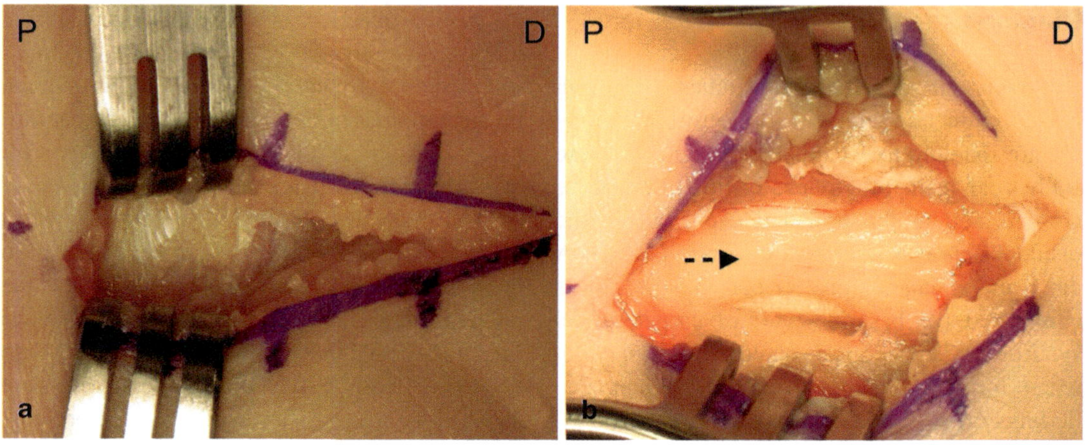

Fig. 16.1 (**a**) Intraoperative view of carpal tunnel release with mini-open technique through a small longitudinal incision (3 cm). (**b**) The median nerve (black arrow) after mini-open carpal tunnel release. P proximal to the wrist, D distal to the wrist

although many randomized controlled studies have been reported. The theoretical advantage of the endoscopic approach is avoidance of a potentially tender palmar incision and lower rate of pillar pain, which can be associated with earlier return to previous activities; therefore, it may be helpful in certain groups such as professional athletes. However, the risk for iatrogenic nerve injuries, tendon injuries, and late recurrence of symptoms due to incomplete release of the carpal tunnel may be higher with the endoscopic release compared to open release [17–20].

The decision of the surgical technique must be based on surgeon's preference and experience. Based on the clinical experience of the senior author (D.G.S.), carpal tunnel release with one mini-open technique is correlated with less risk of transverse carpal ligament incomplete release and less risk of neurovascular injury. Although, a potentially higher incidence of transient pillar pain and a slightly longer incision site, he prioritizes avoidance of a nerve laceration.

Following surgery, patients are encouraged to actively move their fingers from the first postoperative day, while wrist motion is also recommended within the first week. Tenderness over the incision may last for up to 4–8 weeks. Baseball athletes are recommended to wear padded gloves postoperatively to minimize incisional pain and discomfort. A postoperative therapy program, including desensitization, range of motion, and strengthening exercises, is recommended in patients who report difficulty with hand function 3–4 weeks after surgery. The failure rate with patients reporting persistence of symptoms at 1 year after surgery is 2–20%, and the most common causes are incomplete initial release of the carpal tunnel for recurrent carpal tunnel syndrome or misdiagnosis. Recurrence of symptoms, after a distinct symptom-free period, is usually secondary to cicatrix/scarring formation surrounding the median nerve.

Ulnar Tunnel Syndrome (Guyon Canal)

Introduction

Compressive neuropathy of the ulnar nerve in the wrist and hand was first described in 1861 by a French urologist named Jean Casimir Felix Guyon who studied the relevant anatomy of this entity, describing an intra-aponeurotic space which now is known as the distal ulnar tunnel or Guyon's canal [21, 22]. About a century later in 1969, Shea and McClain described three types of compression syndromes of the wrist and hand based on the location of the nerve compression in the wrist and hand [23]. Later, Gross and

Gelberman divided the distal ulnar tunnel into three zones based on the local anatomy of the ulnar nerve as it coursed through the tunnel [24]. There are several different terms used in the literature for ulnar nerve compression in hand and wrist including Guyon canal syndrome, ulnar tunnel syndrome, cyclist's palsy, and handle-bar palsy. Although cyclists are the most common athletes affected by this pathology, repetitive stress over Guyon's canal in other sports such as baseball, racket sports, and karate can also result in this type of ulnar nerve injury. The exact incidence of ulnar tunnel syndrome is not really known, since it is commonly missed or misdiagnosed.

Anatomy

The ulnar nerve (UN) becomes more superficial at the wrist level and travels along with the ulnar artery and the flexor carpi ulnaris (FCU) tendon before entering the narrow distal ulnar tunnel, or Guyon's canal, accompanied by the ulnar artery (UA). At this level, the ulnar nerve is located dorsal and ulnar to the ulnar artery and radial to the FCU tendon. The distal ulnar tunnel is a fibro-osseous tunnel 4–4.5 cm in length, located 1–2 cm proximal, and deep to the distal wrist crease. It includes UN, UA as well as the venae comitantes and connective fatty tissue. It extends from the proximal edge of the volar carpal ligament (VCL) which is the roof of the tunnel, to the fibrous arch of the origin of the hypothenar muscles [24]. The borders of the tunnel are not well defined and distinct throughout the entirety of the canal as the UN and UA take a tortuous path.

There are two main bony landmarks, the pisiform that marks the proximal and ulnar border of the tunnel, and the hook of the hamate that marks the radial and distal border. The entrance of the tunnel is triangular, with a radial apex. The roof of the tunnel is consisted proximally of the volar carpal ligament, and distally of the palmaris brevis and the fatty/fibrous tissue of the hypothenar eminence. The floor of the tunnels is made proximal to distal from the flexor digitorum profundus (FDP) tendons, the transverse carpal ligament (TCL), the pisohamate and pisometacarpal ligaments, and finally the opponens digiti minimi (ODM) muscle. The tunnel is walled radially by the extrinsic flexor tendons and the hook of the hamate while the ulnar boundary is made of the tendon of the FCU, the pisiform, and the abductor digiti minimi (ADM) [24].

In the ulnar tunnel, the UN bifurcates into two branches, the superficial sensory branch which provides sensation to the palmar hypothenar eminence, the small finger and the ulnar aspect of the ring finger, and the deep motor branch [25]. The motor branch originates from the ulnar aspect of the UN and passes distally and radially to the hook of the hamate. It innervates the hypothenar muscles, the ulnar two lumbricals, the interosseous muscles, the adductor pollicis, and one head of the flexor pollicis brevis [26]. In up to 77% of patients, there is a connection between the recurrent motor branch of the median nerve (MN) and the deep motor branch of the UN, called Riche-Cannieu anastomosis. This connection can result in innervation of the thenar muscles by the UN, leading to confusing clinical and electrodiagnostic findings [27].

In order to simplify the diagnosis and treatment of ulnar tunnel syndrome, Gross and Gelberman divided the distal ulnar tunnel into three zones [24] based on the branching of the UN as well as the anatomic structures surrounding it. Zone 1 includes the part of the tunnel proximal to the bifurcation of the UN, zone 2 is the area surrounding the deep motor branch of the UN, and zone 3 is the area surrounding the superficial branch of the UN [24]. In zone 1, the roof of the tunnel is formed by the VCL proximal and the palmaris brevis distal. The floor of the tunnel is made from the FDP tendons, the transverse carpal ligament (TCL), and distally from the pisohamate and pisometacarpal ligaments as the floor. Zone 2 includes the deep branch of the UN and starts at the level of the bifurcation of the UN up to the fibrous arch of the hypothenar muscles [22]. The roof of zone 2 proximally is the palmaris brevis and distally the fibrous arch of the hypothenar muscles. The deep branch of the UN travels in a radial direction around the hamate and dives deep to the fibrous arch, between the

ADM and the FDM, innervating both of these muscles before it pierces and innervates the ODM. The UA is located in zone 2 radial and volar to the UN. Zone 3 starts distal to the bifurcation of the UN and includes the area around the superficial sensory branch of the UN as it travels volar to the fibrous arch of the hypothenar muscles. The roof of zone 3 is formed by the palmaris brevis, the floor by the pisometacarpal ligament and the triquetro-hamate joint capsule, while the ulnar wall is ADM and the radial border zone 2 [24]. As opposed to the deep-dorsal course of the motor branch, the sensory branch takes a volar-ulnar course after the bifurcation. Although is called a sensory branch, there are two motor branches originating from the ulnar nerve and innervate the palmaris brevis within the first 10mm of zone 3, while the rest of the nerve is a purely sensory nerve, becoming the proper digital nerve to the ulnar side of the small finger and the common digital nerve to the web space of the ring and small fingers.

Etiology

The exact location of the compression of the ulnar nerve along its course can be identified by the presenting signs and symptoms. According to Shea and McClain, the common cause for ulnar tunnel syndrome in all three zones of the tunnel is reported to be ganglion cysts (39%) followed closely by occupational neuritis (32%) [23]. Based on more recent studies, ganglion cysts remain the most common identifiable cause; however, in most of the cases, the exact cause of ulnar nerve compression in the wrist and hand cannot be identified [28, 29]. Other less common causes include lipoma, repetitive trauma in athletes, palmaris brevis hypertrophy, hypothenar hammer syndrome, trauma including hook of hamate fractures or pisiform dislocation, and inflammatory arthritis (Fig. 16.2). Rarely the cause can be iatrogenic injury during wrist arthroscopy, opponensplasty, or tendon transfers [23, 27, 29].

In baseball players, repetitive mechanical compression of the ulnovolar portion of the palm and the underlying ulnar nerve within Guyon's canal from the baseball bat can result in ulnar tunnel syndrome. Also, repetitive compression and trauma can result in aneurysmatic enlargement of the ulnar artery and subsequently to compression of the ulnar nerve [27]. In some cases, a single direct impact from an external force during a baseball hit can lead to aneurysmatic formation of the ulnar artery or to a fracture of the hook of the hamate, also leading to compression of the ulnar nerve. While hamate hook fractures are rare fractures constituting approximately only 2% of all carpal fractures, they commonly occur in select athletic populations, such as in baseball players, tennis players, golf players, and hockey players, and on the side of the hand that holds the base of the bat, club, racquet, or stick. If diagnosis is delayed and symptoms persist for long time, the athletic performance of these players is negatively affected [29, 30]. In cyclists, the ulnar palm is compressed on the bicycle handles resulting in chronic and continuous pressure of the nerve usually in zone 2 [31, 32].

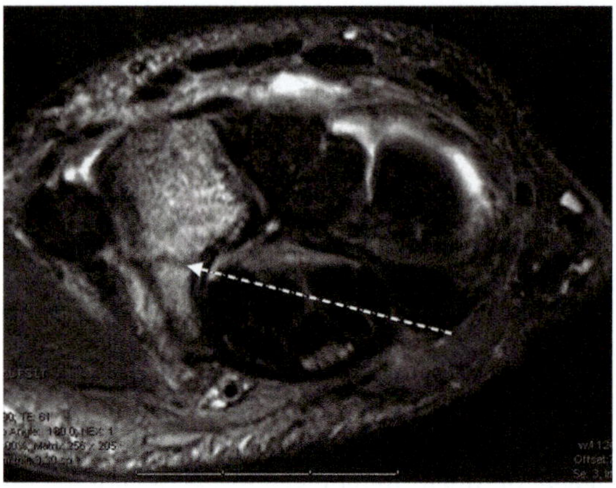

Fig. 16.2 Axial cut of MRI of left wrist showing a non-union of hook of hamate fracture (white arrow)

Compression in zone 1, which is the most common area of compression, usually results in both sensory and motor symptoms since the ulnar nerve is a still mixed nerve at this location. However, purely motor or purely sensory deficits can occur due to the location of the nerve fibers within the nerve [33, 34]. The motor fibers are dorsal while the sensory fibers are volar; therefore, compression from a dorsal lesion within the tunnel can affect isolated motor fibers, while volar lesion may compress only sensory fibers [24, 28]. In zone 2, the UN is usually compressed on the fibrous arch of the hypothenar muscles, with hook of the hamate fractures and a thickened pisohamate ligament being common causes for compression in this zone. Vascular lesions of the ulnar artery, such as thrombosis and aneurysm, are the most common cause of ulnar nerve compression in zone 3 [24].

It is noteworthy that ulnar tunnel syndrome and carpal tunnel syndrome can coexist in many cases. In a study of 53 cases of ulnar tunnel syndrome, positive findings on electrodiagnostic testing for median nerve lesions were evident on 22 cases [35]. Of these 22 cases, 13 had symptoms suggestive of carpal tunnel syndrome [35]. Similarly, the converse has also been shown in other studies. Patients with positive findings for carpal tunnel syndrome on electrodiagnostic testing had also evidence of compression of the ulnar nerve in the ulnar tunnel [36, 37]. In fact, the authors of one study stated that coexistence of carpal and ulnar tunnel syndrome is more common than isolated carpal or ulnar tunnel syndrome [38].

History

It is important to include questions during examination of these patients about their occupation and recreational activities, since these can be suggestive of the etiology of the nerve compression. When ulnar tunnel syndrome is suspected, physical examination should include the entire upper extremity for any other potential causes of ulnar nerve compression, including cervical spine pathology, thoracic outlet syndrome, and cubital tunnel syndrome. Moreover, the contralateral upper extremity should also be inspected and examined for asymmetry and muscle atrophy. Ideally, more proximal compression of the ulna nerve can be ruled out by the history and physical examination [39].

Patients with ulnar tunnel syndrome may develop pure motor, pure sensory, or mixed symptoms based on the location of the nerve compression within the ulnar tunnel. Usually, these patients complain of paresthesia and numbness in the ring and small fingers. Additionally, they can complain of being awakened during the night because of their symptoms while in more severe cases with affected motor function and muscle weakness, patients can state that they noted clumsiness and lack of dexterity.

Physical Examination

Physical examination should include documentation of ulnar nerve sensory and motor integrity, while the patency of the ulnar artery should always be assessed with the Allen test. On physical examination, inspection may reveal wasting of the interosseous muscles between the metacarpals, more prominent of the first dorsal interosseous muscle and clawing of the small and ring fingers with hyperextension of their metacarpophalangeal (MCP) joints [39]. However, these findings are suggestive of severe compression of the motor fibers. Sometimes volar or dorsal wrist masses are visible, indicating presence of space-occupying lesions causing nerve compression, though the majority of ganglia are not visible on physical examination. A positive Tinel sign over the Guyon canal is noted when percussion over the ulnar nerve at the ulnar tunnel provokes paresthesias along the ulnar forearm and hand. Tenderness on palpation over the hook of the hamate is suggestive of fracture or non-union. Neurologic examination for sensation may reveal decreased sensation over the volar surfaces of the small and ulnar side of the ring fingers and over the hypothenar eminence [23]. However, sensation to the dorsal ulnar hand is preserved as sensation to this area provided by the dorsal cutaneous branch of the ulnar nerve, which originates approximately 3–5 cm proximal to the ulnar styloid. The Semmes-Weinstein monofilament test and the two-point static discrimination test are both useful tests for assessment of the severity of the disease. The Semmes-Weinstein monofilament test is more sensitive in measuring a gradual, progressive loss of nerve function as more fibers are lost, while the static and moving two-point discrimination tests are best used for evaluating nerve regeneration. Examination for motor function may reveal decreased grasp and pinch strength due to extrinsic (flexor digitorum profundus of the small finger) and intrinsic (adductor pollicis) muscles weakness. Interossei weakness may also result in weak fingers' abduction and adduction. Testing of muscle strength should always include comparison with the contralateral side. There are several provocative tests for the diagnosis of ulnar tunnel syndrome. A positive Froment sign can be observed due to weak adductor pollicis muscle. As the patient tries to hold a piece of paper placed between the thumb and the index finger, the thumb interphalangeal joint flexes in an attempt to substitute flexor pollicis longus activity for inadequate adductor pollicis strength. Similar to Froment sign, Jeanne's sign is positive when the patient compensates for the inadequate adductor pollicis strength during pinch with MCP joint hyperextension.

Diagnostics

Further evaluation of ulnar tunnel syndrome includes electrodiagnostic and imaging studies. Electrodiagnostic studies are useful to confirm ulnar nerve compression; assess the severity of the nerve damage; differentiate ulnar tunnel syndrome from other compressive neuropathies such as cubital tunnel syndrome, carpal tunnel syndrome, thoracic outlet syndrome, cervical radiculopathy, or even peripheral neuropathy; and locate the area of compression. Electrodiagnostic evaluation includes nerve conduction studies (NCS) and electromyography (EMG) [40]. In cases of ulnar tunnel syndrome, needle EMG may demonstrate isolated denervation of the hypothenar muscles with unaffected FCU function [40]. Decreased sensory responses, increased latency to the first dorsal interosseous and abductor digiti minimi muscles, and preserved conduction velocity across the elbow are typical for nerve compression in zone 1 [41, 42]. Preserved conduction velocity across the elbow, normal latency of the hypothenar muscles, and diminished latency of the first dorsal interosseous are suggestive for lesions in zone 2 injures [41, 42]. Finally, isolated diminished evoked sensory responses are typical for zone 3 lesions [43].

Imaging evaluation includes radiographs, magnetic resonance imaging (MRI), and computer tomography (CT). Standard posteroanterior and lateral wrist radiographs should be always ordered to evaluate for any fractures of the distal radius, ulna, and carpal bones. Carpal tunnel view is also useful to assess for a hook of the hamate fracture. In certain cases, CT should be ordered to identify fracture of the hook of hamate, fracture of other carpal bones, or proximal metacarpals fractures. CT scans can also show ectopic calcifications within the ulnar tunnel. MRI scan can also identify fracture of the hook of hamate (Fig. 16.2) and is the indicated study for the identification of anomalous muscles, and for space-occupying soft-tissue lesions, like ganglion cysts [44, 45]. Furthermore, the branching pattern of the ulnar nerve can be defined in MRI. Ultrasonography is also a noninvasive low-cost method for evaluation of vascular, soft-tissue, and nerve structures [36, 46–48]. Finally, in cases of suspected vascular pathology of the ulnar artery, Doppler examination or arteriography can be ordered [30, 39].

Treatment

In most cases, especially in patients with ulnar tunnel syndrome due to repetitive activities such as in baseball players, tennis players, or cyclists, an initial course of conservative treatment is recommended [27–29]. The mainstay of conservative management includes protective splinting, nonsteroidal anti-inflammatory medications, and activity modification. Softer handlebars can improve symptoms in cyclists, while protective gloves and proper position of the bicycle seat, so as excessive weight on the hands is avoided, can be also extremely beneficiary [31, 32]. Likewise, protective gloves can also help baseball or tennis players. In all these cases, a period of cessation of the causative activities should be advised if previous measures fail [8, 30].

In certain cases when ganglion cysts are the cause, aspiration of the cysts under ultrasound can be successful. However, aspiration without image guidance should not be performed as it can lead to iatrogenic injury of ulnar nerve and artery [48]. After a period of 2–4 months of failed nonsurgical management, surgical treatment is indicated [27, 49, 50]. However, in severe cases with intrinsic muscle atrophy, denervation, or weakness, surgical treatment is advised as initial management [27, 28]. Surgical treatment should focus on the treatment of the causative pathology and on decompression of the entire ulnar tunnel from its proximal to distal boundaries [11].

Surgery can be performed under general, regional, or local anesthesia. However, local anesthetic can obscure the anatomic landmarks of the ulna tunnel; therefore, some authors do not recommend local anesthesia [49]. The pisiform and hook of the hamate are the two palpable bony landmarks, and a longitudinal/oblique 4–5 cm skin incision between these two landmarks is marked. The skin incision begins 1–2 cm proximal to the volar wrist crease proximal and ends 2–3 cm distal to it [26, 28]. The incision is curved over the wrist crease to avoid contracture [27, 28]. The ulnar artery and nerve are exposed after retraction of the FCU ulnarly, proximal to the wrist crease. A palmar cutaneous branch of the ulna nerve can be identified in about 15% of patients [26, 39]. The distal antebrachial fascia over the proximal wrist, the VCL, and the palmaris brevis are incised to decompress and expose the proximal part of the ulnar nerve, proximal to the bifurcation. The ulnar artery and nerve are gently retracted ulnarly to expose the hook of the hamate. The pisohamate ligament and the fibrous arch of the hypothenar muscles can be identified forming the floor of the tunnel hamate [39]. The tendinous origin of the hypothenar muscle is incised close to the hook of the hamate to decompress the deep branch of the ulnar nerve in zone 2. The hook of the hamate should be completely released from all the surrounding fascial attachments [28, 39]. Finally, the ulnar artery should be assessed along its course for any aneurysms or thromboses, while any space-occupying lesions such as ganglion cysts should be removed. Care must also be taken to avoid any iatrogenic injury to the carpal tunnel structures since the ulnar tunnel and the carpal tunnel are adjacent spaces. In cases of symptomatic nonunion of hook of hamate with ulnar neuritis, hook of hamate excision is performed in association with ulnar nerve decompression (Fig. 16.3).

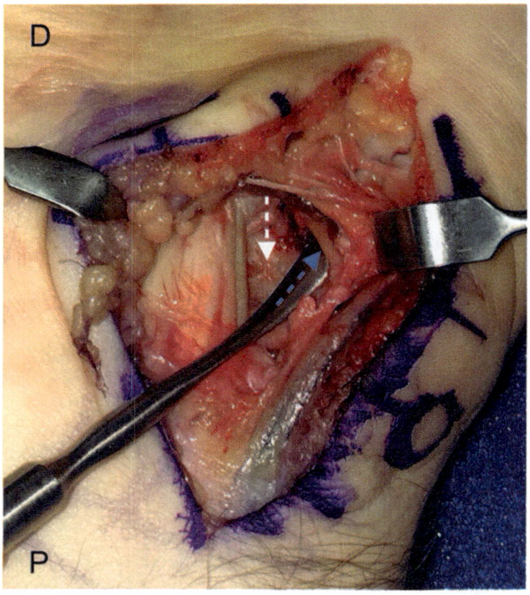

Fig. 16.3 Intraoperative view of excision of hook of hamate nonunion and Guyon canal release with ulnar nerve release. The white arrow is pointing the hamate, while the blue arrow is pointing the motor branch of ulnar nerve. P proximal to the wrist, D distal to the wrist

Good results have been reported following surgical management of ulnar nerve compression at the wrist, although most of the data are associated with case reports. Persistent numbness at the ring and little fingers have been reported postoperatively [29]. However, failure to identify and address a compression site intraoperatively can lead to failed resolution of symptoms.

Summary

Carpal and ulnar tunnel syndromes are the most common compressive neuropathies at the wrist in athletes. A thorough understanding of the anatomy and function of the median and ulnar nerve as well as knowledge of the potential sites of nerve compression can lead to safe surgical management with successful function outcome.

References

1. Zhang D, Collins JE, Earp BE, et al. Surgical demographics of carpal tunnel syndrome and cubital tunnel syndrome over 5 years at a single institution. J Hand Surg Am. 2017;42:929.e1–8.
2. Krivickas LS, Wilbourn AJ. Peripheral nerve injuries in athletes: a case series of over 200 injuries. Semin Neurol. 2000;20:225–32.
3. Mauer UM, Rath SA. Stress-induced carpal tunnel syndrome in athletes–exemplified by 3 kinds of sports. Schweiz Z Sportmed. 1992;40:131–5.
4. Akuthota V, Plastaras C, Lindberg K, et al. The effect of longdistance bicycling on ulnar and median nerves: an electrophysiologic evaluation of cyclist palsy. Am J Sports Med. 2005;133:1224–30.
5. Chammas M, Boretto J, Burmann LM, Ramos RM, Santos Neto FC, Silva JB. Carpal tunnelsyndrome – part I (anatomy, physiology, etiology and diagnosis). Rev Bras Ortop. 2014;49:429–36.
6. Blumenthal S, Herskovitz S, Verghese J. Carpal tunnel syndrome in older adults. Muscle Nerve. 2006;34:78–83.
7. Uzun A, Seelig LL. A variation in the formation of the median nerve: communicating branch between the musculocutaneous and median nerves in man. Folia Morphol (Warsz). 2001;60:99–101.
8. Geoghegan J, Clark D, Bainbridge L, Smith C, Hubbard R. Risk factors in carpal tunnel syndrome. J Hand Surg Eur Vol. 2004;29:315–20.
9. Uchiyama S, Itsubo T, Nakamura K, Kato H, Yasutomi T, Momose T. Current concepts of carpal tunnel syndrome: pathophysiology, treatment, and evaluation. J Orthop Sci. 2010;15:1–13.
10. MacDermid JC, Wessel J. Clinical diagnosis of carpal tunnel syndrome: a systematic review. J Hand Ther. 2004;17:309–19.
11. Williams TM, Mackinnon SE, Novak CB, et al. Verification of the pressure provocative test in carpal tunnel syndrome. Ann Plast Surg. 1992;29:8–11.
12. Zyluk A, Szlosser Z. The results of carpal tunnel release for carpal tunnel syndrome diagnosed on clinical grounds, with or without electrophysiological investigations: a randomized study. J Hand Eur Vol. 2013;38:44–9.
13. Sears ED, Swiatek PR, Hou H, et al. Utilization of preoperative electrodiagnostic studies for carpal tunnel syndrome: an analysis of national practice patterns. J Hand Surg Am. 2016;41:665–672.e1.
14. Fowler J, Munsch M, Tosti R, Hagberg W, Imbriglia J. Comparison of ultrasound and electrodiagnostic testing for diagnosis of carpal tunnel syndrome. J Bone Joint Surg Am. 2014;96(17):e148.
15. Graham B, Peljovich A, Afra R, et al. The American Academy of Orthopaedic Surgeons evidence-based clinical practice guideline on: management of carpal tunnel syndrome. J Bone Joint Surg Am. 2016;98:1750–4.
16. Tang CQY, Lai SWH, Tay SC. Long-term outcome of carpal tunnel release surgery in patients with severe carpal tunnel syndrome. Bone Joint J. 2017;99-B(10):1348–53.
17. Sayegh ET, Strauch RJ. Open versus endoscopic carpal tunnel release: a meta-analysis of randomized controlled trials. Clin Orthop Relat Res. 2015;473(3):1120–32.
18. Murphy RX Jr, Jennings JF, Wukich DK. Major neurovascular complications of endoscopic carpal tunnel release. J Hand Surg [Am]. 1994;19(1):114–8.
19. Schonauer F, Varma S, Belcher HJ. Endoscopic carpal tunnel release: practice in evolution. Scand J Plast Reconstr Surg Hand Surg. 2003;37(6):360–4.
20. Zhang D, Earp BE, Blazar P. Evaluation and management of unsuccessful carpal tunnel release. J Hand Surg [Am]. 2019;44(9):779–86.
21. Guyon F. Note on the anatomical condition affecting the underside of the wrist not previously reported. 1861. J Hand Surg Br. 2006;31(2):147–8.
22. Maroukis BL, Ogawa T, Rehim SA, Chung KC. Guyon canal: the evolution of clinical anatomy. J Hand Surg [Am]. 2015;40(3):560–5.
23. Shea JD, McClain EJ. Ulnar-nerve compression syndromes at and below the wrist. J Bone Joint Surg Am. 1969;51(6):1095–103.
24. Gross MS, Gelberman RH. The anatomy of the distal ulnar tunnel. Clin Orthop Relat Res. 1985;196:238–47.
25. Polatsch DB, Melone CP Jr, Beldner S, Incorvaia A. Ulnar nerve anatomy. Hand Clin. 2007;23(3):283–289, v.
26. Mackinnon SE, Novak CB. Compressive neuropathies. In: Wolfe SW, Hotchkiss RN, Pederson WC, Kozin SH, Cohen MS, editors. Green's operative hand surgery. Seventh ed. Philadelphia: Elsevier; 2017. p. 921–58.
27. Earp BE, Floyd WE, Louie D, Koris M, Protomastro P. Ulnar nerve entrapment at the wrist. J Am Acad Orthop Surg. 2014;22(11):699–706.
28. Waugh RP, Pellegrini VD Jr. Ulnar tunnel syndrome. Hand Clin. 2007;23(3):301–10.
29. Murata K, Shih JT, Tsai TM. Causes of ulnar tunnel syndrome: a retrospective study of 31 subjects. J Hand Surg [Am]. 2003;28(4):647–51.
30. Yuen JC, Wright E, Johnson LA, Culp WC. Hypothenar hammer syndrome: an update with algorithms for diagnosis and treatment. Ann Plast Surg. 2011;67(4):429–38.
31. Capitani D, Beer S. Handlebar palsy – a compression syndrome of the deep terminal (motor) branch of the ulnar nerve in biking. J Neurol. 2002;249(10):1441–5.
32. Patterson JM, Jaggars MM, Boyer MI. Ulnar and median nerve palsy in long-distance cyclists. A prospective study. Am J Sports Med. 2003;31(4):585–9.
33. Dupont C, Cloutier GE, Prevost Y, Dion MA. Ulnar-Tunnel Syndrome at the Wrist. A report of four cases ulnar-nerve compression at the wrist. J Bone Joint Surg Am. 1965;47:757–61.

34. Boyes JH. Repair of the motor branch of the ulnar nerve in the palm. J Bone Joint Surg Am. 1955;37-A(5):920–4.
35. Seror P. Electrophysiological pattern of 53 cases of ulnar nerve lesion at the wrist. Neurophysiol Clin. 2013;43(2):95–103.
36. Ginanneschi F, Filippou G, Reale F, Scarselli C, Galeazzi M, Rossi A. Ultrasonographic and functional changes of the ulnar nerve at Guyon's canal after carpal tunnel release. Clin Neurophysiol. 2010;121(2):208–13.
37. Ginanneschi F, Milani P, Mondelli M, Dominici F, Biasella A, Rossi A. Ulnar sensory nerve impairment at the wrist in carpal tunnel syndrome. Muscle Nerve. 2008;37(2):183–9.
38. Kiylioglu N, Akyildiz UO, Ozkul A, Akyol A. Carpal tunnel syndrome and ulnar neuropathy at the wrist: comorbid disease or not? J Clin Neurophysiol. 2011;28(5):520.
39. Bachoura A, Jacoby SM. Ulnar tunnel syndrome. Orthop Clin North Am. 2012;43(4):467–74.
40. Grundberg AB. Ulnar tunnel syndrome. J Hand Surg Br. 1984;9(1):72–4.
41. Werner RA. Electrodiagnostic evaluation of carpal tunnel syndrome and ulnar neuropathies. PM R. 2013;5(5 Suppl):S14–21.
42. Campion D. Electrodiagnostic testing in hand surgery. J Hand Surg [Am]. 1996;21(6):947–56.
43. Cavallo M, Poppi M, Martinelli P, Gaist G. Distal ulnar neuropathy from carpal ganglia: a clinical and electrophysiological study. Neurosurgery. 1988;22(5):902–5.
44. Andreisek G, Crook DW, Burg D, Marincek B, Weishaupt D. Peripheral neuropathies of the median, radial, and ulnar nerves: MR imaging features. Radiographics. 2006;26(5):1267–87.
45. Andreisek G, Burg D, Studer A, Weishaupt D. Upper extremity peripheral neuropathies: role and impact of MR imaging on patient management. Eur Radiol. 2008;18(9):1953–61.
46. Harvie P, Patel N, Ostlere SJ. Prevalence and epidemiological variation of anomalous muscles at guyon's canal. J Hand Surg Br. 2004;29(1):26–9.
47. Ginanneschi F, Filippou G, Milani P, Biasella A, Rossi A. Ulnar nerve compression neuropathy at Guyon's canal caused by crutch walking: case report with ultrasonographic nerve imaging. Arch Phys Med Rehabil. 2009;90(3):522–4.
48. Nakamichi K, Tachibana S. Ganglion-associated ulnar tunnel syndrome treated by ultrasonographically assisted aspiration and splinting. J Hand Surg Br. 2003;28(2):177.
49. Kim DH, Han K, Tiel RL, Murovic JA, Kline DG. Surgical outcomes of 654 ulnar nerve lesions. J Neurosurg. 2003;98(5):993–1004.
50. Almeida V, de Carvalho M. Lesion of the deep palmar branch of the ulnar nerve: causes and clinical outcome. Neurophysiol Clin. 2010;40(3):159–64.

17 Vascular Injuries of the Hand and Wrist

Elizabeth A. Helsper and Charles A. Goldfarb

Baseball players are at risk for acute and chronic injuries to their upper extremity, potentially resulting in time off from play. Several sports injury surveillance systems have been performed to record injury trends in order to guide injury prevention measures [1, 2]. Although there is a general understanding of the vascular injuries in baseball players, the incidence of vascular injury is not well understood or well quantified despite recent epidemiology studies [1, 2].

Mechanism of Injury

Vascular injury in baseball players is rare but is more common compared to athletes in other sports. This is true because baseball players are exposed to repetitive hand trauma with each catch of the ball or swing of the bat [3]. In particular, the hypothenar region of the gloved hand in catchers and the fingertips of pitchers are subject to repetitive trauma [4]. This exposure has, on rare occasions, been documented to lead to ischemia of the hand and digits often with symptoms of pain, cold intolerance, and numbness [5, 6].

The repetitive trauma experienced by baseball players occurs not only during the course of a game but also in frequent practices, in warm-up sessions, and over many years of play. Ginn et al. [3] indicated catchers may receive up to 150 pitches per game at speeds over 90 mph. Additionally, catchers must receive warm-up and practice pitches, potentially resulting in over 300 impacts to the gloved hand per day [3].

While hand and digital ischemia has been reported in older, symptomatic baseball players [3], more recent studies [1] have confirmed microvascular changes in the hands of young, asymptomatic players. The prevalence of hand symptoms and vascular abnormalities was greater in catchers than in other positions players [3]. Compared to catcher's mitts of the past, modern-day gloves have less padding and more flexibility which facilitates one-handed catching and easier ball manipulation. When the two-handed catching technique can be avoided, the catcher is able to keep his dominant hand out of harm's way protecting it from inadvertent injury. Despite the use of well-padded mitts, often with additional padding, vascular changes in the gloved hand of asymptomatic catchers have been reported, suggesting that modern glove designs do not adequately protect the hand from repetitive trauma [3]. The authors of this study recommended

E. A. Helsper
Department of Orthopaedic Surgery, University of Kansas School of Medicine-Wichita, Wichita, KS, USA

C. A. Goldfarb (✉)
Department of Orthopaedic Surgery, Washington University School of Medicine, Barnes Jewish Hospital, Saint Louis, MO, USA
e-mail: goldfarbc@wudosis.wustl.edu

G. M. Lourie (ed.), *Hand and Wrist Injuries in Baseball*,
https://doi.org/10.1007/978-3-030-81659-9_17

studies on glove design to improve hand protection and long-term, longitudinal studies of professional baseball players to determine the natural history of vascular injury and to mitigate the risk factors for injury.

Anatomy

A thorough understanding of arterial anatomy is necessary when evaluating vascular pathology of the hand and wrist. The vascular supply of the hand is a complex network of vessels. The radial and ulnar arteries provide the main blood supply to the wrist and hand, and anastomose at several levels to form vascular arches that supply the digits [7, 8]. The superficial palmar arch is supplied mainly from the ulnar artery and generally gives rise to three or four common digital arteries. The deep palmar arch is supplied largely by the radial artery and provides three to four palmar metacarpal arteries (Fig. 17.1) [9].

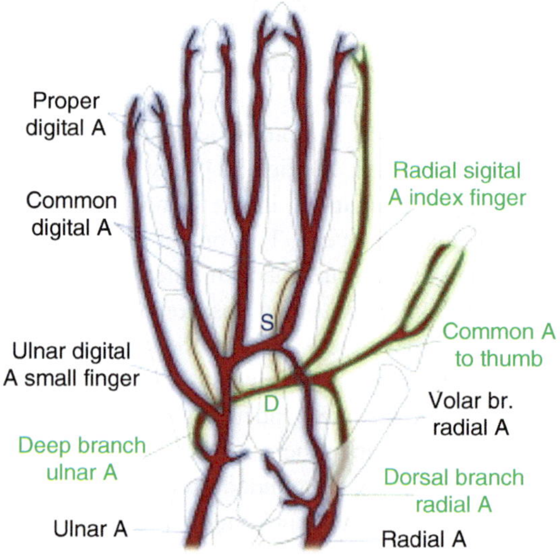

Fig. 17.1 Schematic demonstrating hand arterial anatomy. Deep palmar arch (D) system from dorsal branch of radial artery contributes to radial index finger, thumb, and branches to the common digital arteries of the second, third, and fourth web space. Superficial palmar arch (S) system from the ulnar artery contributes to ulnar digital artery and common digital arteries of the second, third, and fourth web space. (Reproduced from Wong et al. [9])

At the level of the distal forearm, the ulnar artery lies radial to the ulnar nerve and flexor carpi ulnaris. At the entrance of Guyon's canal, the ulnar artery remains radial and slightly volar to the ulnar nerve. Guyon's canal is triangular shaped, bound ulnarly and proximally by the pisiform, deep by the transverse carpal ligament and the pisohamate ligament, and radially by the hook of the hamate. In Guyon's canal, both the ulnar nerve and ulnar artery bifurcate into superficial and deep branches (Fig. 17.2) [6]. The superficial branch of the ulnar artery runs across and superficial to the hypothenar musculature. This branch, protected only by skin and muscle fibers from the palmaris brevis before penetrating the palmar aponeurosis to become the superficial palmar arch, is especially vulnerable to trauma as it exits Guyon's canal [6].

The superficial palmar arch is defined as complete when there is a direct connection with the radial artery, deep palmar arch, or median artery, as occurs in 78% of hands [6, 10–12]. The superficial palmar arch, which is located distal to the deep palmar arch, often gives rise to a deep branch that supplies the deep palmar arch, the ulnar digital artery of the small finger, and three common digital arteries (Fig. 17.1) [9]. Although the anatomy may vary, the superficial palmar arch is most often completed by the superficial branch of the radial artery. Arterial variations potentially may influence clinical symptomatology and operative outcomes [6, 11]. Coleman et al. [13] noted approximately 80% of hands studied had a complete palmar arch from which all digital arteries arise. In the remaining 20% of hands, which had incomplete arches without anastomosis, compromise of one of the feeding arteries (ulnar, radial, or median) may jeopardize vascular supply to the digits [14].

The radial artery divides at the level of the radial styloid into dorsal and volar branches. The dorsal branch crosses the anatomic snuffbox and travels deep to the first dorsal compartment and in the first dorsal web space, traversing from dorsal to volar to form the deep palmar arch by joining the ulnar artery [7, 15]. The deep palmar arch travels across the palm, lying deep to the flexor

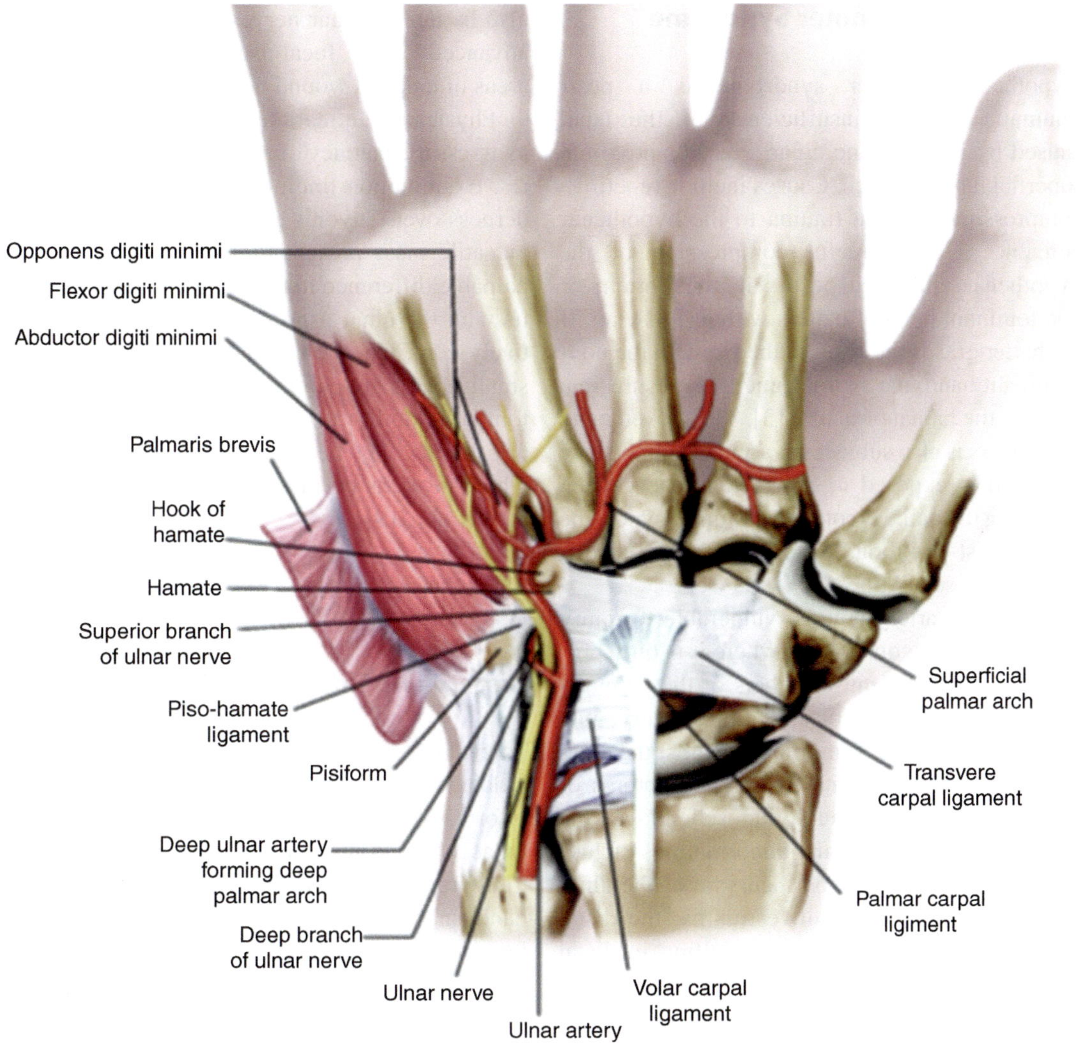

Fig. 17.2 Anatomy pertinent to understanding hypothenar hammer syndrome. Note proximity of ulnar artery to hook of the hamate. (Reproduced from Yuen et al. [11])

tendons and proximal to the superficial arch. The deep palmar arch gives rise to the digital arteries to the thumb, the radial digital artery to the index finger, and also gives branches to the three common digital arteries in the second, third, and fourth web spaces (Fig. 17.1) [9]. The volar branch of the radial artery supplies the thenar musculature and may join the ulnar artery to from a complete superficial palmar arch as discussed above [7, 15, 16].

The arterial system of the digits begins as the common digital arteries in the palm and divides into proper digital arteries in the web spaces. The ulnar three digits and the ulnar aspect of the index digit are supplied largely by the ulnar artery and the superficial palmar branch. The radial aspect of the index digit is supplied by the radial artery and the deep palmar arch. In addition, the arterial system of the thumb is supplied by the radial artery and the deep palmar arch. The deep palmar arch gives rise to the common digital artery of the thumb before becoming radial and ulnar digital branches to the thumb (Fig. 17.1) [16].

Hypothenar Hammer Syndrome

Hypothenar hammer syndrome is a post-traumatic vascular insufficiency of the hand caused by injury to the ulnar artery or proximal superficial palmar arch. Causes include repetitive compression or blunt trauma to the hypothenar eminence [17]. Forceful compression of the hypothenar eminence occurs in the bottom or nondominant hand of batters with each swing. If the batter grasps the knob of the bat with the non-dominant hand, the swing sometimes results in a hook of the hamate fracture [3]. The gloved hand of catchers is also subject to vascular injury, since the hand is exposed to repeated impacts when receiving the ball. Hypothenar hammer syndrome is the most common cause of vascular insufficiency in baseball players.

The ulnar artery is most vulnerable to injury just distal to Guyon's canal, where it is only protected by skin and muscle fibers of the palmaris brevis. The poorly protected ulnar artery may also be traumatized from impact against the adjacent hook of the hamate [6, 17]. Symptoms of hand or fingers including digital ischemia are the result of traumatic vascular abnormalities including spasm, thrombosis, or aneurysm of the ulnar artery. With minor repetitive trauma, the distal ulnar artery may vasospasm, resulting in distal vessel occlusion if prolonged. Damage to the vessel intima may lead to thrombus formation and the generation of microemboli [6, 17]. Chronic damage to the intima gives the artery a classic corkscrew configuration on angiography. Injury extending to the vessel media leads to aneurysm formation [17].

Symptoms of hypothenar hammer syndrome include acute pain in the fingers and over the hypothenar eminence which is exacerbated by repetitive use [6, 17]. Typically, pain is localized to the ulnar three digits [10]. Hypothenar hammer syndrome tends to be progressive with ischemic symptoms developing over weeks to months after thrombus formation [18]. Additionally, patients may experience more chronic symptoms including cold intolerance, blanching or discoloration of the fingertips, claudication, cyanosis, and pallor [14]. Paresthesia, pain, and numbness may also be due to ulnar nerve irritation [10, 17]. In advanced cases, focal ischemic ulcerations or areas of delayed wound healing may be seen [6].

Physical examination includes the Allen test to assess the patency of the radial and ulnar arteries. Examination findings may also include tenderness over Guyon's canal, occasionally with a pulsatile mass present [6, 17]. There may be a palpable difference in the temperature of the digits with the ulnar aspect of the hand being relatively cool. Cool, pale, and discolored ring and small fingers are common. However, due to anatomic variability of the superficial palmar arch, any finger may be involved except the thumb which depends on the radial artery for its blood supply [17, 19].

Assessment

History and Differential Diagnoses

To evaluate vascular injuries in baseball players, a detailed medical history is obtained including information on previous hand injuries and tobacco use. Annotation is made whether symptoms are present in the throwing hand, the gloved hand (more common), or both. Pertinent history includes age, skill level (correlating with intensity of play), position, and specific painful activities during play. Questions about the type of equipment utilized, including glove type, should be considered. Different bat types describing the knob end of the bat, including squared or tapered, are obtained but are likely not a major risk factor for vascular injuries [3].

Differential diagnoses include Raynaud's disease or phenomenon, clotting or vascular disorders, tobacco or recreational drug use, vasculitis, diabetic neuropathy, collagen vascular disease, arterial emboli from cardiac or proximal arterial source, thromboangiitis obliterans (Buerger disease), atherosclerosis with secondary thrombosis, trauma, thoracic outlet syndrome, or connective tissue disease (scleroderma, systemic lupus erythematosus, rheumatoid arthritis, hand-arm vibration disease) [6, 17, 19]. Additionally, the effects of repetitive blunt trauma through hammering objects or the use of vibratory tools should be considered [15].

Physical Examination

Physical examination to assess vascularity includes inspection of the hands and wrists for evidence of repetitive trauma, including changes in skin color, callosities, ulcers, edema, loss of skin wrinkles, deformity, and finger hypertrophy [3, 4, 17]. If any finger demonstrates hypertrophy, a standard ring-sizing device or simple tape measure can be used to compare with the corresponding finger on the contralateral hand. Ginn et al. [3] illustrated index finger hypertrophy occurring in the gloved hand in catchers. The hypertrophied digits demonstrated enlargement of the soft tissue overlying the proximal phalanx and proximal interphalangeal joint. On average, the digit was 5 mm greater in diameter than the index digit on the throwing hand. None of the pitchers, infielders, or outfielders in their study demonstrated finger hypertrophy [3].

Grip strength testing, range of motion of the wrist and fingers, and neurovascular assessment should be performed. Two-point discrimination or Semmes Weinstein testing is performed. The Allen test, used to assess the patency of the radial and ulnar arteries, is carefully performed. The technique involves the examiner tightly compressing both radial and ulnar arteries of the patient's supinated wrist to completely obstruct arterial flow to the hand. Then the patient is asked to clench their fingers into a fist and unclench repeatedly for about 30 s until the hand is pale. The examiner then relaxes compression on the ulnar artery only while observing the hand for color change. Normal hand color shoulder return within 5 s indicating that the ulnar artery is patent. If pallor remains until the radial artery is subsequently released, then occlusion of the ulnar artery is suspected [17]. Patency of the radial artery should be similarly tested. The digital vessels of each finger can also be tested in a similar fashion by occluding the radial digital and ulnar digital arteries [20]. Hypothenar hammer syndrome affects the digits primarily supplied by the superficial palmar arch (ulnar three digits), while the radial digits are less likely involved. Therefore, digital ischemia of the thumb is uncommon [11].

A handheld, pencil-tipped Doppler device may be utilized to assess the patency of the radial and ulnar arteries, the palmar arches, and each of the digital arteries [16]. The normal Doppler signal can be checked with and without compression testing. Absence of biphasic signals within a digit suggests an arterial insufficiency. A dynamic examination by an experienced clinician is a crucial part of the vascular examination of the hand.

Imaging

The use of noninvasive imaging should follow physical examination in the setting of suspected vascular insufficiency. Sonography has been established as the first imaging modality to confirm a diagnosis of hypothenar hammer syndrome, often with the combination of gray scale ultrasound and color Doppler. Sonography will identify both aneurysms and segmental thrombosis of the ulnar artery [11]. In the patient with significant digital ischemia in need of urgent treatment, digital subtraction angiography may be obtained.

Angiography remains the gold standard test for the diagnosis of hypothenar hammer syndrome, especially if surgical exploration is anticipated [11, 15]. Most agree that angiography is needed to exclude proximal embolic events, confirm the location of the ulnar artery involvement, evaluate the digital arteries distally, and define the anatomy of the palmar arches. Angiography can serve as an anatomical road map prior to any operative intervention (Fig. 17.3) [11]. Recognizing the pathognomonic angiographic "corkscrew appearance" of the ulnar artery adjacent to the hamate should raise suspicion of hypothenar hammer syndrome [11].

Other specialized testing to evaluate for vascular injuries includes digital brachial indices (DBIs), computed topography angiography (CTA), and magnetic resonance angiography (MRA). DBIs have been described for the

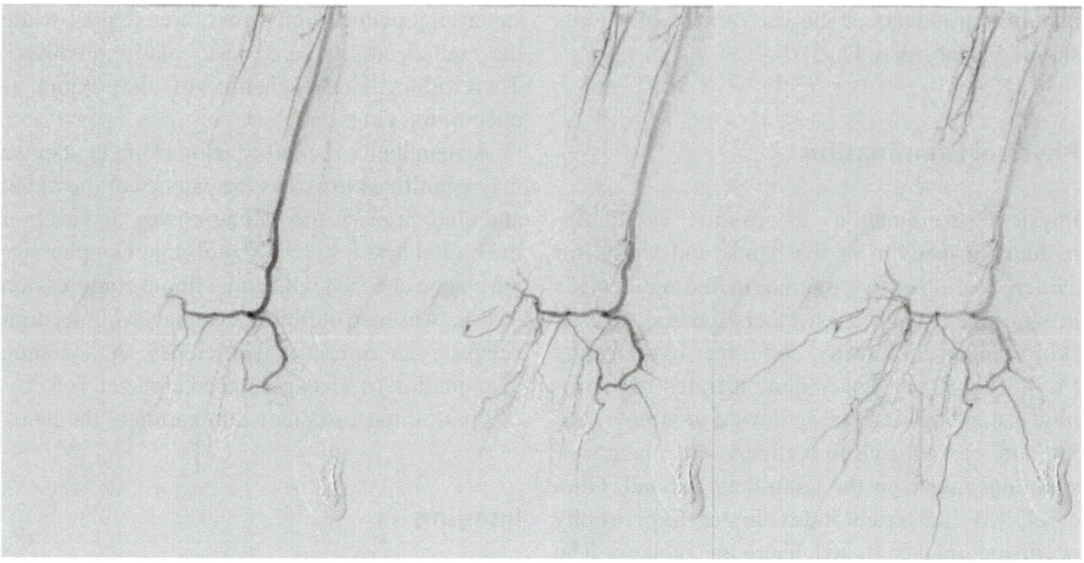

Fig. 17.3 Digital subtraction angiogram (DSA) showing occlusion of ulnar artery in the distal forearm with absent ulnar vascular flow in the wrist and hand. (Copyright, Dr. David Brogan, Washington University, St. Louis, MO)

evaluation of chronic arterial insufficiency of the fingers or hand with an index of less than 0.7 indicating significantly decreased blood flow [21]. However, the utility of DBI in the setting of acute thrombosis is uncertain [15]. In cases where a diagnosis of thrombosed aneurysm has been made on ultrasound and digital ischemia is not evident, multi-slice CTA of the wrist is preferred as a less invasive complementary imaging method to arteriography (Fig. 17.4) [11, 15]. CTA is a valuable diagnostic modality if the pathology is proximal to the digital arteries [11]. MRA is infrequently used to evaluate arterial insufficiency in the hand given its limitation depicting vessels 1.0 mm or smaller within the distal extremities [15, 16].

Treatment

Conservative Treatment

Several conservative treatment regimens have been recommended for hypothenar hammer syndrome. The therapeutic strategy remains controversial due to limited studies and variability of patient presentation [11]. Environmental modification including cessation of smoking, avoidance of cold exposure, limitation of activities that precipitate symptoms, and increased protective equipment should be encouraged [11, 22]. Some of these are, of course, more easily implemented than others.

Lowrey et al. [23] evaluated 20 professional baseball players, one collegiate player, and a former major league player. Based on modified digital Allen's test and Doppler flow, only nine of these 22 athletes had normal circulation in the left index finger, compared with 21 of 22 having normal circulation in the right hand. All nine players who had normal circulation in the left index finger used either a thick golf glove when batting or a handball glove beneath the catcher's mitt for additional padding. In the athletes with impaired circulation, almost half utilized no additional padding [23]. This supports the recommendation of Ginn et al. [3] that glove design modifications are needed to protect the hands of professional baseball players, especially catchers.

Medical management is aimed at mitigating the sympathetic hyperactivity in vasospastic and occluded arteries. Medications include oral vasodilators, platelet aggregation inhibitors, tricyclic

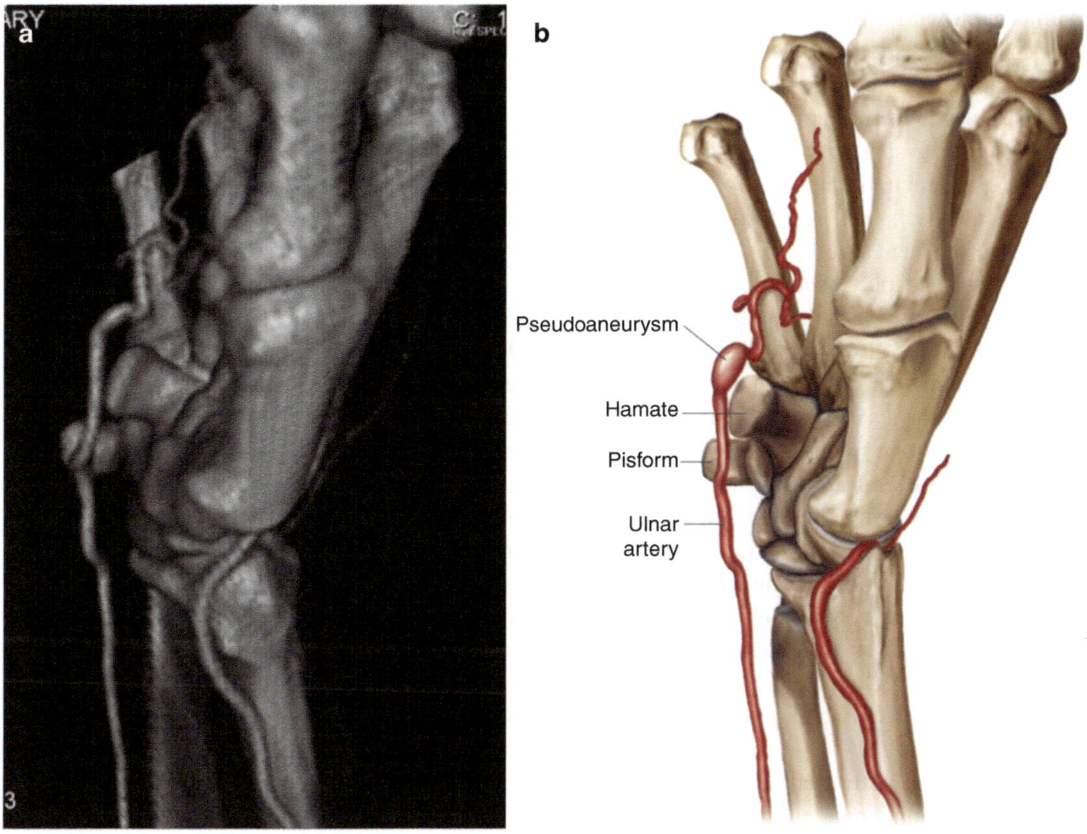

Fig. 17.4 (**a**) CTA demonstrating pseudoaneurysm of the ulnar artery. (**b**) Schematic of pseudoaneurysm in correlation to CTA. (Reproduced from Yuen et al. [11])

antidepressants, selective serotonin reuptake inhibitors, and intravenous prostacyclin analog (iloprost) [10, 11, 16, 22, 24]. However, no clear recommendation exists on the optimal medication use or duration of vasodilators, antiplatelets, or anticoagulants [20].

Marie et al. [22] reported on three patients with hypothenar hammer syndrome with ischemic digital ulcers who partially responded to oral vasodilators (calcium channel blockers). They were subsequently treated with a 5-day course of intravenous prostacyclin analog (iloprost) which resulted in complete healing [23]. In patients with hypothenar hammer syndrome who received conservative measures alone (calcium channel blockers often in combination with platelet aggregation inhibitors ((aspirin, clopidogrel, ticlopidine)), their results demonstrate digital necrosis healing at a median 1.6 months [22]. In summary, the authors recommended initiating vasodilating agents (calcium channel blockers) and platelet aggregation inhibitors (aspirin, clopidogrel) in patients with hypothenar hammer syndrome without digital ischemia / necrosis. In patients with digital ischemia / necrosis, they recommended hemodilution with dextran, intravenous heparin, low-molecular weight heparin, or prostacyclin analog.

Nuber et al. [14] reported on 13 athletes with hand ischemia, including nine professional baseball catchers, one first baseman, a pitcher, a national champion frisbee player, and an amateur handball player. The catchers complained predominately of symptoms in the index digit of their catching hand. The first baseman and the frisbee player required hospitalization due to severe hand ischemia. Arteriograms demonstrated the first baseman had an incomplete palmar arch with ulnar artery occlusion and the frisbee player had occlusion of the superficial palmar arch. Both athletes received a vasodilator infusion of papaverine chloride during arteriography to relieve spasm, followed by intravenous heparin and dextran infusion for 2 to 4 days. Once acute ischemia resolved, both athletes noted improvement at follow-up examination and both returned to play. The first baseman added padding to his glove and the frisbee player started wearing a padded glove while competing [14].

Angiography can also be therapeutic if endovascular fibrinolysis is needed. Sharma et al. [25] reported a case of hypothenar hammer syndrome treated with several boluses of nitroglycerin, verapamil, papaverine administered into the brachial artery, with repeat angiography demonstrating improved filling of the digital arteries. They report the patient's symptoms improved over 24 h and did not recur; the patient was discharged on a regimen of subcutaneous dalteparin for 5 days and oral aspirin, clopidogrel, and nifedpine [25].

Bakhach et al. [26] used intra-arterial fibrinolysis via cannulation of the radial artery when digital ischemia failed to respond to resection of the thrombosed ulnar artery and vein graft reconstruction. Abdel-Gawad et al. [11] used tissue plasminogen activator via a microcatheter placed in the ulnar artery. However, fibrinolysis is advocated only for treatment in acute onset digital ischemia, less than 2 weeks from the occurrence of occlusion [20].

Surgical Treatment

The ideal surgical treatment for hypothenar hammer syndrome is unclear. Surgical management is typically recommended for thrombotic hypothenar hammer syndrome that fails conservative measures, is associated with aneurysm formation, or is associated with distal ischemia and digital survival is threatened [18]. Possible surgical interventions include segmental resection and arterial reconstruction or excision and ligation of the involved segment. If adequate collateral blood flow exists, surgical treatment with resection and ligation of the thrombosed artery is reasonable [12]. Ligation is considered with proven adequate collateral circulation with a DBI ≥ 0.7. Ligation of the diseased distal ulnar artery prevents distal embolic events, eliminates the painful mass, relieves ulnar nerve compression, and removes the thrombus that initiated the vasospastic reflex [8].

In patients who have inadequate collateral blood flow or in those for whom the arterial Doppler confirms poor blood flow, arterial reconstruction is warranted. The DBI in these cases is typically less than 0.7. End-to-end ulnar artery repair is appropriate in well-defined small aneurysms as long as the arterial ends can be brought together without tension; this is rarely possible. If repair cannot be performed without tension, segmental grafting is required. Ulnar artery reconstruction with interposition vein graft is perhaps most common, but long-term patency is a concern. Reverse vein grafts may be harvested from the distal saphenous vein or from the forearm using the cephalic or basilic veins [8].

Chloros et al. [21] reported graft patency in 10 of 13 patients (77%) treated with reverse interpositional vein grafting for ulnar artery thrombosis at minimum 2-year follow-up. Endress et al. [27] noted a high incidence of graft occlusion, reporting 14 of 18 grafts (78%) occluded at mean follow-up of 9.8 years. This was higher than previously reported. Despite the high percentage of occlusion, patients remained satisfied with low functional disability overall. Patients with occluded grafts likely benefited from the sympathectomy effect of segmental excision, which also would remove a source of emboli [27]. However, these reports did not include high-performance athletes.

Improved patency rates using arterial grafts have been shown in coronary artery bypass grafting, attributed to both the anatomic properties and physiologic responses of arterial grafts compared to reverse vein grafts [27]. Arterial interposition grafts may be harvested from the inferior epigastric or lateral femoral circumflex artery (LFCA) (Fig. 17.5). Advocates for arterial grafts have demonstrated improved long-term

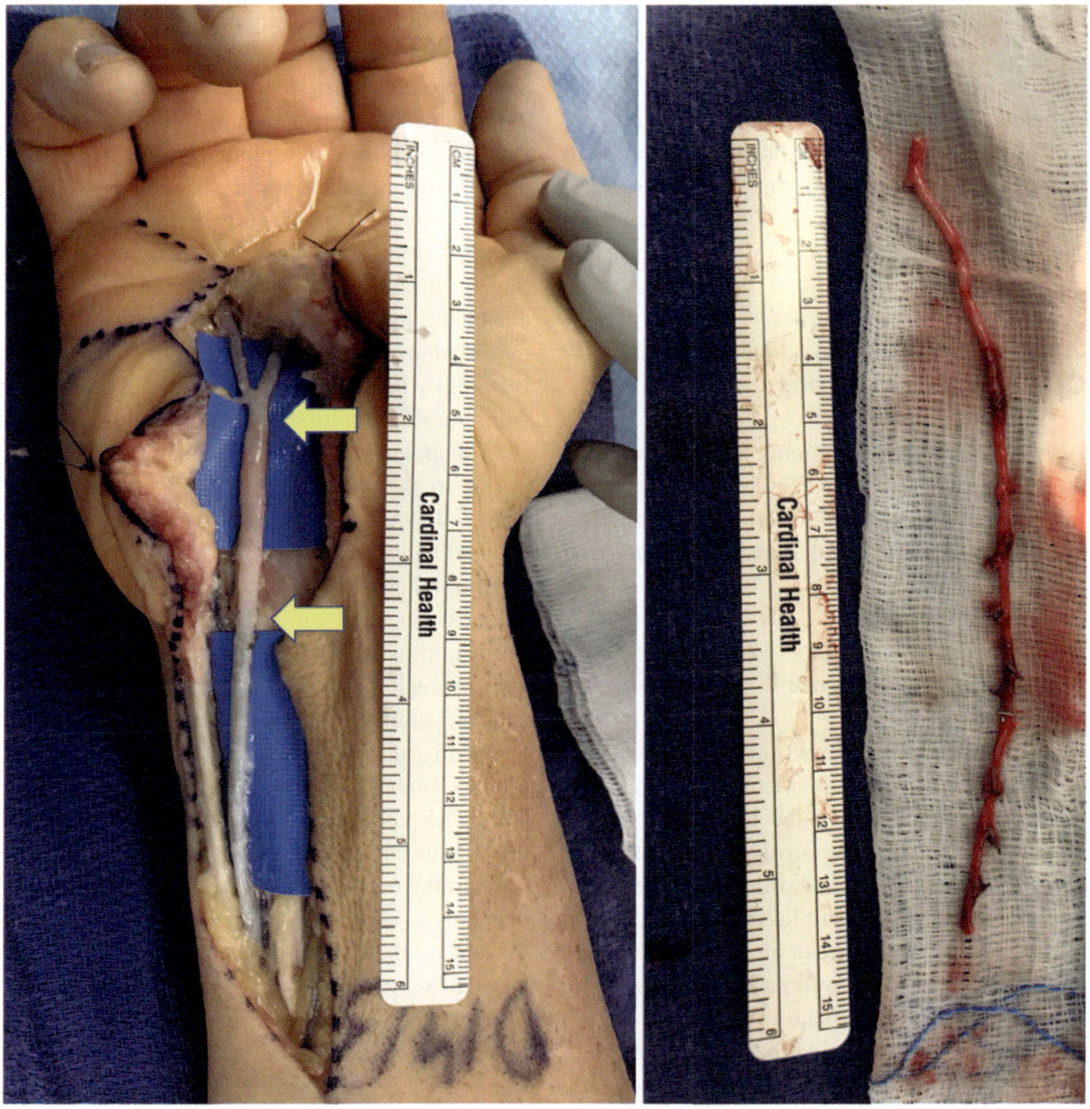

Fig. 17.5 Left, surgical exposure of occluded ulnar artery at the level of the wrist, filled with thrombus between the arrows. Right, harvest of the descending branch of the lateral femoral circumflex artery. (Copyright, Dr. David Brogan, Washington University, St. Louis, MO)

patency rates compared with venous grafts. For example, 11 ulnar artery reconstructions done with an autologous LFCA by a single surgeon were all patent at mean 63 months follow-up and 9 of the 11 reported improvement in their symptoms [28].

Resection and ligation of the lesion is the simplest option, and no anticoagulation is necessary postoperatively. The hand is protected for 2–6 weeks, and no restrictions are necessary after 6 weeks. Conversely, patients managed with interposition graft reconstruction are ideally managed as inpatients with 3 to 5 days of anticoagulation therapy. Protection of the graft is important long term and using the hand as a hammer is forbidden. Cold sensitivity and palmar tenderness are expected as long-term sequelae. A return to baseball is not recommended, but may be considered for some demonstrating long-term patency of an arterial graft [12].

Complications

Complications of unresolved hand and digital ischemia include ulceration, infection, gangrene, and loss of the digit(s). Complications of surgical intervention include, but are not limited to, graft occlusion and persistence of symptoms such as cold intolerance, pain, tingling, numbness, and cyanosis [8].

Other Vascular Injuries

Although hypothenar hammer syndrome is the most common vascular disorder, other vascular injuries to occur in baseball players include digital artery ischemia, digital artery entrapment, and proximal emboli.

Digital Artery Ischemia

Players in other infield positions, commonly first base, have an increased incidence of digital ischemia, generally affecting the index digit of the gloved hand [5, 23]. The strongest impact as the ball strikes the gloved hand occurs at the metacarpophalangeal (MCP) joint level of the index and middle fingers. Sugawara et al. [5] reported eight cases of digital ischemia in baseball players with numbness and cyanosis the most common findings. Angiography revealed that the site of occlusion of the digital arteries was most frequently distal to the proximal interphalangeal (PIP) joint. The probability of developing digital ischemia related to years of accumulated playing time. In contrast to hypothenar hammer syndrome where the ulnar artery is occluded in the region of repetitive impact, digital artery ischemia results from arterial occlusion distal to the point of repetitive impact, possibly due to the vibration effect of ball impacting the gloved hand [5].

Digital Artery Entrapment

Itoh et al. [29] reported cases of digital artery entrapment in the throwing hand of baseball pitchers. In all cases, patency of the superficial palmar arch and ulnar artery was confirmed by angiography, differentiating the malady from hypothenar hammer syndrome. In one case, the PIP joint and distal interphalangeal (DIP) joint of the middle finger could be hyperextended approximately 30° with forced extension, reproducing coldness and numbness at the tip of the finger. Pulsation of the proper digital arteries was detectable up to the middle aspect of the proximal phalanx but was undetectable distal to the PIP joint when the joint was held in hyperextension. Surgical exploration revealed the neurovascular bundle was entrapped just proximal and dorsal to the PIP joint by Cleland's ligament. Relief of symptoms occurred with the release of Cleland's ligament.

In another case, symptoms of numbness and coldness occurred while the hand was held in an intrinsic plus position (flexion of the MCP joint and extension of the interphalangeal joints). Digital subtraction angiograms demonstrated narrowing of the first and second intermetacarpal arteries branching from the superficial palmar arch. The pathology was in the lumbrical canal, the region where the digital nerves and arteries run parallel on the superficial layer of the lumbrical muscle. The roof of the lumbrical canal is formed by the palmar aponeurosis palmarly and vertical septa on the radial and ulnar sides. Treatment included releasing the thickened palmar aponeurosis [29].

Emboli

Proximal causes of digital emboli must be considered. While outside the scope of this chapter, aneurysms of the axillary artery branches may occur in athletes who practice repetitive rotatory movements of the shoulder girdle. Kee et al. [30] reported cases of arterial emboli in the digits of the throwing arms of two professional baseball pitchers with aneurysms of axillary artery branches. In one case, surgical exploration revealed an occluded posterior circumflex artery with a 1.5 cm diameter aneurysm containing thrombus. In the second case, arteriography confirmed the presence of an aneurysm of the subscapular artery. The branch artery was resected and the axillary artery was repaired in both cases.

References

1. Camp CL, Dines JS, van der List JP, Conte S, Conway J, Altchek DW, et al. Summative report on time out of play for Major and Minor League Baseball: an analysis of 49,955 injuries from 2011 through 2016. Am J Sports Med. 2018;46(7):1727–32.
2. Rhee PC, Camp CL, D'Angelo J, Desai VS, Shin SS, Sheridan D, et al. Epidemiology and impact of hand and wrist injuries in major and minor league baseball. Hand. 2019:1558944719864450.
3. Ginn TA, Smith AM, Snyder JR, Koman LA, Smith BP, Rushing J. Vascular changes of the hand in professional baseball players with emphasis on digital ischemia in catchers. JBJS. 2005;87(7):1464–9.
4. Trehan SK, Weiland AJ. Baseball and softball injuries: elbow, wrist, and hand. J Hand Surg Am. 2015;40(4):826–30.
5. Sugawara M, Ogino T, Minami A, Ish S. Digital ischemia in baseball players. Am J Sports Med. 1986;14(4):329–34.
6. Porubsky GL, Brown SI, Urbaniak JR. Ulnar artery thrombosis: a sports-related injury. Am J Sports Med. 1986;14(2):170–5.
7. Tan RES, Lahiri A. Vascular anatomy of the hand in relation to flaps. Hand Clin. 2020;36(1):1–8.
8. de Mooij T, Duncan AA, Kakar S. Vascular injuries in the upper extremity in athletes. Hand Clin. 2015;31(1):39–52.
9. Wong VW, Katz RD, Higgins JP. Interpretation of upper extremity arteriography: vascular anatomy and pathology. Hand Clin. 2015;31(1):121–34.
10. Koman LA, Urbaniak JR. Ulnar artery insufficiency: a guide to treatment. J Hand Surg Am. 1981;6(1):16–24.
11. Abdel-Gawad EA, Bonatti H, Housseini AM, Maged IM, Morgan RF, Hagspiel KD. Hypothenar hammer syndrome in a computer programmer: CTA diagnosis and surgical and endovascular treatment. Vasc Endovascular Surg. 2009;43(5):509–12. https://doi.org/10.1177/1538574409334346. Epub 2009 Jul 29.
12. Wolfe SW, Hotchkiss RN, Pederson WC, Kozin SH. Green's operative hand surgery. Elsevier Health Sciences; 2017.
13. Coleman SS, Anson BJ. Arterial patterns in the hand based upon a study of 650 specimens. Plast Reconstr Surg. 1962;29(1):85–6.
14. Nuber GW, McCarthy WJ, Yao JS, Schafer MF, Suker JR. Arterial abnormalities of the hand in athletes. Am J Sports Med. 1990;18(5):520–3.
15. Iannuzzi NP, Higgins JP. Acute arterial thrombosis of the hand. J Hand Surg Am. 2015;40(10):2099–106.
16. Chang J, Neligan PC. Plastic surgery, vol. 6. Elsevier Health Sciences; 2012.
17. Taj S, Malamis AP, Lomasney LM, Bednar MS. Radiologic case study. Orthopedics. 2010;33(5):286–365.
18. Kasitinon D, Dimeff RJ. Dropping the hammer: an uncommon case of right-hand pain in a professional hockey player. Sports Health. 2019;11(3):238–41.
19. Nitecki S, Anekstein Y, Karram T, Peer A, Bass A. Hypothenar hammer syndrome: apropos of six cases and review of the literature. Vascular. 2008;16(5):279–82.
20. Parekh A, Jaladi R, Sharma S, Van Decker WA, Ezekowitz MD. Images in cardiovascular medicine. The case of a disappearing left atrial appendage thrombus: direct visualization of left atrial thrombus migration, captured by echocardiography, in a patient with atrial fibrillation, resulting in a stroke. Circulation. 2006;114(13):e513.
21. Chloros GD, Lucas RM, Li Z, Holden MB, Koman LA. Post-traumatic ulnar artery thrombosis: outcome of arterial reconstruction using reverse interpositional vein grafting at 2 years minimum follow-up. J Hand Surg Am. 2008;33(6):932–40.
22. Marie I, Hervé F, Primard E, Cailleux N, Levesque H. Long-term follow-up of hypothenar hammer syndrome: a series of 47 patients. Medicine (Baltimore). 2007;86(6):334–43.
23. Lowrey CW, Chadwick RO, Waltman EN. Digital vessel trauma from repetitive impact in baseball catchers. J Hand Surg Am. 1976;1(3):236–8.
24. St-Pierre F, Shepherd RF, Bartlett MA. Diagnosis of hypothenar hammer syndrome in a patient with acute ulnar artery occlusion. BMJ Case Rep. 2019;12(9):e230963.
25. Sharma R, Ladd W, Chaisson G, Abben R. Hypothenar hammer syndrome. Circulation. 2002;105(13):1615–6.
26. Bakhach J, Chahidi N, Conde A. Hypothenar hammer syndrome: management of distal embolization by intra-arterial fibrinolytics. In: Annales de chirurgie de la main et du membre supérieur. Elsevier; 1998. p. 215–20.
27. Endress RD, Johnson CH, Bishop AT, Shin AY. Hypothenar hammer syndrome: long-term results of vascular reconstruction. J Hand Surg Am. 2015;40(4):660–5.
28. De Niet A, Van Uchelen JH. Hypothenar hammer syndrome: long-term follow-up after ulnar artery reconstruction with the lateral circumflex femoral artery. J Hand Surg Eur Vol. 2017;42(5):507–10.
29. Itoh Y, Wakano K, Takeda T, Murakami T. Circulatory disturbances in the throwing hand of baseball pitchers. Am J Sports Med. 1987;15(3):264–9.
30. Kee ST, Dake MD, Wolfe-Johnson B, Semba CP, Zarins CK, Olcott C IV. Ischemia of the throwing hand in major league baseball pitchers: embolic occlusion from aneurysms of axillary artery branches. J Vasc Interv Radiol. 1995;6(6):979–82.

Part IV

Special Topics

Baseball Injuries in Children and Adolescents

18

Allan E. Peljovich

Driven adolescents who hope to play at the next level, develop apprehension about losing their starting role on a team, or the desire to gain the respect of their coaches often feel a pressure to work through pain as they acculturate to the sports culture that sometimes rewards athletes for their 'toughness.' This pressure can be reinforced, intentionally or unintentionally, by their parents/families who have likely devoted considerable resources and time to their child's sport and training. Recognition of the potential for injury and the wide spectrum of injuries is the key to treating baseball-related hand injuries in children and adolescents. Traumatic arthritis, related to chronic scaphoid malunion, avascular necrosis, and even digital pseudoaneurysms occur in children (Fig. 18.1). Identifying and treating acute injuries and sound knowledge regarding various acute and chronic/acquired injuries are critical. Developing relationships with coaches and athletic trainers and educating them on distinguishing real injury from normal activity-related soreness can help mitigate the potential impact of an injury and create an environment that minimizes the time lost from sport.

Baseball-related injuries to the hand have important implications for participation. The hand, specifically, is among the most common, if not the most commonly, injured body parts [1–3]. These injuries occur at an average around 11–13 years of age in reports that account for all ages of children and adolescents [1, 3]. One large high-school-based surveillance study found that nearly 30% of injuries are game ending [4]. Approximately 37% are able to return to sport within 1 week, but about 17% are out of sport for at least 3 weeks. Fractures, sprains, and contusions make up the majority of acute hand injuries [1, 2, 4]. Perhaps one reason for the lost time from participation following injury is that hand fractures require surgery (22%) more commonly than fractures in other locations [2]. Acute hand injuries in baseball most often result from a player making contact with a baseball apparatus. This particular mechanism, whether player contact with ball or bat, for example, accounts for 60–87% of hand injuries [3, 4]. Falling on outstretched hand, whether during a slide, a collision between players, or during a defensive play, accounts for 10–25% of hand injuries. And, catchers and infielders seem to experience hand injuries most frequently, while pitchers are least likely to sustain a hand injury [5].

A. E. Peljovich (✉)
The Hand & Upper Extremity Center of Georgia, Atlanta, GA, USA

The Hand & Upper Extremity Program, Children's Healthcare of Atlanta, Atlanta, GA, USA

WellStar Atlanta Medical Center Orthopaedic Surgery Residency Program, Atlanta, GA, USA

The Hand & Upper Extremity Program, The Shepherd Center, Atlanta, GA, USA
e-mail: drp@handcenterga.com

G. M. Lourie (ed.), *Hand and Wrist Injuries in Baseball*,
https://doi.org/10.1007/978-3-030-81659-9_18

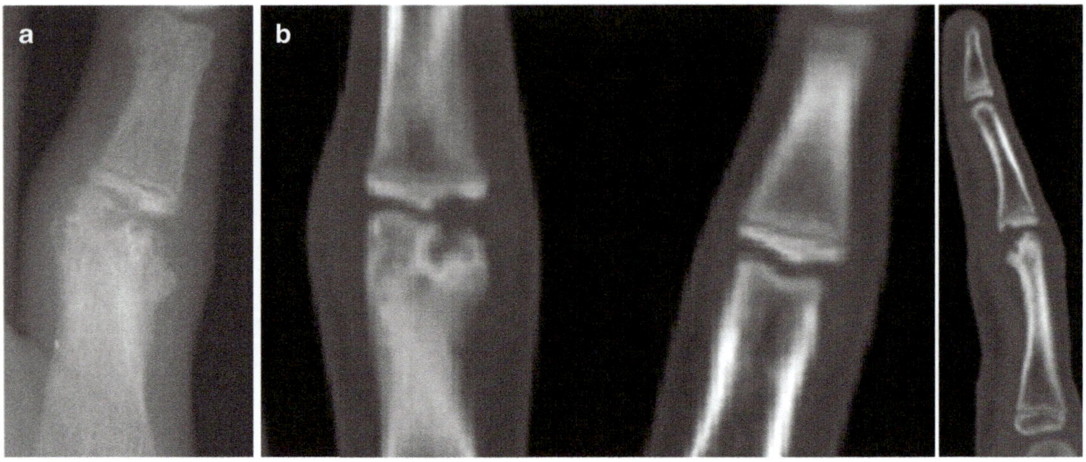

Fig. 18.1 Examples of finger injuries resulting in traumatic arthritis. In both cases, the injury was felt to be a 'jammed' finger and not evaluated until pain and swelling persisted for a few weeks. (**a**) Malunited, intra-articular PIP fracture. (**b**) CT scan of avascular necrosis following a PIP dislocation

'The Arm' argued that the high intensity of baseball participation, training combined with the pursuit of scholarships, has led to a rise in early specialization and adult-like upper extremity injuries [6]. Scientific publications have found that early sports specialization increases the risk of upper extremity injury by 1.6–1.8 times compared to nonspecialized youth athletes [7–9]. Post et al. found that high-school baseball players who spend >8 months/year playing baseball were two times more likely to sustain an upper extremity injury [10]. The same study found that those who specialize and pitch were 3.8 times more likely to sustain an upper extremity injury. Specialization has a negative impact on pre-adolescent baseball players too. Arnold et al. evaluated baseball injuries in one community among 9- to 12-year-old athletes. The rate of injury was 2.2/1000 athlete exposures and all were specialized [11].

What Sets Children and Adolescents Apart

Children are not little adults, and their distinct musculoskeletal system has a strong impact on evaluation and decision making. The thick periosteal sleeve and presence of a physis at younger ages can confound the radiographic assessment of acute injuries. The occasional presence of pseudoepiphyses on the opposite end of the bone from the primary physis in the metacarpals and phalanges can further confuse plain film interpretation (Fig. 18.2) [12–14]. Diagnosing carpal injuries can prove difficult during childhood and pre-teen years as some bones will not be fully ossified. Carpal fractures can be particularly difficult to spot on plain radiographs. Incomplete ossification also affects the ability to assess carpal alignment [15]. Since there is an inherent bias that bad things do not happen to children or that only certain injuries, that is, scapholunate tears, happen in adults, some injuries in children are overlooked [16–20]. Negative X-rays in the presence of a positive exam warrant attention and is an indication for advanced imaging. Given the pressure young athletes feel to avoid missing games, physicians should have a high index of suspicion for fractures and ligamentous injuries even when radiographs are normal, be familiar with other conditions that are often unique to children, and recognize the need to utilize advanced imaging. At the same time, the surgeon should not be too dependent upon advanced imaging and allow it to replace sound clinical assessment. Such is the case with Triangular Fibrocartilage Complex (TFCC) injuries in children where the MRI is not as sensitive a study as in adults [16].

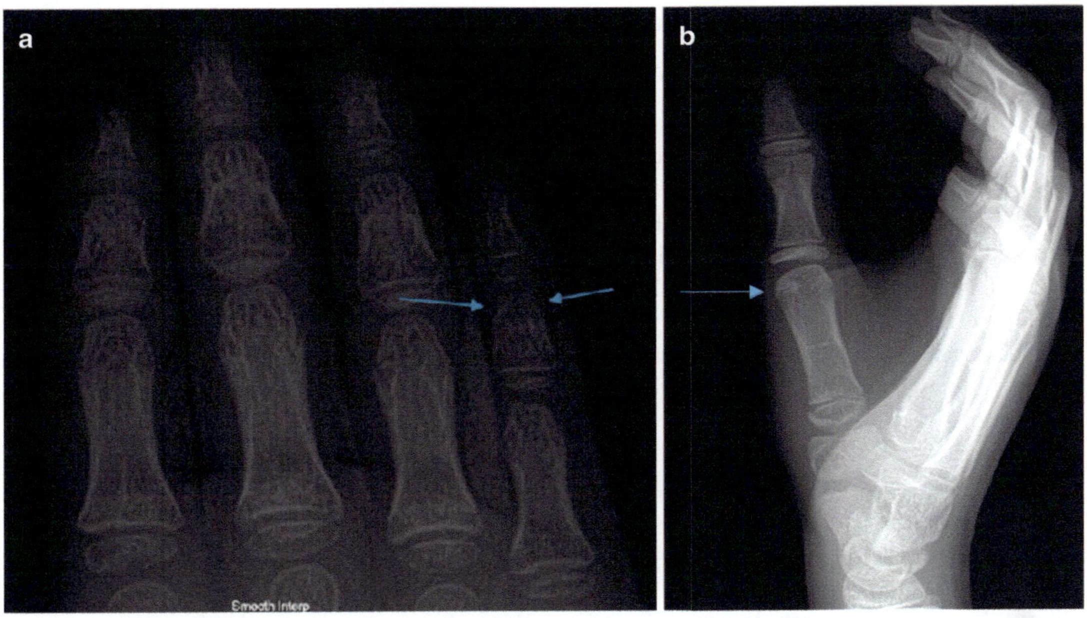

Fig. 18.2 Examples of pseudarthrosis confounding the evaluation of injured hands. (**a**) Small finger, middle phalanx. (**b**) Thumb, proximal phalanx

The approach to treatment of children and adolescents with hand injuries can also be distinct from adults at times. Unstable fractures occur less frequently; therefore, all extra-articular fractures merit a manual reduction if displaced given the inherent stability afforded by the thick periosteal sleeve and physis. Physeal remodeling potential also impacts treatment decisions. Remodeling in the flexion/extension plane depends primarily upon age and can be extensive. Malrotation never sufficiently remodels over time, and there is a limit to coronal plane correction. An extra-articular thumb metacarpal fracture with a >30° flexion angle, for example, can be treated nonoperatively in younger children with an expectation of correction over time even if reduction proves suboptimal. Articular fractures and displaced carpal fractures generally warrant more aggressive treatment including surgical reduction and fixation just like their adult counterparts. Then, too, as with sports-related injuries in the adult, treatment can be directed toward the quickest path back to the playing field, especially in the case of high-school age athletes who may be in a recruitment period.

The intensity of youth baseball starts even at the youth level and increases into the high-school ages. Scholarships and the lofty aspirations of many pediatric athletes, and their families, add additional stress to the patient in their recovery from injuries. There is pressure to quickly return to play. The treating physician must appreciate these dynamics in their assessment and treatment plans. Whenever possible, children and teens are cleared to return to sport, sometimes with restrictions, that is, certain defensive positions, hitting only, or pinch running. We tend to treat young children and pre-teens with a bit of an extra conservative touch making as certain as we can there is limited to no negative consequence associated with return. As children get into teenage years, and the implications of sport become important to them, return to play is treated as they were an adult, but, not like a professional. Teenagers and their families are always advised of the potential negative consequences of early return should they exist, but older teens with injuries that can be stabilized for sport can be allowed to return. A 7-year-old with a phalangeal fracture might be cleared only after 2–3 weeks. A 11th grade high schooler with a similar phalangeal fracture might be cleared with a 'play splint' if the fracture is stable. Furthermore, an indicated surgery can potentially be delayed until the end of a season provided their issue can be stabilized for play without negative consequences. A ball player with a TFCC injury that can be adequately treated with a wrist wrap, for example, can be cleared for sport and the injury addressed surgically if indicated at the end of the season. On the other hand, one with a fracture dislocation of the proximal interphalangeal (PIP) needing surgery will not be cleared for play with the injured hand for potentially several weeks.

Evaluating the Child's Hand

Getting to the diagnosis of a child's baseball injury, like any other sports injury, will sometimes require negotiating around some of the expectations and pressures that are on the child to return to sport. Familiarity with the sport, the defensive positions, hitting, and even base running will ultimately help advise return to play criteria. The two goals of the history are to help arrive at a diagnosis and understand the impact of the issue on the player's 'world.' It is certainly important to determine whether the pain/problem is discretely located or regional, if the issue is the result of a discrete injury or acquired/chronic, if there are associated neurovascular symptoms, and modifying factors that both intensify and relieve the issue. Then, too, it is critical to appreciate the impact on the ability to play, what sort of season the player is in (school versus club), are there critical games/opportunities and/or recruiting events forthcoming. Does the issue affect a 9th grade ball player at the beginning of his/her junior varsity season with a full summer of club tournaments planned? Is this a rising junior/senior in the middle of summer baseball with important recruiting events in the near future?

Imaging the young athlete's hand merits some discussion. Plain film evaluation is almost standard in the evaluation of an athlete's injury. Critical to such evaluations is familiarity, or at least appreciation, of how the radiographic appearance of a child's hand is determined by normal growth and development. Much of the phalangeal heads and articular surfaces of the phalanges, for example, are initially cartilaginous and gradually ossify, and become more visible on plain films, with growth. Developing an understanding of when the carpal ossification centers first tend to appear, for example, and how this influences the measurements of carpal angles, distances, and carpal height helps to reconcile the plain film with the young athlete's signs and symptoms (Fig. 18.3) [21]. Evaluating the plain film for pediatric metacarpal and phalangeal injury requires the ability to distinguish the occasional pseudoepiphysis on the opposite end of the primary physis from a true fracture line [13]. A line drawn along the volar phalangeal cortex will intersect the condylar head more dorsally as children age and stabilizes to intersecting the middle third of the condylar heads after 9 years of age (Fig. 18.4) [22]. This understanding helps interpret alignment of phalangeal neck fracture. The physes of the metacarpals and phalanges can obscure a fracture.

Advanced imaging, often in the form of MRI, is employed when examination and plain film imaging fall short of a clear diagnosis. MRI, as opposed to a CT scan, can help sift through

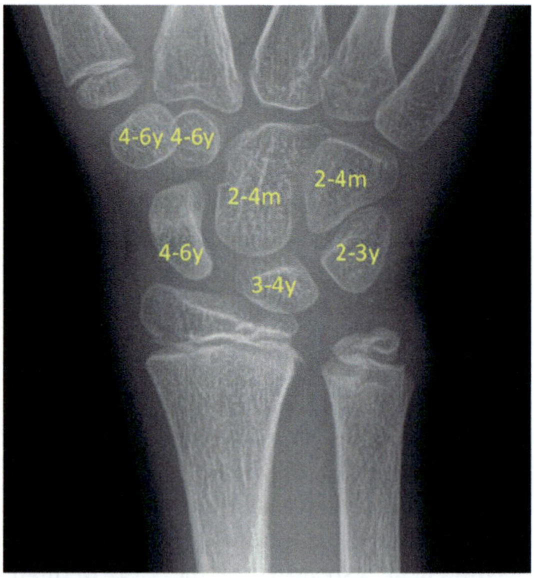

Fig. 18.3 Wrist radiograph with the age at onset of ossification labeled

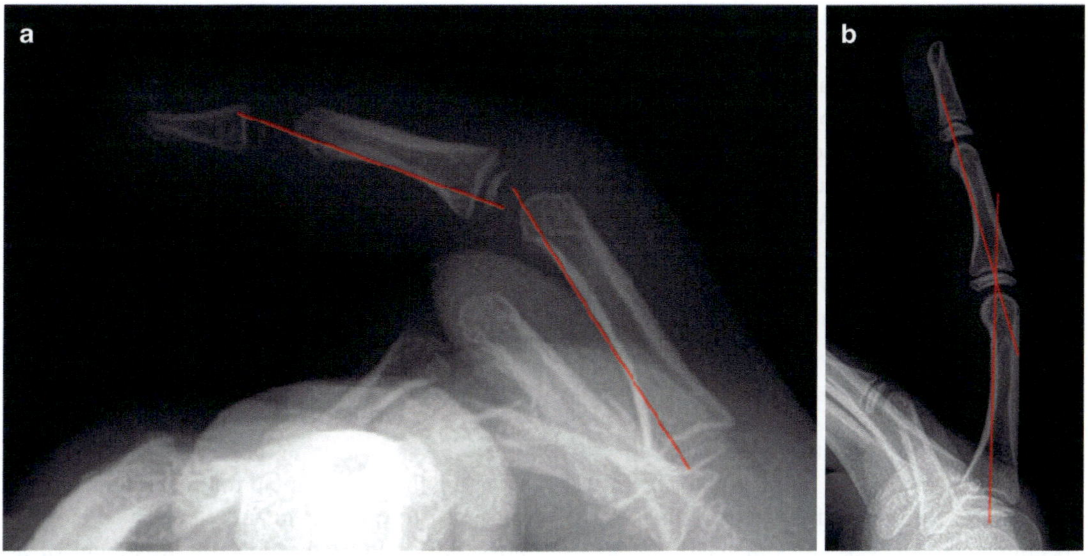

Fig. 18.4 The volar phalangeal line (VPL) is a radiographic measure that can help the clinician assess alignment after treating a fracture of the phalangeal neck. Nearly all lines drawn along the volar cortex of the proximal and middle phalanges will intersect the volar third of the phalangeal head up until 9 years of age, after which the VPL tends to intersect the middle third of the phalangeal head. (**a**) The VPL of the proximal and middle phalanges of this 2-year-old intersects the volar third of the phalangeal head. (**b**) The VPL in this 10-year-old intersects the middle third of the phalangeal heads

differential diagnoses, soft tissue injury, and identify otherwise impossible conditions, that is, bone contusion [23]. This is especially important if a quick return to play has the potential to negatively affect outcomes, that is, occult scaphoid fracture. But there are findings on a child's wrist MRI that are normal variants and can mislead and result in unnecessary treatment plans. Cortical depressions, which can appear like erosions from inflammatory arthritis except they are sometimes covered with cartilage, exist in up to 60% of wrist studies and 70% of proximal metacarpals [24, 25]. The metacarpal depressions, in fact, seem to be correlated to sports participation. Other changes noted in normal, asymptomatic pediatric wrists include pockets of joint fluid >2 mm (50%), ganglions (24%), and single bone signal changes similar to edema (40%) [26]. The critical point is to use MRIs to further assess a child's hand and wrist based upon a thorough history and physical examination, thus allowing the clinician to both dismiss normal variant findings that do not correlate with the athlete and not jump to MRI as the study that will guide treatment [18]. At the same time, upward of 35% of pediatric wrist MRIs ordered for pain are negative for relevant findings; yet, wrist arthroscopy for persistent pain and findings demonstrate pertinent pathology almost all the time [20, 27]. In other words, do not let a negative MRI wrongfully lead to no treatment when an athlete's symptoms, signs, and physical findings suggest a discrete problem.

Anomalous Carpals and Muscles

Evaluation of young athletes also requires an awareness of uncommon congenital differences that at times present with pain and at times mislead. Bipartate carpals, though rare, can lead to the misdiagnosis of fracture [28]. The scaphoid and lunate each develop, sometimes, from two ossification centers that fail to unite [29]. Clinical context is key, as an official report for a bipartite carpal could easily be interpreted as a chronic nonunion. Extra bones of the wrist have been described. The "os centrale carpi" is an accessory bone sometimes located in the direct proximity of the scaphoid and has been misdiagnosed as a scaphoid fracture on plain films (Fig. 18.5). An astute observer will recognize an unusual difference to the X-ray and confirm, with advanced imaging, that it is actually a separate carpal located somewhere between the capitate, trapezoid, and scaphoid [30].

Anomalous muscle around the hand and forearm are rare but known entities. The extensor digitorum brevis manus (EDBM) is perhaps the best-known example in the wrist that can have associated symptoms. It is an anomalous muscle found in the dorsum of the wrist and frequently mistaken for a mass like a ganglion or boss [31]. A cadaveric study found this muscle in 2.3% of specimens, and it was in both hands in 26.3% [32]. The muscle is found within the fourth dorsal compartment where the tendons of the extensor digitorum communis and extensor indicis proprius are located. It originates along the dorsal wrist capsule with attachments extending proximally to the radius and dorsally along the metacarpals. It inserts along the index or long extensor mechanism and becomes most clinically prominent with finger extension. When symptoms are present, they are exacerbated during finger extension and often in the setting of repetitive activity. Recognition of this anomaly helps with diagnosis, and advanced imagining with MRI or Ultrasound will demonstrate that its characteristics are like nearby muscles. Rarely symptomatic, treatment can include physiotherapy and surgery if symptoms do not abate.

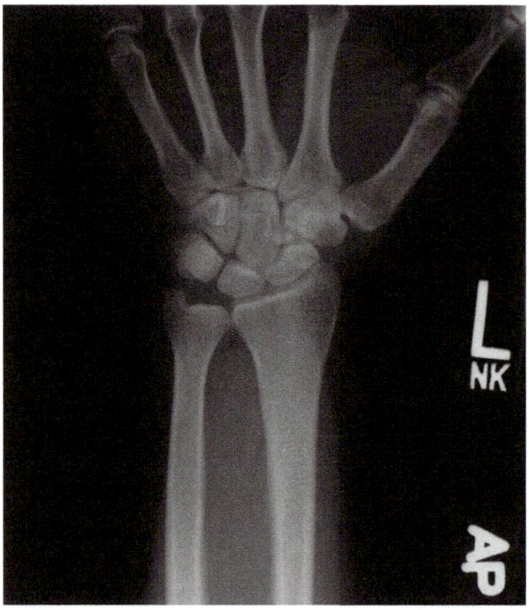

Fig. 18.5 This radiograph depicts an ossific carpi centrale located on the ulnar side of the distal scaphoid. This anatomic variation is often mistaken as either an acute fracture or non-union of a previous fracture

Treating the Child's Hand

Creating the environment for healing that results in return to premorbid function, or as close as possible, remains the goal for treatment of all injuries. Many, if not most, fractures either present in sufficiently appropriate alignment (accounting for remodeling) or can be manipulated into appropriate alignment and treated closed. The presence of open physes, and the inherent remodeling potential they imbue, allows the hand surgeon to exceed adult thresholds of alignment, barring articular displacement, and still expect an excellent outcome. The treating physician should not be lulled into the expectation that the developing phalanx can overcome all deformities nor that children will always have good outcomes. Phalangeal fractures in children and adolescents can certainly result in permanent deformity, instability, stiffness, and even traumatic arthritis (Fig. 18.1). Some displaced peri-articular fractures in incompletely ossified phalanges can be overlooked and undertreated due to the small size of the ossified fragment leading to potentially poor outcomes (Fig. 18.6).

Knowledge of phalangeal remodeling potential is growing and still not fully appreciated. That bones only remodel well when the deformity is in the plane of motion, the displacement is 'close' to the location of the physis, and there is 'enough' time left prior to natural physeal closure is understood; however, there is still a paucity of data that provide guidance regarding the boundaries between acceptable and unacceptable alignment. A coronal angulation limit of 10° or sagittal

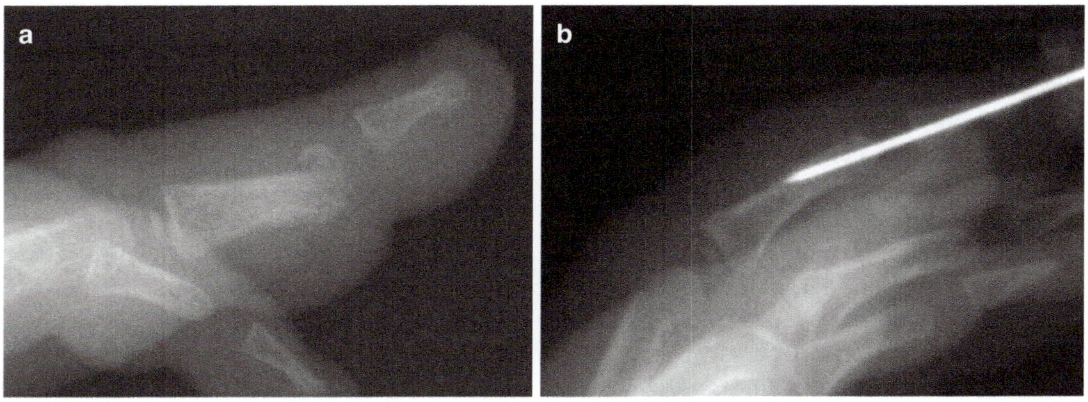

Fig. 18.6 Lateral radiographs of a phalangeal neck fracture in an infant. (**a**) The initial lateral suggests a small fragment that is displaced. (**b**) But, as shown after surgical fixation, the small fragment represents the incompletely ossified phalangeal head illustrating the importance of interpreting radiographs in children

angulation limits of 15–25°, for example, are boundaries based upon opinion and dogma [33–36]. In reality, the child's phalanx probably has a greater remodeling capability than is traditionally assumed, and new data support this notion. Phalangeal neck/distal condyle fractures felt to have poor remodeling potential due to its distance from the primary physis have, in fact, demonstrated a capacity to remodel in the plane of motion [37]. Al-Qattan recently demonstrated that coronal angulation up to around 20–25° in the coronal plane (out of plane of motion) remodels [38]. These 'newer' concepts provide the treating clinician with more scientifically based information upon which to help guide treatment plans.

Regarding the articular surface, all phalangeal head fractures that involve the condylar surface should be stabilized in anatomic alignment either by closed or by open methods. Avulsion fractures off the proximal epiphysis, that is, volar plate or collateral ligament avulsion fractures, do not need to heal in anatomical position provided the fragments are small (remains undefined) and the joint remains stable even though these may technically be Salter-Harris III fractures (Fig. 18.7). Indications for surgical fixation of these epiphyseal fragments are ambiguous, but larger fragments that involve >25–30% of the articular surface, with significant gapping and instability, may require attention.

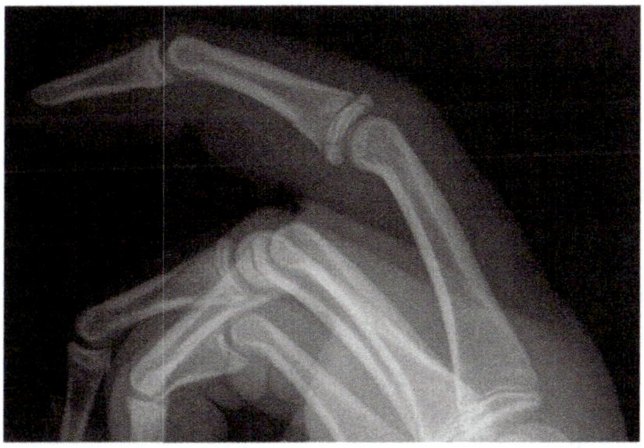

Fig. 18.7 A 12-year-old sustained 'jammed' finger sliding into base head first. Lateral radiographs confirm avulsion-type fractures of the volar plate and central slip; both are technically Salter-Harris III variants

An overriding principle in sports medicine to help the injured athlete quickly return to sport has filtered from professional and college athletes to the level of high-school athletics. Parents of younger athletes will often choose conservative treatment of phalangeal fractures when available but high-school athletes may aspire playing at a collegiate or professional level. Injuries that occur to upper classmen can be particularly stressful if they are hoping to be recruited to the next level. In such situations, and assuming the athlete can return to their sport and position with an injured finger, the hand surgeon can offer options for treatment that provide the quickest return to sport. Dual methods of protection for athletic activity and nonathletic activities, like play casts, rigid orthoplastic splints, and digital splinting, are employed. Whenever possible, early mobilization during nonathletic time is encouraged to hasten the return of mobility and dexterity. In surgical cases, these principles are still utilized. Some injuries, like those involving the TFCC, can be nursed along during season and addressed in the off-season. When surgery is performed in acute fractures, implanted pins are buried under the skin to minimize the risk of infection, configured to potentially allow for some early protected mobilization, and overprotection during sport if appropriate. The athlete's compliance with care is paramount, and parents need to assume some oversight.

It is important to consider the types of injuries other than the common fractures, sprains, and strains. Two, in particular, are worth highlighting, especially in children and adolescents. Stress fractures and bone contusions are the kinds of injuries diagnosed when they are considered.

Stress Injury

Stress fracture should be included in the differential diagnosis when a young athlete presents with a history of insidious and worsening activity-related pain in the wrist. A thorough history and physical examination will likely reveal a consistency of location and findings that may seem nonspecific but include focal tenderness, some trouble with mobility, and perhaps relative weakness. Most importantly, there is an absence of a true, discrete injury though the athlete and their family will likely describe one. Signs of other issues like tendinosis and synovitis are likely to be lacking. Secondary gain is also a diagnosis that needs consideration. Plain films will be important to obtain, and even if negative, advanced imaging should be considered. The authors certainly advocate for MRI when pain has been present for months and worsening, and stress fracture is a consideration. Once diagnosed, treatment depends upon whether the physician believes that rest and cessation from practice and play will allow the bone to heal. Case studies in the literature point to the scaphoid as the most commonly reported carpal with stress fracture, but the hook of hamate has also been involved and should always be considered in the differential diagnosis of injuries to the hook [39–44]. These reports concerning carpal stress fractures in children and adolescents illustrate some consistencies in presentation: insidious onset of pain, males aged 15–18 years, and regular daily training of multiple hours per day in their sport. Findings on examination included discrete carpal tenderness, reduced range of motion compared to the contralateral wrist, and reduced strength compared to the contralateral hand. There is a similar pattern of stress injury that affects the proximal interphalangeal (PIP) joint in children between 13 and 16 years of age. The stress injury affects the base of the middle phalanx and presents with a few weeks of PIP discomfort and stiffness, but not typically an effusion [45–48]. Radiographs may present either a Salter-Harris 2 or 3 nonunion and be mistaken for an acute fracture except there is no history of discrete injury. Advanced imaging is always indicated in the presence of a history of persistent discomfort and will reveal the injury. Rest is the mainstay of treatment, but surgery can also be contemplated in particular circumstances, that is, failure to respond to rest or radiographic findings suggesting chronic nonunion [44, 47].

Incomplete carpal coalitions are also susceptible to repetitive stress injury that can disrupt both the bone and cartilaginous connections. Incomplete 'separation' among the carpal bones during the fourth to eight weeks of fetal development leads to varying degrees of connection called carpal coalitions. These coalitions may be categorized by their completeness and the nature of the connection: fibrous, cartilaginous, or bony. Nearly every combination of possible connections has been reported, but by far coalitions of the lunate-triquetrum, the capitate-hamate, and the capitate-trapezium are the most common [49–52]. As with any other stress fracture, awareness of the possibility is critical to making the diagnosis, but diagnostic algorithms that include advanced imaging for persistent pain will almost always lead to the diagnosis once the imaging is obtained. Their overall prevalence has reportedly varied from 0.5% to 8.8% of study populations, though relatively more prominent in African American children, and are usually incidentally diagnosed through radiographs taken for other purposes [52, 53]. Complete coalitions are typically painless, incomplete coalitions, especially those with fibrous connections are prone to pain secondary to the presence or formation of pseudarthroses that results from the repetitive stress demands of sport [54, 55]. These can occasionally present acutely after a discrete injury, a fall during an attempted fielding play, for example, though a careful history might uncover a history of low-level chronic discomfort that never interfered with sport before the injury [49, 56, 57].

Ball players will present with insidious onset of pain in the region of the coalition. Careful assessment of tenderness may tip off to the possibility of a coalition as the area will be intercarpal. It may be mistaken for a sprain, occult fracture, stress fracture, bone contusion, or some vague form of tendinitis. Examination is usually only remarkable for focal intercarpal tenderness and pain from stressing the carpal bones in the tender area [58]. Sometimes the examination is completely negative [55]. In the case of piso-hamate incomplete coalitions, the pain is ulnar, can mimic piso-triquetral arthritis, ulno-carpal impaction syndrome, or a TFCC tear, and has been reported to present with symptoms of ulnar neuropathy [59–62]. Radiographs are the first line of imaging, but the coalition is easily missed. Sometimes the only hint on a radiograph is a focal area between carpal segments where the space narrows. The 'carpal C-sign' refers to the unique appearance of a piso-hamate coalition on a standard lateral plain film [63]. Advanced imaging is typically required to confirm the diagnosis. CT scan will often demonstrate a focal irregularity at the coalition and may reveal atypical spacing of the specific carpal interval. An MRI is the preferred study since it can reveal a fibrous coalition in the cases where a bony connection is not present, can assess reactive edema, and can help sort through the differential diagnosis.

Treatment should initially consist of some combination of rest, bracing, and temporary cessation of activity. Gradual return to sport is initiated after an asymptomatic period. Ball players should progress through deliberate advancement of activities from swinging a bat to hitting and transition from a throwing program to fielding. Taping the involved wrist can aid during the transition and even help manage low-level discomfort during the course of a season. Surgery is indicated when nonoperative treatment proves insufficient in allowing a player the ability to effectively participate in sport. The nature of surgery depends upon which carpals are involved. 'Completing' an incomplete coalition of the lun-triquetral or capitohamate joint via arthrodesis is one approach. Such children often already have a reduction in wrist mobility they have adapted too [49, 51, 54]. Carpectomy is another method to treat the pain as in the case of piso-hamate coalitions [62].

Bone Contusions

Distinct from either stress fractures or traumatic fracture, a bone contusion represents an intermediate skeletal injury: enough acute energy to injure but not fracture. Never visible on plain films, this diagnosis is made from a combination of the clinical history detailing pain from a discrete injury and advanced imaging demonstrating a discrete area of edema within the bone in the absence of a fracture line or other findings that could support vascular necrosis and stress response [64]. These injuries are most often discovered when unresolving pain following an injury is pursued in the ball player even though radiographs appear normal, especially pain that affects the child's ability to play. The differential diagnosis includes ligamentous injury, cartilaginous injury, and occult fracture. Bone contusions also occur in concert with injuries to ligaments and cartilage [65]. The challenge in treating these injuries once recognized, other than supportive care, is the length of time for pain resolution which can be months. And, while unsettled and unexplained, there is one prospective study that evaluated scaphoid contusions in which 1 of 50 converted to a true fracture [66].

Diagnosing this injury is the challenge and starts with recognition. The young athlete will have presented either acutely or after weeks of pain relatable to a single memorable event. Radiographs will be normal, and examination will reveal a discrete area of tenderness unless multiple bones are involved. Diagnosis requires an MRI, though a bone scan will also be positive, and this study should be obtained acutely to help rule out a more significant injury based upon examination after a few weeks without improvement despite supportive treatment (Fig. 18.19). While casts to protect scaphoid contusions have been reported, it is unclear that anything more than supportive bracing and patience is required for treatment [66–68]. Follow-up plain films and MRI are warranted if pain worsens or persists.

Specific Acute Injuries

Fingertip Injuries

Among the most common injuries a ball player sustains is to their fingertip. It is exposed on the throwing hand during defensive plays, while sliding back to a base, and when on the receiving end of an errant pitch. Young ball players are taught to field balls with an open palm, slide head first with hands in a fist, and turn inward on an errant pitch to protect their face and hands but the injuries nonetheless occur with regularity. An injury to the tuft with or without nailbed involvement is among the most common subtypes of fingertip injuries, but so too are injuries affecting the extensor mechanism of the distal interphalangeal joint (DIP) [69]. The thumb, middle, and ring are the most commonly affected [69, 70]. Two particular injury subtypes will be reviewed: mallet injuries and Seymour fractures.

Mallet Injuries

Injuries that affect the terminal tendon of the finger may very well be the most common finger injury representing upward of 33% of childhood distal phalangeal injuries [69]. Far from a benign injury, the negative consequences associated with this injury, especially when associated with a fracture, have been reported in as high as 45% of children and include reduced mobility, swan-neck deformity, deformity, and wound problems associated with treatment/splints [69, 70]. Most of these issues are fortunately minor but should not be overlooked.

Mallet injuries result from an acute, forced flexion moment upon the tip of the finger. Concomitant axially directed force, and perhaps the degree of that force, is what can lead to a simultaneous fracture. Pure tendon injuries tend to be relatively painless, and these children present with an obvious extensor lag to the DIP. Mallet fractures, on the other hand, lead to more dramatic presentations, that is, pain, dorsal swelling proximal to the nailfold, and bruising. The degree of lag may not be great as with tendon injuries, but the appearance of the finger should serve as notice of injury. Both presentations can result in compensatory swan-neck posturing from unbalanced PIP extension. All children with such presentation should be referred for an appropriate evaluation that includes radiographs and should be provisionally splinted with the DIP in extension until then. Findings on examination in the acute setting include dorsal DIP tenderness and an extensor lag. The mallet fractures more often present with more swelling and ecchymosis. In fact, some children with mallet fractures that are minimally displaced seem to retain some active extension and can fool the examiner, save a radiograph which illustrates the injury. Wehbé and Schneider have classified these injuries based upon the presence of DIP subluxation, physeal involvement, and the size of the articular fragment [71]. The diagnosis should be straightforward, though this injury is often overlooked by children, their parents, and their coaches leading to significantly delayed presentation in 15–25% of cases [70, 72]. This injury has also been mistaken for paronychia and treated with antibiotics to no affect [73].

In 1984, Wehbé and Schneider published a landmark paper concerning the treatment of mallet fractures in which the data analysis found no benefit in outcome to operative treatment [71]. Many authors, nonetheless, advocate such treatment if the injury results in either DIP subluxation or the fragment involves greater than 30% of the articular surface [74]. In such a series concerning adolescents, nearly all those who underwent closed pinning using the Ishiguro method regained full extension, while the cases that did not were in children who presented in a delayed fashion [74]. In a similar cohort where children were treated with splints, 14% healed with a slight extensor lag averaging 2° (all had mallet fracture) [70]. Outcomes compared favorably with the reports of operative treatment, and the study included children with subluxation and significant articular fragments. A recent report retrospectively compared closed pinning to nonoperative treatment that included bone stimulation [75]. Outcomes were quite similar, though the children who underwent pinning experienced stiffer DIP joints when the pins were left for more than 5 weeks.

Closed treatment is the preferred treatment of pediatric and adolescent mallet injuries, even those that include large fragments and/or DIP subluxation (Fig. 18.8). Surgical treatment is relatively indicated in situations where the child/adolescent has difficulty with full-time splinting, and in this case, simple DIP extension pinning is sufficient, though one can consider one of the methods described to reduce and secure the fracture, that is, the Ishiguro method. Open treatment should be avoided for fear of infection. A child presenting with a true fracture dislocation is another matter, and this injury warrants operative fixation.

In situations where children present late, it is important to first recognize that overall prognosis is already negatively impacted to some degree. There is still success with treating as an acute injury even as late as 8–9 weeks [70]. For those children who truly fail primary treatment, or present well beyond the hope of primary treatment (>3–4 months), and are experiencing functional issues with the finger, estimated to exist when the extensor lag is >40°, treatment is probably warranted. If radiographs suggest arthrosis, there is contracture, or there is DIP pain, arthrodesis and chondrodesis are appropriate surgical options. If full motion remains, and the joint is otherwise pain free and without arthrosis, options include tenodermodesis, scar overlapping suture, central slip tenotomy, and even spiral oblique retinacular ligament reconstruction. Reports for the latter two techniques, commonly described in adult series, include older adolescents rarely and not enough to derive any conclusions. Tenodermodesis has been reported as an effective technique for failed treatment in supple, pain-free DIP joints in children [76–78]. The 'scar overlapping' suture technique was recently described as an alternative reconstructive technique similar in principle to tenodermodesis, but without tightening the skin [79]. The authors posit that by leaving the skin untensioned, one can avoid the potential problems of creating DIP stiffness, especially over time as the finger grows, though those concerns have not been clearly manifest in the limited reports concerning tenodermodesis.

Seymour Fracture

The juxtaepiphyseal fracture of the distal phalanx was first described by Seymour as a distinct pediatric injury in 1966 [80]. A number of reports since serve as cautionary tales regarding this uncommon and underappreciated sports-related injury with the potential for serious complication that occurs in children averaging 8–11 years of age [69, 81–87]. Failure to treat this injury acutely is associated with infection, including osteomyelitis, with rates ranging from 35% to 76% [86–88]. Other complications include nail dystrophy, premature physeal arrest, stiffness, and deformity from malunion [69, 84, 85, 87].

The injury, like a mallet fracture, occurs from direct impact that is both axially directed and pushes the tip of the finger into flexion but affects the bone with an open physis different than with closed. Diving into a base head first, errant fielding of a hit ball, and getting hit by a pitched ball are all mechanisms of injury. The impact leads to a Salter-Harris 1–2 physeal fracture with a flexion deformity (Fig. 18.9). To the naked eye, the

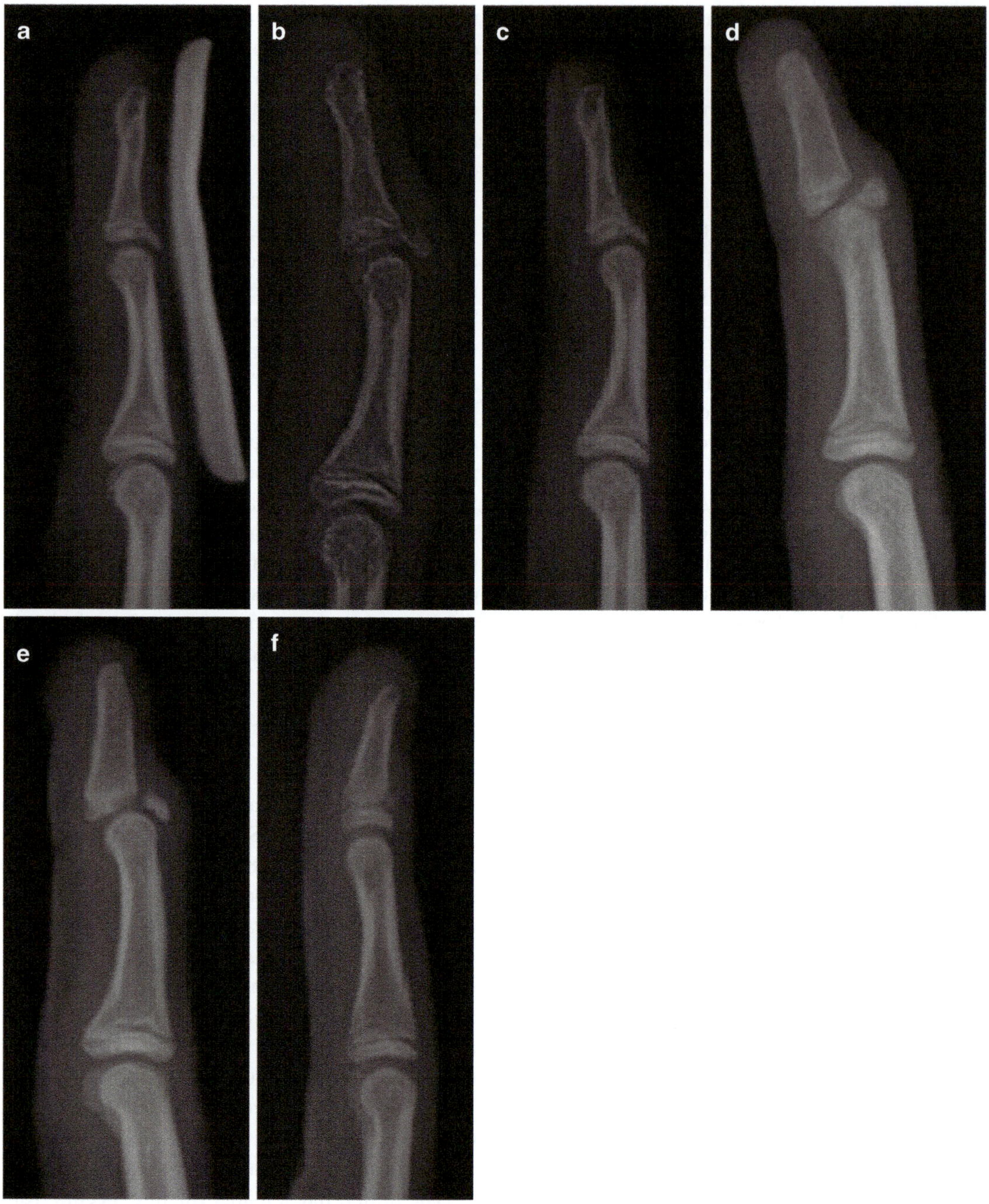

Fig. 18.8 Mallet fractures (**a**–**c**). (**a**) A 15-year-old infielder presents after mishandling a ground ball hitting the tip of his ringer finger. Initial key radiograph demonstrates mallet fracture with congruent DIP joint. (**b**) This was treated with a full-time extension splint, and (**c**) clinically healed by 6 weeks with maximal extension of near neutral. (**d**, **e**) A 14-year-old infielder with similar injury to the long finger. (**d**) Key radiograph confirms mallet fracture with some joint incongruency. (**e**) After 6 weeks of full-time extension splinting, clinically healed and painless with near neutral extension and >60° flexion. (**f**) It is important to distinguish a mallet fracture from the common Salter-Harris 2 fracture of the distal phalanx. The fragment in this case is off the dorsal metaphysis, as opposed to the epiphysis

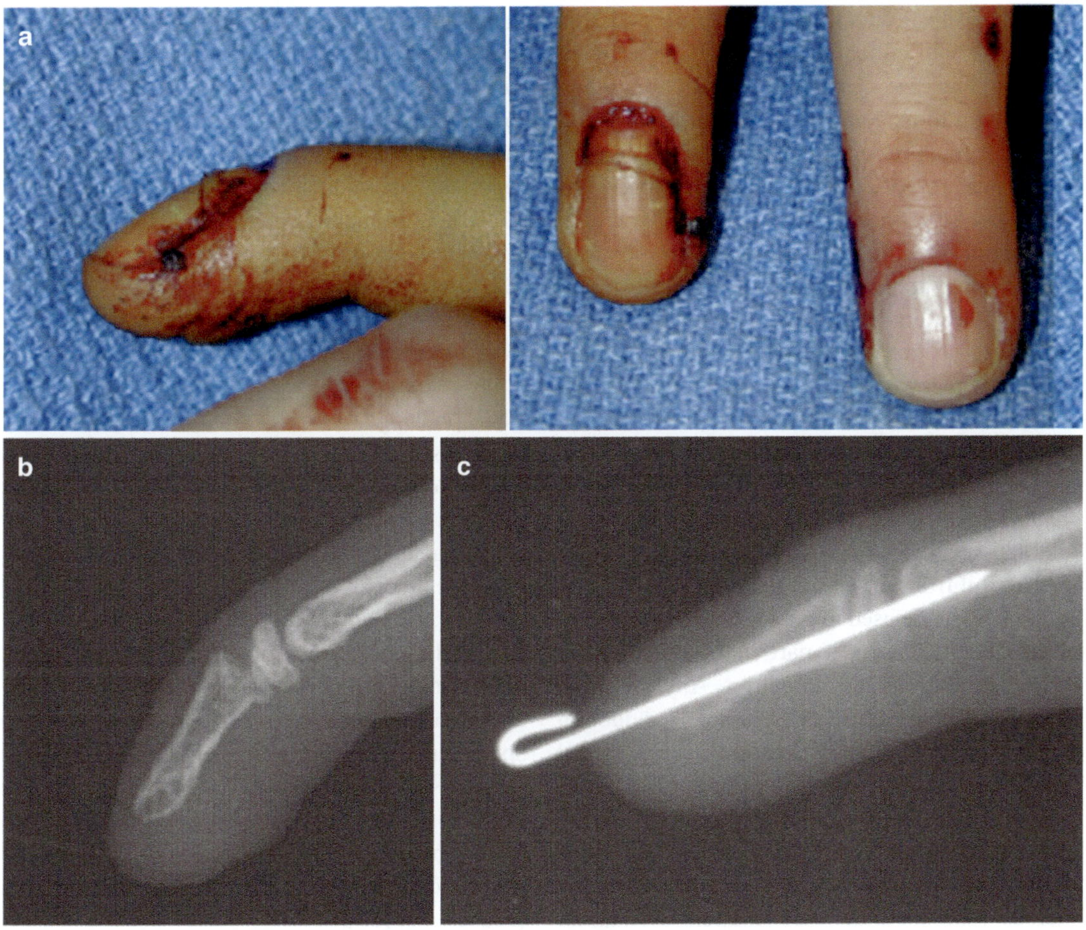

Fig. 18.9 The clinical photographs of this 10-year-old athlete who injured the tip of his finger from an errant pitch while at bat. (**a**) The picture is that of a nail root avulsion. Note the flexion deformity of the finger and the bleeding. (**b**) Radiographs confirm an underlying displaced Salter-Harris 2 fracture of the distal phalanx displaced in flexion. This is a Seymour fracture (open distal phalanx fracture with associated nail matrix injury). (**c**) Proper treatment includes infection prevention with irrigation/antibiotics and open reduction and fixation in order to extrude the enfolded nail matrix and allow for an anatomic repair

injury can look like a subungual hematoma, and/or a laceration near the eponychial fold, and/or any degree of nail plate avulsion [88]. The significance of the injury is occasionally not recognized and the focus of treatment is based on the distal phalanx with the soft tissue component dismissed as associated and incidental, and the result is delayed presentation in 20–35% of cases [86–88]. In reality, this is an open fracture of the distal phalanx. The nail is the other critical component of the injury often underappreciated, especially when the finger presents with partial or complete nail avulsion. There is nearly always a laceration at the level of the germinal matrix with interposed nail matrix in the fracture site that has been reported to exist in 47% of cases [88]. Inappropriate treatment whether by lack of direct repair or simple reduction without removing the interposed tissue inevitably results in nail dystrophy.

Appropriate treatment begins with recognition of the potential significance of severe injury. A laceration near the nail fold, bleeding, subungual hematoma, or nail avulsion should not be dismissed as a simple injury without radiographs. Children who sustain this injury during sport should be substituted out of the game and sent immediately to either an emergency department or an urgent care center for prompt treatment. When plain films confirm the presence of a juxtaphyseal fracture, management begins with the administration of intravenous antibiotics as would be the case for any open fracture. Appropriate treatment then includes removal of the nail plate and exploration of the nail matrix and/or laceration. The fracture is identified and thoroughly irrigated with sterile saline. The nail matrix, if interposed, is extruded from the fracture site. The fracture is reduced, and the nail matrix is repaired with fine (6-0) absorbable suture. If the nail plate was intact, it is thoroughly cleaned and placed back under the eponychial fold and secured with absorbable suture (4-0–5-0). The foil from the suture pack or a plastic nail prosthesis can be used as an alternative to the nail plate. The final critical part of treatment is to assess stability of the reduction. Any sense of instability with associated loss of reduction should be addressed by fixation accomplished with k-wire or even a hypodermic needle of sufficient girth. While managing this injury in an operating room is always appropriate, management in the emergency department is equally efficacious [85, 86, 88]. What matters is that all components of the injury are addressed. If the surgeon prefers treatment in the operating room on a delayed basis, then immediate treatment with antibiotics, nail plate removal, and irrigation/debridement of the open fracture must occur. Such acute, partial treatment is not associated with an increased risk of infection [86, 87].

Following definitive treatment, the fingertip is dressed, along with the fixation wire if applied, in such a method as to still allow observation of skin for perfusion. Immobilization should be robust and comfortable, and extensive if a wire is applied, that is, cast or rigid hand/forearm-based splint. Antibiotics can be continued orally for up to 3 days. Immobilization is continued until radiographs and clinical exam confirm healing typically around 3–4 weeks postoperatively. Children can return to play once the wounds and fracture are healed and any fixation is removed. Any soreness/sensitivity can be addressed with a distal interphalangeal splint or taping that leaves the proximal joints free. The fingertip is still followed with radiographs for the next 2–4 months to monitor motion, nail growth, and physeal integrity. With acute, appropriate treatment, reported complications include infection (0–10%), premature physeal closure (0–20%), and nail dystrophy (1–25%) [69, 84–88].

Phalangeal Neck Fracture

The phalangeal neck fracture (alternatively labeled subcondylar, distal condylar, or subcapital) is somewhat unique to children and peaks between the toddler and skeletally immature adolescent ages. They are the result of axial loading and occur with relative frequency in younger children. An awkward ground or fly ball, a head-first slide, and an attempted tag are the typical circumstances that will lead to this injury. The situations, and mechanisms, are very similar to a sprain, and this injury is often assumed to be a sprain as the displacement is very subtle and the joint is stiff and painful. And these injuries do not always result in ecchymosis or significant swelling which also lends itself to underrecognition (Fig. 18.10) [89].

Determining rotational alignment and coronal angulation are key to the physical examination. These parameters can be established with a careful and gentle examination, but any doubts can be resolved with a local anesthetic digital block and re-examination. The examination is truly the best method to assess rotation which is the critical data point in treatment algorithms. Inspection of radiographs involving any fracture of the phalangeal head and neck warrants appreciation that much of the head is cartilaginous in younger children, and small osseous fragments represent large cartilaginous portions. Any confusion is often settled with contralateral radiographs. Fragments are also occasionally rotated greater than 90°, and appreciating the 'normal' radiograph is critical for anatomical reduction [89, 90].

Children with nondisplaced phalangeal neck fractures are traditionally treated with rigid cast-

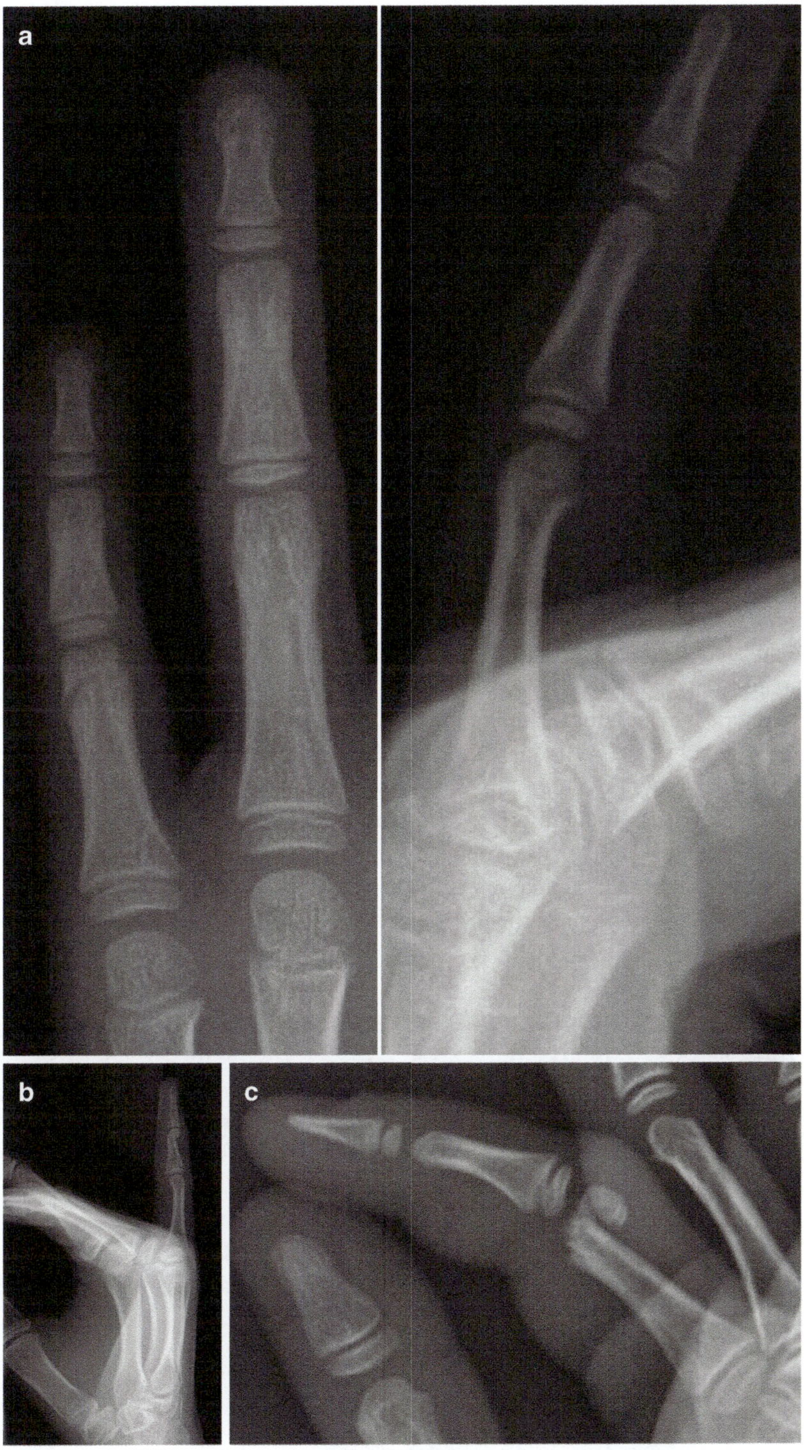

Fig. 18.10 Radiographic examples of pediatric phalangeal neck fractures. (**a**) Nondisplaced, Type 1, phalangeal neck fracture. (**b**) Displaced, Type 2, phalangeal neck fracture. (**c**) Completely displaced, Type 3, phalangeal neck fracture

ing due to inherent instability with this pattern. Park et al. recently challenged this notion a comparative study detailing that simple buddy taping of even mildly displaced phalangeal neck fractures resulted in outcomes similar to operative reduction and stabilization at an average of 17 months given the remodeling that occurred in the nonoperative group [91]. This fracture generally heals with sufficient stability to allow for return to sport with buddy straps by 3–4 weeks until pain free. This transition should be confirmed first by both the absence of clinical tenderness and the presence of radiographic healing. Most children do not require formal physiotherapy after cast removal.

Of the displaced varieties, type 2 phalangeal neck fracture (dorsal angulation and translation) is the typical subtype encountered by hand surgeons. Manipulation can be attempted in type 2 displaced fractures provided the family understands that upward of 60% will re-displace within a week. A successful manipulation should be re-evaluated every 7–10 days until healed. It is important to obtain X-rays out of the cast to avoid the potential confounding of overlapping fingers and cast material given the small size of the fracture. Any loss of alignment warrants consideration for surgical management (Fig. 18.11).

The remodeling potential for these fractures was once thought minimal necessitating operative treatment for any displaced pediatric phalangeal neck fracture, but it is greater than originally thought. In the largest series, Puckett et al. found that all malunited phalangeal neck fractures (type 2) remodeled fully in the sagittal plane and partially in the coronal plane (Fig. 18.12) [37].

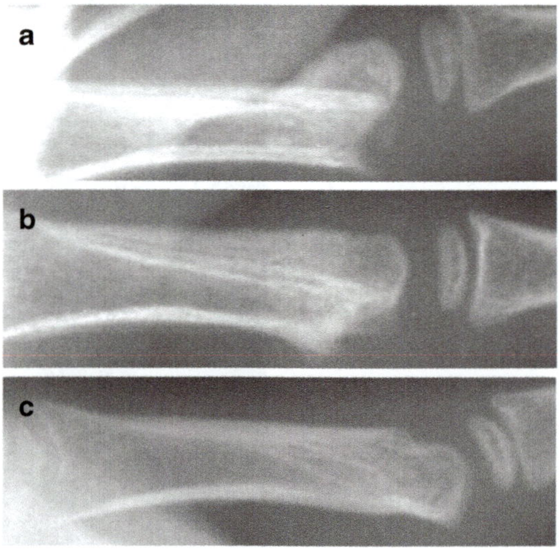

Fig. 18.12 A series of lateral radiographs of a Type 3 pediatric phalangeal neck fracture remodeling over the course of 9 months. (**a**) Initial radiographic healing. (**b**) 5 months later. (**c**) 9 months later

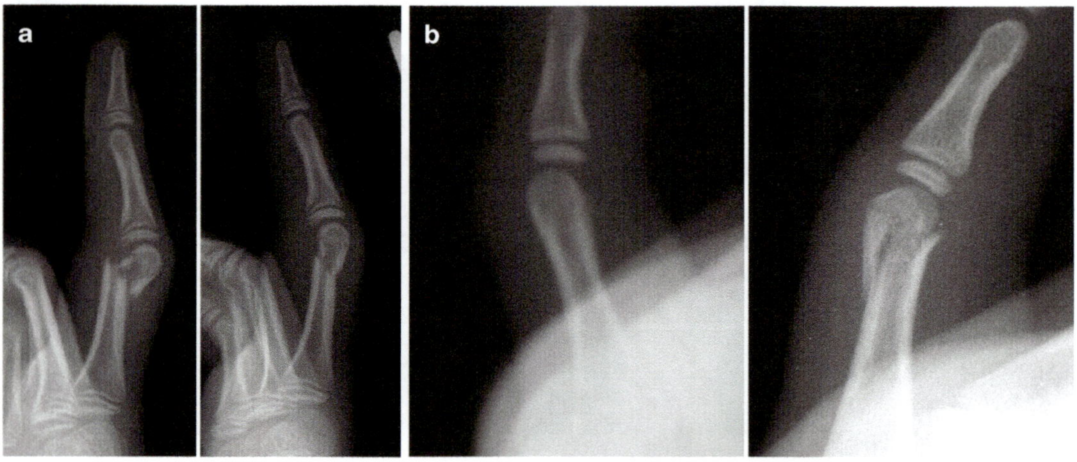

Fig. 18.11 Closed treatment of phalangeal neck fractures. (**a**) Closed reduction can successfully realign a displaced phalangeal neck fracture as demonstrated in these pre- and postreduction lateral plain films. (**b**) At the same time, successfully reduced phalangeal neck fractures need close observation as demonstrated in this clinical example where alignment was lost 1 week after a successful closed reduction

Matzon and Cornwall introduced an algorithm that allowed healed displaced phalangeal neck fractures (sagittal plane deformity, no rotational deformity, with sufficient growth remaining) to remodel; otherwise, displaced fractures were treated through a combination of manipulation, pinning, and open reduction as needed to gain alignment [92].

While acute displaced fractures still benefit from interventions, malunited fractures can potentially be allowed to remodel depending upon the age of the child and the wishes of the family. Malrotation, clinically visible coronal deviation (>15°), or insufficient growth remaining (<1 year) mandates anatomic alignment. A family choosing nonoperative treatment of acceptably displaced phalangeal neck fractures must understand that months will need to pass before mobility returns. In the less likely event of insufficient remodeling, a secondary subcondylar resection arthroplasty can help restore flexion [93]. Parents of athletes, musicians, and other physically active children often choose surgery as motion is restored faster, whereas parents of young children may be more likely to choose casting to avoid surgical procedures and general anesthesia.

Most can be reduced with flexion after first correcting coronal and rotational alignment. The hand surgeon should be familiar with various techniques of closed reduction and pinning for phalangeal neck fractures (Fig. 18.13) [94–97]. Children who present 2 to 3 weeks after injury with a displaced fracture will not be amenable to simple closed reduction due to partial healing. In these circumstances, closed osteoclasis becomes an attractive surgical option especially if criteria for remodeling are not met or there is desire for quicker return of mobility (Fig. 18.14) [98]. With this technique, a relatively large Kirschner wire (0.045–0.062) is introduced percutaneously and manually manipulated to disrupt the immature callus. Once loosened, the fragment is either reduced manually or with the aid of an intrafocal pin to 'hinge' the fragment into alignment; fixation is then achieved using percutaneously placed pins. Anatomic alignment is not necessary provided it is acceptable or in a position to remodel. Osteoclasis can sometimes be accomplished up to 5–6 weeks following injury before full healing has occurred [92]. Only an open osteotomy would suffice once callus is sufficiently mature (>5 weeks), and this is a last resort in order to avoid its associated risks: stiffness and avascular necrosis of the fracture fragment. If required, the neck is approached dorsally with a longitudinal or gently curved incision, and accessing the fracture either around the side of the lateral band or in between the lateral band and extrinsic extensor. The surgeon must avoid the collateral ligaments and surrounding soft tissue as best as possible to avoid devascularizing the phalangeal head, place the K-wires such that the ligaments are not captured, and start physiotherapy in a functional splint at 2–3 weeks' time to minimize loss of mobility. Gentle dissection techniques and avoiding soft tissue stripping can still reduce an already tenuous blood supply and create the environment for postoperative stiffness. Anatomic alignment may need to be sacrificed in favor of acceptable alignment (rotationally and coronally aligned, partial restoration of the sagittal alignment) in order to avoid these complications and anticipate a staged subcondylar reconstruction if motion proves insufficient. An open approach is sometimes necessary, but the author will at times alternatively allow the malunion to mature, wait until remodeling, and then correct later malrotation or coronal deviation [99].

Proximal/Periphyseal Phalangeal Fracture Including Avulsion Fractures

Periphyseal, juxtaepiphyseal, and metaphyseal fractures are discussed together as treatment principles are very similar. Periphyseal fractures are the most common fracture type in children affecting the proximal phalanx, especially the thumb, and in particular Salter-Harris 2 fractures; though in a separate series concerning fractures of the fingers published by Al-Qattan, the juxtaepiphyseal pattern is equally common [100, 101]. Juxtaepiphyseal fractures, classified by Al-Qattan as either type 1 (transverse on the metaphyseal side within 2 mm of physis) or type 2 (with an

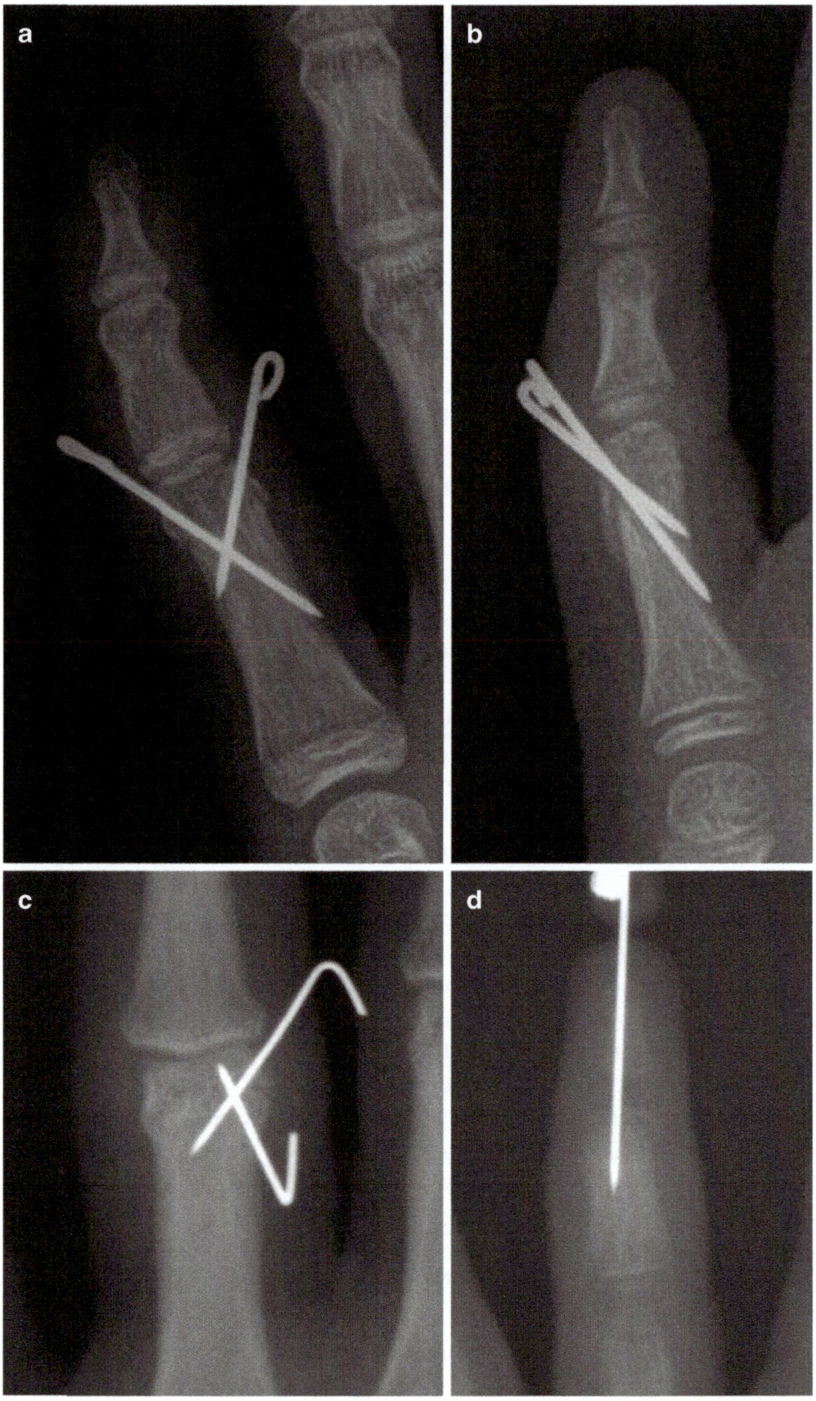

Fig. 18.13 Radiographic examples of various pinning configurations for displaced phalangeal neck fractures. (**a**) Standard crossed pinning through the collateral recesses. (**b**) For coronal oblique neck fractures where there is little purchase on one side, two divergent pins can be placed unilaterally. (**c**) For coronal oblique neck fractures where there is little purchase, a second antegrade pin can provide rotational stability, with casting providing further support. (**d**) For the smallest of fragments, middle phalangeal neck fractures, and young children, a single retrograde pin can prove sufficient

associated 'Thurston-Holland' fragment), are the next most common pattern of phalanx fracture (Fig. 18.15). Most paraphyseal fractures in children are stable after reduction. As children become adolescents, however, these fractures are more commonly unstable and need to be reduced and surgically stabilized. Nonetheless, any displaced paraphyseal fracture in the young ball

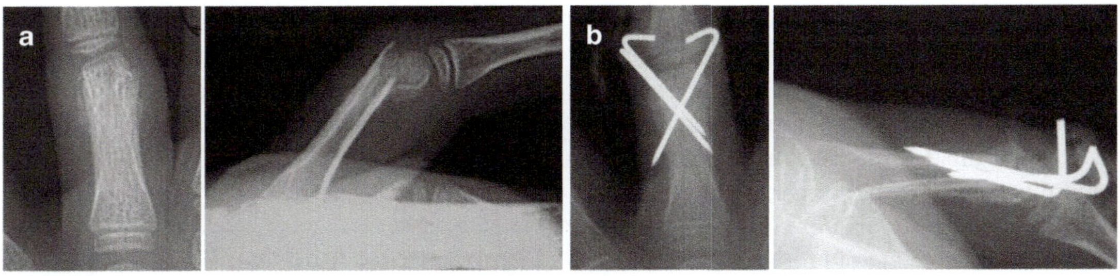

Fig. 18.14 A subacute Type 2 phalangeal neck fracture with poor alignment. (**a**) Initial radiographs demonstrate immature callus formation. (**b**) A closed, percutaneous, osteoclasis is performed, which allows manipulation of the fracture into acceptable, albeit not anatomic, position

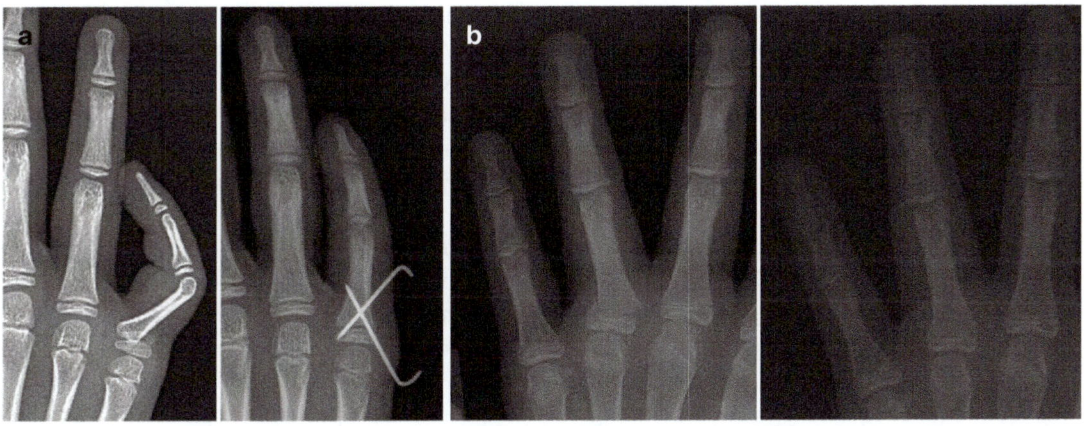

Fig. 18.15 Juxtaepiphyseal fracture subtypes. (**a**) Type 1 juxtaepiphyseal 'extra-octave' small finger proximal phalangeal fracture pre- and posttreatment. (**b**) Type 2 juxtaepiphyseal ring finger proximal phalangeal fracture with the 'Thurston-Holland' metaphyseal fragment pre- and postmanual reduction

player should initially be treated with a closed manipulation, and surgery, typically closed percutaneous pinning, reserved for the uncommon unstable or irreducible displaced fracture.

'Extra-octave' Other Physeal/ Juxtaepiphseal Fractures

The apex radial, ulnarly angulated paraphyseal fracture involving the proximal phalanx of the little finger is among the most common phalangeal fractures in children. Known as the 'extra-octave' fracture, it serves as a good model for paraphyseal fractures involving any of the digits including the thumb. Alignment is primarily judged by clinical exam, and children who can adduct the finger next to its 'neighbor' generally will have an acceptable degree of coronal plane angulation (within about 15°). Up to 20–25° can be accepted in skeletally immature children provided parents understand remodeling may be incomplete. Any rotational deformity or unacceptable angulation is initially treated with manipulation. Sagittal plane angulation is typically within remodeling parameters, but greater than about 30° ought to be reduced. Fractures that re-displace (approximately 5–10%) or prove irreducible are treated with surgical fixation (Fig. 18.15) [36]. Closed reduction and percutaneous pinning are primary means of fixation with open reduction rarely required.

Irreducible fractures suggest the possibility of entrapped soft tissue including extensor tendon in the case of dorsally displaced fractures, and these rare circumstances necessitate open reduction. The irreducible periphyseal fracture is approached either dorsally or midaxially on the side of the metaphyseal/epiphyseal fragment. The extensor hood in the proximal phalanx and the central slip for the middle phalanx require careful handling. In the former, then the interval between the sagittal band/extrinsic extensor and lateral band can be incised for access. This interval is repaired prior to formal skin closure. Access to the middle phalanx is usually achieved by retracting the lateral bands after releasing the transverse retinacular ligament. Since the central slip inserts on the epiphysis, it can be left undisturbed. As with open treatment of phalangeal neck fracture, the peri-articular soft tissues must be respected, and every attempt made to avoid their dissection. This includes not simply the nearby ligaments which carry important vascular supply, but the physis itself which can be damaged with aggressive handling. The important principle to bear in mind in skeletally immature ball players is that the final alignment needs only to be 'sufficient,' with or without considering remodeling potential, especially if anatomic reduction would require aggressive handling of the critical soft tissues. Children with displaced phalangeal base/shaft fractures that present late with callus on radiographs warrant particular mention. Extra-physeal fractures can be surgically treated closed using percutaneous osteoclasis techniques to improve alignment provided the surgeon is particularly careful around the physis. True incipient malunions of physeal fractures, on the other hand, should be considered for later osteotomy to avoid possible iatrogenic physeal injury incurred during percutaneous or open 'take-down' of the periphyseal callus.

Ligamentous Avulsion Fractures of the Fingers

Soft tissue avulsion fractures of the phalangeal bases are very common injuries, especially as children get closer to skeletal maturity. The volar plate avulsion fragment of the base of the middle phalanx is perhaps the most frequent pattern which also includes lateral collateral avulsion fragments and dorsal central slip avulsion fractures (Fig. 18.16) [102]. Treatment of these injuries is straightforward and is dependent upon whether ligament or tendon is injured. Volar plate and lateral collateral avulsion fractures represent ligament-equivalent injuries. They are first assessed for joint stability which is rarely compromised. Early motion is initiated with buddy straps utilizing rigid digital splints only for sport and only as needed [103–107]. Prolonged immobilization encourages early stiffness and prolongs the pain and recovery associated with these injuries. Full active range of motion is typically achieved within 2–3 weeks from the injury; if it is not, formal hand therapy is advisable. It is quite helpful to advise patients and families that swell-

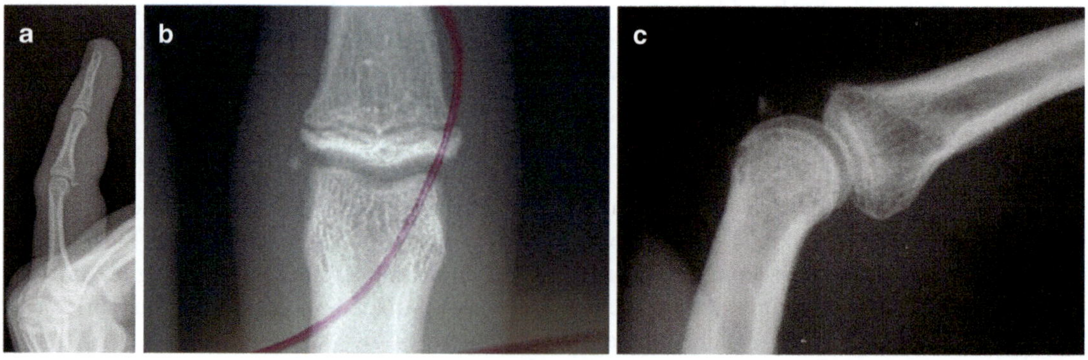

Fig. 18.16 Examples of digital avulsion fractures. (**a**) The volar-plate avulsion fracture off the insertion of the base of the phalanx is an epiphyseal fragment. (**b**) The collateral ligament avulsion fracture off the insertion of the ligament is another epiphyseal fragment. (**c**) The central-slip avulsion fracture is another epiphyseal fragment but includes the tendinous insertion of the extensor mechanism

ing and soreness can last for many months following this injury, especially in adolescents. This education can eliminate unnecessary concern and follow-up visits.

Dorsal avulsion fractures off the base of the middle phalanx are central slip-equivalent injuries akin to an acute boutonniere injury. These are immobilized full time for 3–4 weeks to protect the extensor mechanism by only holding the PIP joint in extension (MCP and DIP joints are free (Fig. 18.16)). Rigid, conforming, and moldable materials can be applied for games/practice by a trainer or therapist. Once the injury is no longer tender and/or radiographs demonstrate bony healing, the player is advanced into a removable PIP extension splint and allowed to slowly regain flexion with intermittent daily exercises. Active flexion is gradually increased provided active extension is maintained, and splinting can usually be discontinued within 2–3 weeks of this transition. Rarely a player sustains a combined dorsal and volar avulsion fracture resulting from a combination of hyperextension injuring the volar side and axial compression injuring the dorsal side. In this situation, the dorsal fracture, which contains the central slip insertion, is prioritized and is treated as just outlined. The difference is counseling the player and family that restoration of mobility will likely take much longer.

Ligamentous Avulsion Fractures of the Thumb

The thumb proximal phalanx is a frequently injured bone and becomes increasingly so in the teenage years as the physeal space narrows. Collateral ligament avulsion fractures, in particular, become more common, especially on the ulnar side. The fragments vary in size and need to be assessed on X-rays, paying attention to coronal angulation of the joint, and the location of the fragment on the lateral view, as volar-lateral fragments indicate involvement of the collateral ligament insertion, whereas strict capsular avulsions are more mid-lateral. Assessing stability is one of the critical factors in determining treatment. This must be accomplished with physical examination because neither the radiographic size of the fragment nor its degree of displacement predicts stability. A gentle exam in different degrees of flexion to test the proper and accessory collateral ligaments using the contralateral uninjured thumb as a template will accomplish this assessment. Anatomically aligned and stable fractures are casted for 3–4 weeks and then allowed to move in the flexion/extension axis without stress for another 3–6 weeks until the fragment is clearly healed. Thumb MCP stiffness is typically transient and is not nearly as much of a functional concern as an incompetent ulnar collateral ligament from an unhealed fracture, so it is generally advisable to err on the side of longer immobilization to ensure healing. Smaller fragments are more common, and sometimes these fragments seem rotated or displaced. These smaller avulsion fractures typically heal well with nonoperative treatment leaving surgery for injuries with either acute instability or failed casting (Fig. 18.17) [108–110].

It is also important to pay attention to the size of the fragment and the degree of displacement. These are, in skeletally immature athletes, Salter-Harris 3 equivalent injuries, and physeal preservation is part of treating this injury. Gapping of greater than 2 mm and a fragment larger than 25% of the articular surface traditionally warrant reduction and fixation (Fig. 18.18). Additionally, any rotation of the fragment implies fracture instability and dictates operative reduction and stabilization. Surgical reduction can be achieved percutaneously with a penetrating bone reduction clamp, although care should be taken not to crush the branches of the superficial sensory radial nerve. Open reduction is often required. The surgical approach involves a straight or curvilinear midaxial incision on the side of the fragment along the thumb metacarpophalangeal joint (MCP). Careful dissection through the soft tissues should protect branches of the superficial sensory radial nerve going to the dorsal thumb. On the ulnar side, dissection proceeds to the level of the adductor pollicus aponeurosis and extensor hood. On the radial side, dissection proceeds to the abductor pollicus aponeurosis and extensor hood radially. Incising the

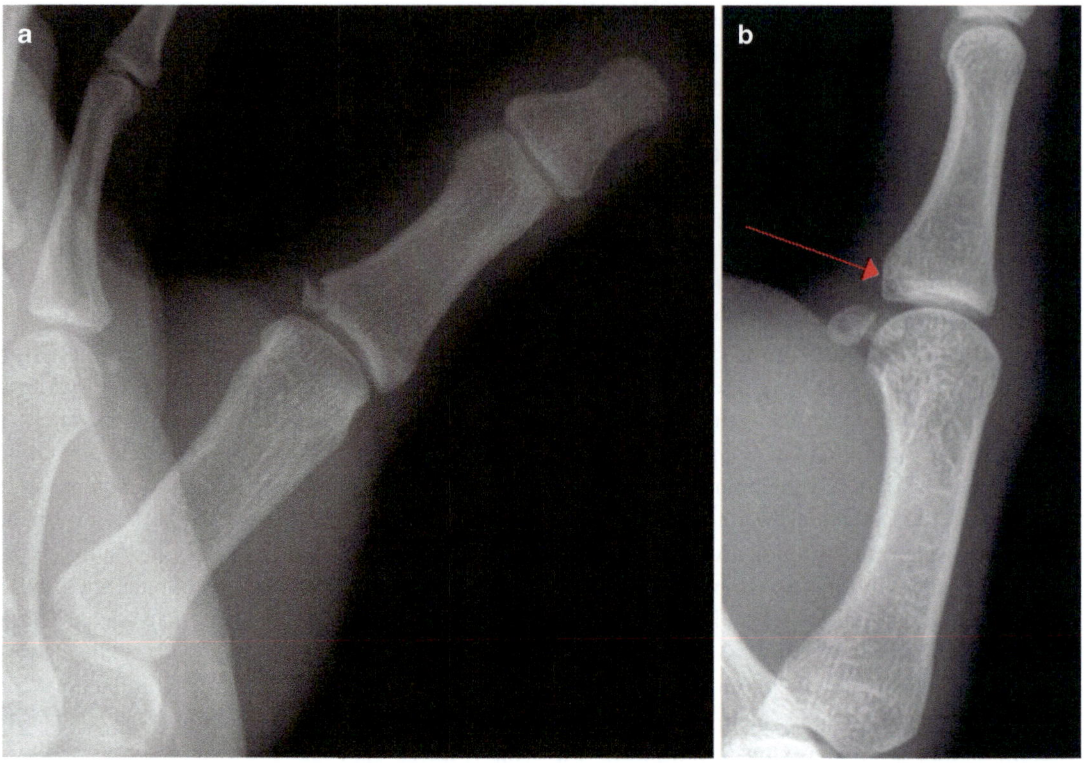

Fig. 18.17 Radiographs of a 17-year-old catcher who 'jammed' his right thumb trapping a low pitch. The thumb MCP was clinical stable, though tender along the ulnar side. (**a**) PA of the right thumb demonstrating a small, but rotated fragment off the ulnar base of the proximal phalanx. The MCP joint looks congruent. (**b**) The lateral view demonstrates a congruent joint. The arrow points to the fragment, which is volar, consistent with an avulsion fracture of the ulnar collateral ligament (bony gamekeeper's injury)

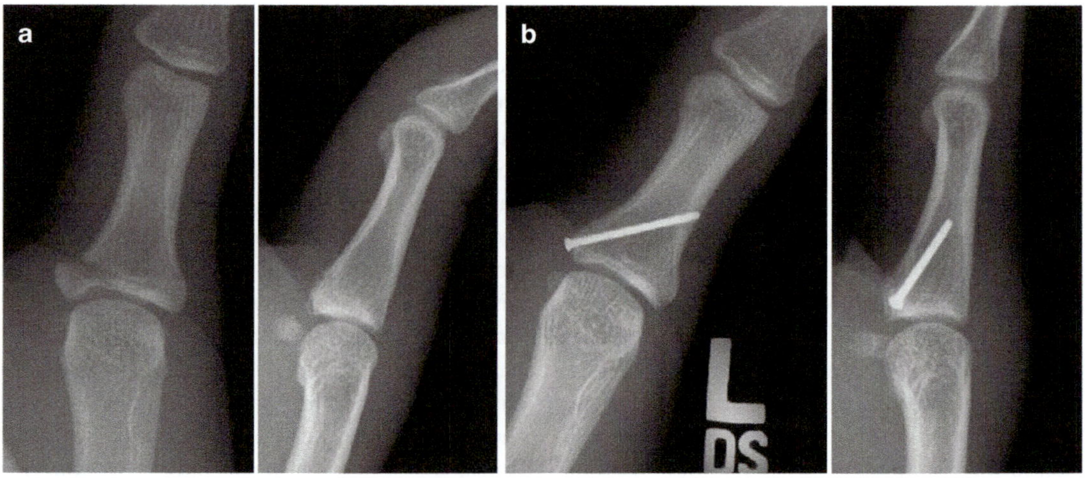

Fig. 18.18 Radiographs from a 17-year-old who sustained a displaced bony gamekeeper's injury sliding head first back to base to avoid a pick off. (**a**) The fragment, about 33%, is off the volar/lateral corner and displaced. (**b**) Radiographs following open reduction and fixation with screw fixation

interval, repaired prior to closure, provides access to the fracture fragment. The MCP capsule can be incised while protecting the collateral ligament to gain greater visualization of the fracture fragment if needed. It is important to maintain the ligamentous attachment to the fragment to maintain vascularity. Once the fragment is appropriately reduced, fixation method is based on the size of the fragment and the age of the child. Smaller fragments and bones with 'wide open' physes are best treated with k-wires, while larger fragments in nearly or completely mature children can be managed with mini-screw fixation.

Scaphoid Injury

The most frequently fractured carpal bone is the scaphoid, even in children. Series exploring the relative frequency among carpal fractures has repeatedly found that 80–90% of the fractures involve the scaphoid [111, 112]. Still, scaphoid and other carpal injuries make up a small percentage of hand and wrist injuries in the younger age groups ranging from 1% to 6% [112, 113]. In pediatric series, upward of 35–40% of the fractures result from sports-related trauma [114, 115]. Peak incidence of fracture in children occurs between 13 and 15 years of age averaging earlier for girls than boys, and fractures within the first decade of life are particularly rare [112, 116–121]. In fact, skeletal maturity is cited as one factor associated with scaphoid fractures in children and adolescents [121]. As if emblematic of sports injuries in children, the pattern of scaphoid fractures transitions from predominantly distal fractures at the younger ages to waist fractures in adolescents who are not only larger but also participate in adult-like sports activities [115, 122]. Proximal pole fractures represent 1–9% in children and adolescents [111, 117, 118, 121–123].

The scaphoid becomes radiographically visible between 4 and 6 years of age and completes ossification by around 15 years of age [117]. Like its primary blood supply, ossification starts distally and proceeds in a retrograde direction, and this may explain the predominance of distal fractures in younger age groups [124].

Postinjury radial wrist pain requires sifting through a variety of possible diagnoses. Scapholunate ligament or other radial sided carpal ligament injury will present with tenderness near and sometimes at the level of the scaphoid. Fractures of the distal radius, especially the radial styloid, nearby carpals, and metacarpal base fractures of the thumb, index, and long will all present with tenderness in the vicinity of the scaphoid [111]. Scaphoid contusion requires advanced imaging to diagnosis and presents very similar in history and examination to a scaphoid fracture [67, 111]. Diligence in pursuing a diagnosis ultimately leads to advanced imaging which demonstrates bone edema (Fig. 18.19). Though very little is published regarding this injury, the possibility of conversion to complete fracture means respecting this injury and treating it cautiously [66]. The possibility of extensor tendinitis, that is, De'Quervain's and second compartment, dorsal radiocarpal impaction, and flexor carpi radialis tendinitis, though not typically from acute trauma, need to be evaluated when assessing the young athlete. Stress fractures of the scaphoid in adolescent and young adult elite athletes are another repetitive stress injury that requires diligent evaluation as advanced imaging is required to confirm this diagnosis [39, 40, 42, 44, 125].

Diagnosis of this injury is critical due to the potentially deleterious consequences of an ununited scaphoid which extend beyond persistent pain and limited athletic participation and to premature traumatic arthritis. The initial fall on an outstretched rotated wrist sliding into a base or diving for a ball in the field is not always recognized as a significant injury. Athletes will often either continue playing with pain or return to play once the wrist is taped or rested presuming a sprain. In fact, many children and adolescents present for treatment with a chronic injury 20–70% of the time (Fig. 18.20) [114, 121, 123]. The consequence of delayed presentation is not just the potential for painful arthritis; it is also the reality that union rates are slower and lower in children who present with an established non-

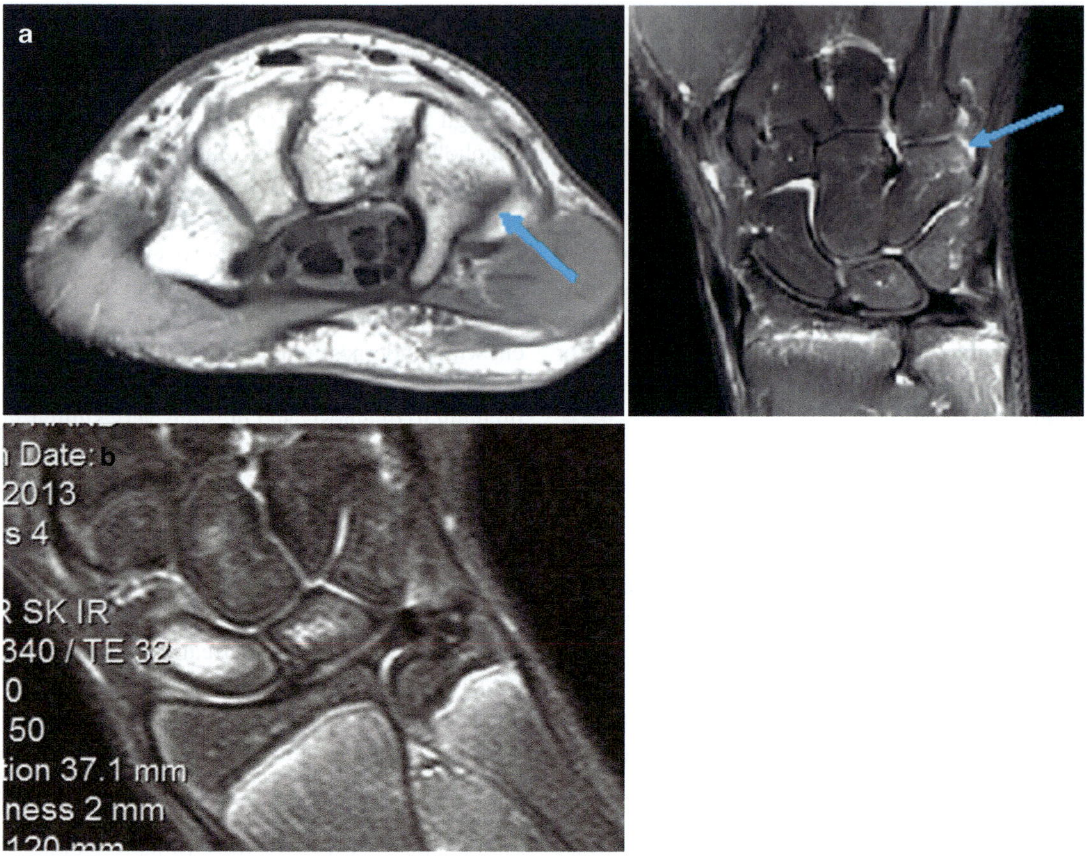

Fig. 18.19 Bone contusions. (**a**) A 17-year-old sustained injury from direct contact along the ulnar/proximal palm at bat. Tenderness over the hook of the hamate was present. MRI demonstrates contusion along the distal hamate body that extends to the junction of the body with the hook, but no fracture. (**b**) Scaphoid and lunate contusion in a 14-year-old sustained during an awkward fall diving for a fly ball in the outfield

union and surgery is nearly always necessary [117, 121, 123].

The challenge with diagnosis of pediatric scaphoid fractures is that, like their adult counterparts, recognition is not straightforward, and plain film evaluation has a false-negative rate ranging from 15% to 54% (Fig. 18.21) [111, 117, 123]. A high index of suspicion is critical to making the acute diagnosis. Important physical findings on examination include distal pole tenderness, snuffbox tenderness, radial wrist pain with axial load, and radial pain with wrist motion [126–130]. Routine PA and lateral plain films often prove insufficient, and an additional pronated lateral and ulnar deviated PA round out the 4-view series that should be obtained to evaluate for scaphoid fracture [131–134]. The 'pencil-grip' view is another important view to consider given that scapholunate ligament injury is within the differential diagnosis of posttraumatic radial wrist pain (Fig. 18.22) [135]. Establishing the diagnosis does not stop with negative initial radiographs in the young athlete. Traditional recommendations of provisional immobilization of suspected fractures and early re-evaluation are a proven strategy in children. Evenski et al. found 30 confirmed scaphoid fractures of a cohort of 104 adolescents with suspected fracture, but 2 weeks from injury was required for the X-ray positivity in 45%, while the rest took between 5 and 7 weeks for the fracture to become 'visible' [117] (Fig. 18.21). An alternate strategy for the elite adolescent ball player is to proceed with advanced imaging to improve the accuracy of the diagnosis. MRI and

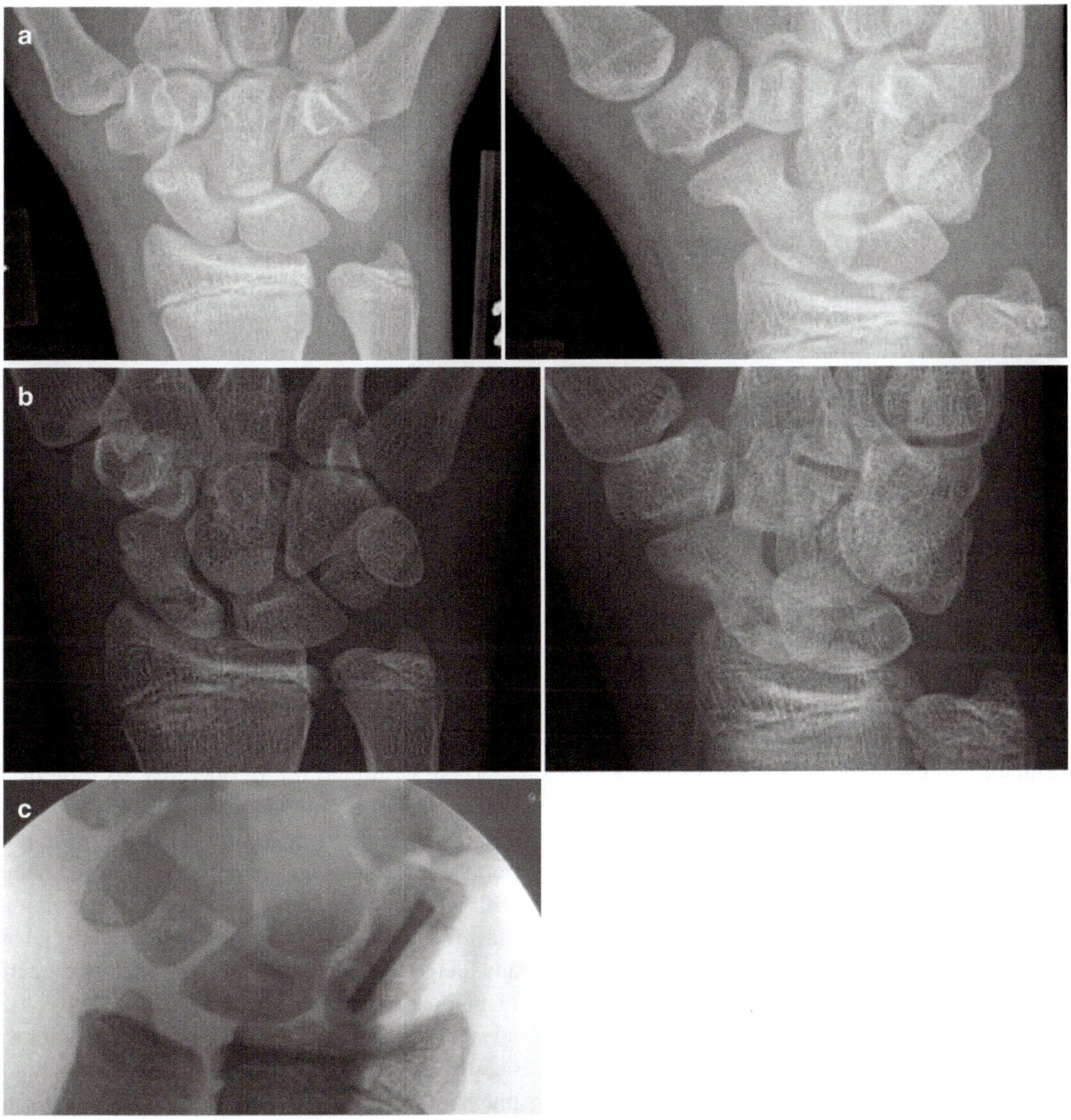

Fig. 18.20 Scaphoid nonunion. A 14-year-old male presented with worsening radial wrist pain during winter baseball practice. He sustained a wrist injury during fall season falling on outstretched hand. (**a**) Representative initial radiographs in the urgent care center were read as normal and he was dismissed with wrist brace. (**b**) Three months later, the same radiographic views reveal chronic proximal pole nonunion. (**c**) The fracture went on to union after open treatment including a headless compression screw and autograft

CT scan both have been shown to improve the sensitivity of diagnosis and are recommended if the athlete strongly desires immediate return if the bone is not fractured (recruiting opportunity, important event) (Fig. 18.23). MRI is probably the second study to obtain for diagnosis given its ability to sift through the differential diagnosis better than other studies given its ability to visualize soft tissues. CT scan is more useful in assessing bony alignment and healing, but both are effective imaging modalities to specifically look for the possibility of occult scaphoid fracture [133, 134, 136–141]. MRI finding of bone bruising without fracture should still be treated as a fracture, as 2% can progress to complete fracture even with immobilization [66].

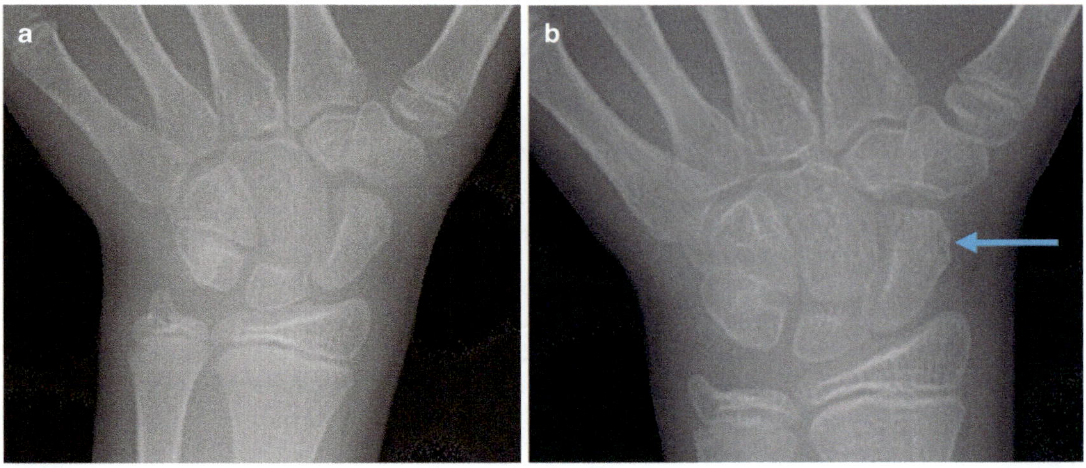

Fig. 18.21 A 13-year-old presents acutely after tripping over second base as he was rounding to third. He had distinct snuffbox tenderness and distal pole scaphoid tenderness. (**a**) Representative initial radiographs did not reveal scaphoid fracture. (**b**) Repeat radiographs in approximately 2 weeks revealed a distal waist fracture

Cast immobilization is the treatment of choice of nearly all acute, non-displaced scaphoid fractures. Displacement ranges about 10% of all presenting acute scaphoid fractures and remains the primary surgical indication [114, 115, 118, 121, 142]. Casting acute, nondisplaced, scaphoid fractures in children and adolescents reliably achieves union greater than 96% of the time, with unions occurring in 100% in a couple of series [114, 115, 118, 121, 123, 142]. Gholson et al. found that healing time varied by fracture location [115]. Distal pole, waist, and proximal pole fractures healed at an average of 6, 9, and 15 weeks, respectively, but this included children who presented greater than 6 weeks with nondisplaced fractures. Other series predominated by factors that delay healing include displacement and osteonecrosis; the latter also being a negative prognostic factor regarding outcomes [115, 121]. Consistent with adult series, healing rates have not been affected by short- versus long-arm casting [142]. The author's preference is a long- to short-arm cast with interosseous molding to reduce rotation and incorporate the thumb across the MCP joint only. The other controversy applies to both nonoperative and operative treatment and involves the radiographic assessment of union. The author's preference is to obtain a CT scan unless the plain films and examination are clear. In the latter situation, the authors also schedule a return visit within a month to confirm clinical improvement and repeat radiographs after return to activities as tolerated.

There is limited use to operative fixation of a nondisplaced scaphoid waist fracture in the young baseball player. Young ball players are not going to be able to return to the field or the lineup with a cast on. Perhaps, the only role for such a player would be pinch-running, but to what advantage for the young athlete? Operative treatment of a nondisplaced fracture does have the advantage of allowing early mobilization prior to healing, and this may reduce the overall return to play time once the bone is healed compared to cast treatment; but this has never been vetted in studies to date. It is important to note that early surgery requires the athlete to assume the risks of surgery and does not seem to improve the healing rate or the time to union [115]. In the end, the decision to operate on the young ball player with a nondisplaced scaphoid waist fracture should be considered carefully and after thorough discussion with the athlete and their families.

Acute, nondisplaced proximal pole fractures are a relative indication for surgical fixation. Gholson et al. found that 95% of their acute, nondisplaced proximal pole fracture healed with casting alone at an average of 15 weeks in chil-

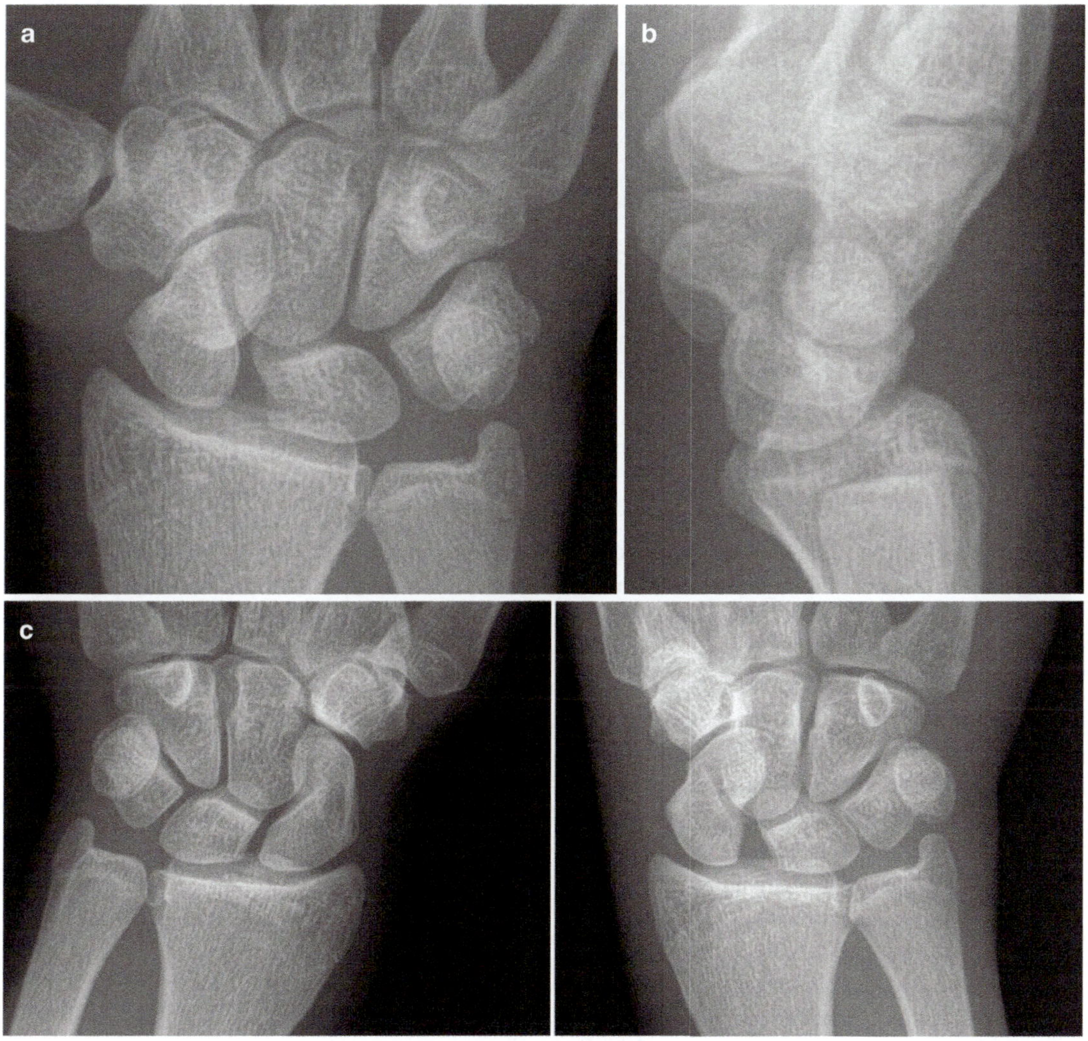

Fig. 18.22 A 17-year-old outfielder injured his right wrist diving for a fly ball. Radial wrist pain ended his game, and it persisted for over 1 week. (**a**) Standard PA of the wrist demonstrating an irregularly positioned scaphoid. (**b**) Standard lateral without significant malalignment of the carpus. (**c**) Pencil group demonstrates asymmetric widening of the SL interval on the injured wrist, confirming SL injury

dren [115]. Grewel et al. found that cast treatment resulted in 90% union at an average of 14 weeks in their cohort of 53 patients averaging 30 years of age at injury [143]. Given the lengthy time to healing, the primary reason to consider surgical fixation is to limit time in cast, not the time to healing, in the hopes of reducing overall time to recovery and return to play.

Acute, displaced fractures, defined as ≥1 mm of displacement and/or altered carpal alignment, should be treated with surgical reduction and fixation. There are potential risks of problems associated with malunion regarding carpal mechanics and risk of arthrosis. The primary issue, though, is the union rate for closed treatment of acute displaced fractures is low, less than 30% for displaced waist and proximal locations and 87% for distal levels [115]. With successful closed reduction, fixation can be secured with a percutaneously placed headless screw, or Kirschner wires, from either the volar or the dorsal approach depending upon fracture location. Open reduction

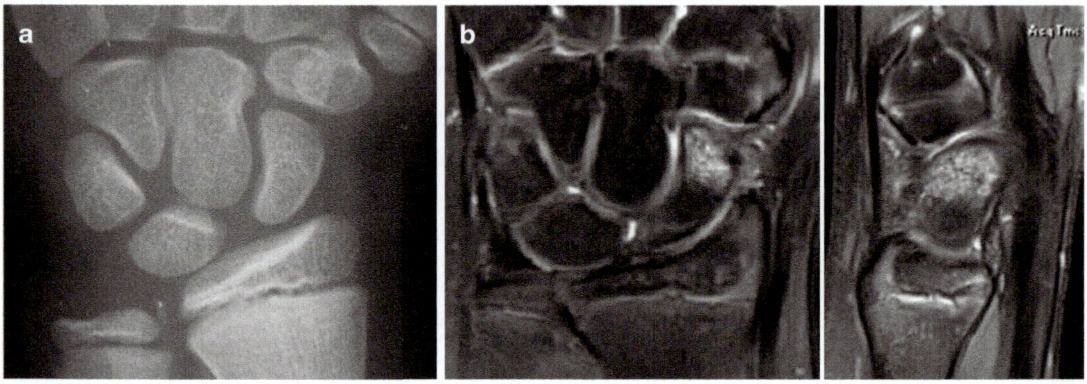

Fig. 18.23 A 9-year-old presented with radial wrist pain following a fall playing defense during practice. The next game, a championship game, was deemed important to parents and an MRI was obtained. (**a**) Representative radiograph taken within a couple of days of injury. (**b**) MRI in similar pain reveals a distal waist fracture

is needed if closed reduction fails to reduce the fracture and correct carpal alignment. Union rates for surgical treatment of displaced fractures is reported as >96% [115, 121, 142]. Location of the fracture influences time to union as for cast treatment of nondisplaced fracture. One series found that the time to union was dependent upon the particular headless compression screw implanted, but not the overall union rate [115].

In the relatively frequent presentation of a chronic fracture (>6 weeks from injury), union rates with appropriate treatment are still excellent overall with rates >95% [115]. Time to healing is substantially increased for chronically presenting pediatric scaphoid fractures by an estimated 0.65–2.25× with cast treatment and 0.3× with surgical treatment [115, 123]. Casting can be considered for chronic presenting nondisplaced fractures, though union rates are lower, more so for proximal and waist fractures and particularly if displaced [115]. In young athletes, surgery is the favored treatment for all chronically presenting scaphoid fractures, with the possible exception of chronic nondisplaced distal pole fractures (Fig. 18.20). Even for chronic nondisplaced fractures, surgery affords reduced overall healing and rehabilitation time compared to cast treatment.

Outcomes for children with scaphoid fractures are generally excellent. Reviews have described excellent functional scores in >95% of children [118, 121]. Poor outcomes are rare and primarily related to the development of osteonecrosis or chronic nonunion [114, 121, 144–147]. While there are case reports of pediatric scaphoid nonunion healing with immobilization alone, the generally accepted recommendation for athletes is surgical fixation often with bone graft, and possible low-intensity pulsed ultrasound, to stimulate healing with excellent union rates [120, 144, 148, 149].

Return to play for children with scaphoid fractures can be in stages. Children with surgical secured acute fractures, for example, can consider returning as a pinch runner with a protective splint at least 3–4 weeks following surgery depending upon comfort. The need for free bilateral wrist movement and strength means that a healed fracture is, at a minimum, required before returning to the lineup and the field. This translates, in older adolescents, to a minimum of 6–10 weeks lost to sport while healing in a cast, and this time is expected to approach 3–4 months with proximal pole fractures. Though not vetted in any published research, stable surgical fixation can allow for mobility rehabilitation at a much earlier time than if casted and may represent a relative indication for surgery in the 'right' athlete.

Other Carpal Injuries

Baseball-related injuries involving the other seven carpals are uncommon, with the exception of the hamate. In one community emergency department, over the course of the year, 6% of the hand fractures in children involved the carpals (1.6% of all pediatric fractures), but that percentage dropped to 0.7% when scaphoid fractures were excluded [112]. In another series, it took 3 years to identify 12 carpal injuries in children <18 years (48 scaphoid fractures identified in the same time) [111]. The common mechanism of injury is either a sliding, diving while fielding a ball, or a direct blow to the hand as can occur at bat and errant fielding. Focal tenderness and appreciating the possibility of such an injury is the key to diagnosis given that initial plain films can be negative in up to 90% of cases [150]. Special views may be required and should be directed by physical examination. Tenderness over the pisiform after being struck by a ball should be assessed with a supinated lateral. Tenderness over the hook of the hamate should be evaluated with both a carpal tunnel view and a radially elevated supinated lateral view (Fig. 18.24). A 'Robert's' AP of the thumb will profile both the trapezium and the trapezoid, while a pronated lateral aids in assessing tender-

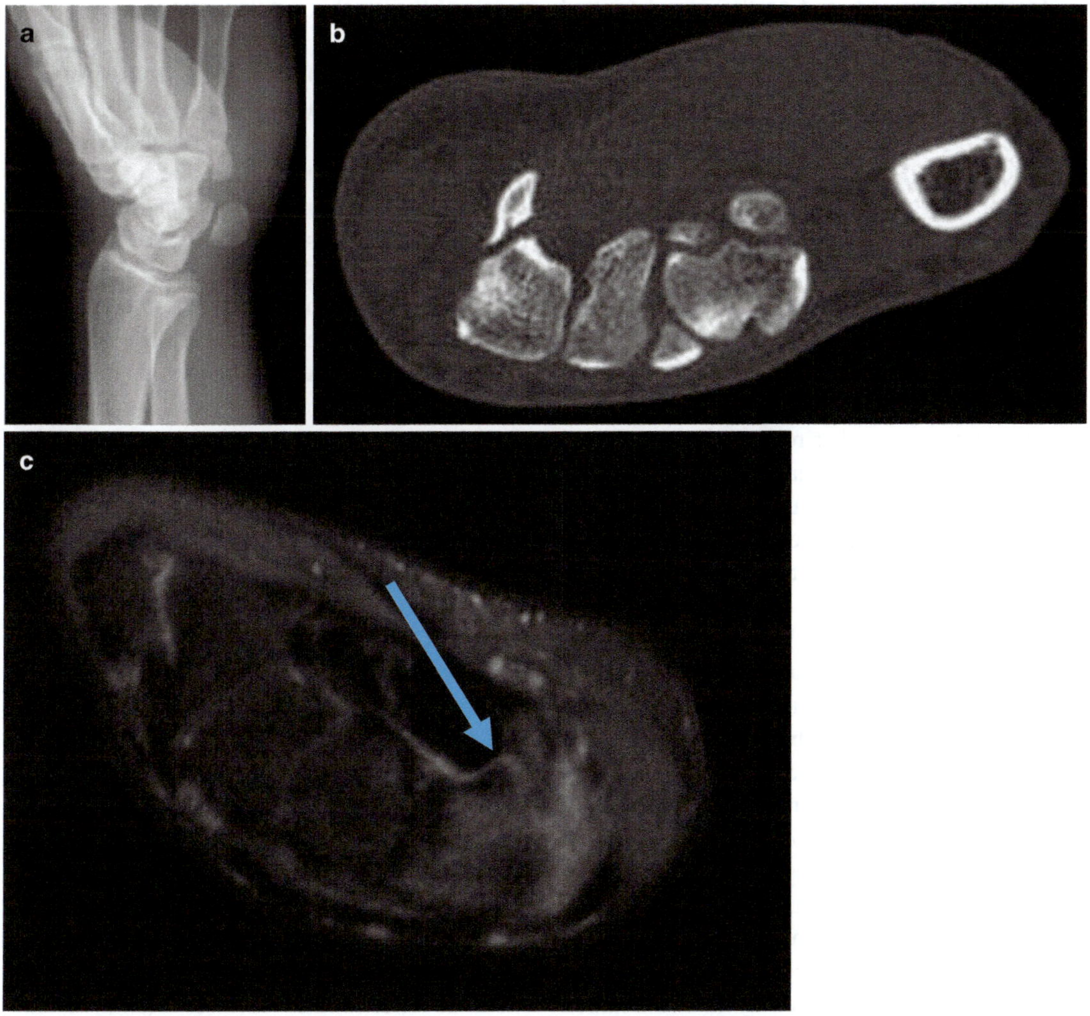

Fig. 18.24 Hook of hamate fracture evaluation. (**a**) A radially elevated supinated lateral X-ray, shown here, is a particularly sensitive view to evaluate suspected hook of hamate fractures. (**b**) CT scan with axial view confirming an acute hook of hamate fracture. (**c**) MRI confirming an acute hook of hamate fracture with associated bone edema

ness over the dorsum of the triquetrum and hamate. A bone contusion or intercarpal sprain is among the other diagnoses to consider. Diagnosing these injuries ultimately requires diligence and persistence, which means advanced imaging with a young ball player presents with persistent, focally tender, wrist pain that does not quickly resolve in the setting of normal plain films. And advanced imaging should be obtained whenever there is tenderness over multiple carpals even when one of them has a visible fracture on plain films due to the common occurrence of multiple simultaneous carpal injuries (Fig. 18.24).

Treatment varies based on the carpal injured and the severity of injury. Stable avulsion-type injuries of the triquetrum might only require a removable splint, while nondisplaced fractures should be casted until osseous union. Capitate fractures, especially at the neck, warrant consideration for surgical fixation whenever there is associated injury or displacement due to the risk of nonunion and avascular necrosis. Young baseball players, like their adult counterparts, are at risk for injuries to the hook of the hamate. These injuries should be treated similarly (elsewhere covered in another chapter) with surgical excision to allow for quicker return to sport. Carpal fractures occur in combination with both other carpals and with distal radius fractures [111, 151, 152]. A thorough physical exam when faced with a young athlete with either a distal radius fracture or any carpal tenderness is critical to avoid missing such a combination. The potential consequences of this injury are considerable, and aggressive treatment is often warranted. 'Fenton's syndrome,' otherwise labeled 'scaphocapitate syndrome,' occurs when the capitate impinges on the distal radius and fractures in the setting of a scaphoid fracture [111, 153, 154]. This combination is also thought to represent a greater arc perilunate injury suggesting significant trauma to the wrist. Trapezial fractures may be seen in thumb carpometacarpal joint injuries. Pisiform fractures and dislocations have been seen in combination with distal radius fractures in 12- and 13-year-old patients and healed with closed reduction and immobilization [155]. It remains important to recognize these possibilities so to fully appreciate the injury and thus administer the optimal treatment options.

Sprains

Sprains, or ligamentous injuries, are likely much more common than appreciated. Many physeal fractures and torus fractures of the distal radius are often misdiagnosed clinically as a wrist sprain; however, real injury involving the ligaments of the wrist is not uncommon.

Intercarpal Ligament Injury, Including Scapholunate Tears

Radiographic assessment of potential soft tissue injuries in young athletes requires knowledge of how the growing wrist and hand affects imaging. Since the scaphoid ossifies from distal to proximal, for example, the scapholunate interval, which seems very wide at young ages, closes radiographically as children skeletally mature. Kaawach et al. analyzed 119 radiographs of children aged 6–14 years and found that the typical adult scapholunate interval of 2 mm is not reached by girls until age 11 and by boys until age 12 [15]. Recent studies confirm that intercarpal distances and even intercarpal angles trend downward with increasing age until puberty [156, 157]. Then, too, other indices like carpal height change in growing children increasing until puberty, when it achieves adult values. Assessing the young athlete for a soft tissue injury, therefore, is helped by looking at contralateral wrist films and advanced imaging. Advanced imaging is particularly advantageous when an athlete is experiencing difficulties transition back to sport or playing games because of wrist pain despite negative radiographs (Fig. 18.25). The reality is that bad injuries do occur in young athletes, and this includes perilunate injuries (Fig. 18.26) [158–161].

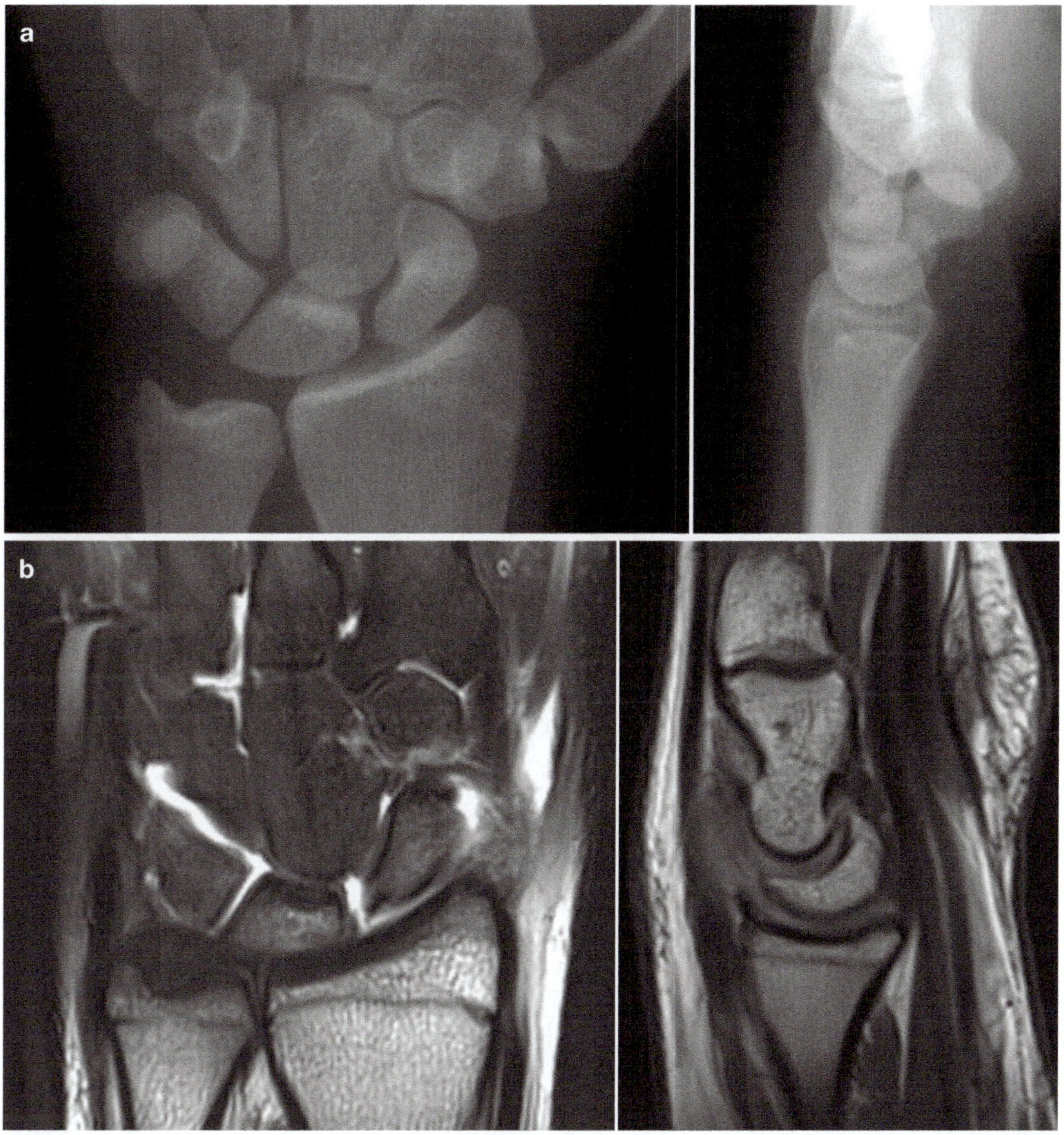

Fig. 18.25 Severe wrist sprain. A 17-year-old outfielder collided with a teammate during a defensive play injuring his wrist. (**a**) Initial radiographs suggest increased scapholunate angle consistent with the finding of dorsal scapholunate tenderness. (**b**) MRI confirmed complete scapholunate tear with associated dorsal intercalated segment instability (DISI) pattern

Triangular Fibrocartilage Complex (TFCC) Tears

Ulnar-sided wrist pain in the young athlete can result from a number of issues as there is a lot of anatomy in this area susceptible to injury given the loads experienced in the ball player's wrist as it rotates and deviates during sport. The extreme loads during a swing especially demand integrity to the soft tissues that support ulnar load and stabilize the distal radio-ulnar joint (DRUJ). Probably the most common ligamentous injury occurs within the TFCC, which is a fibro-ligamentous structure with various components

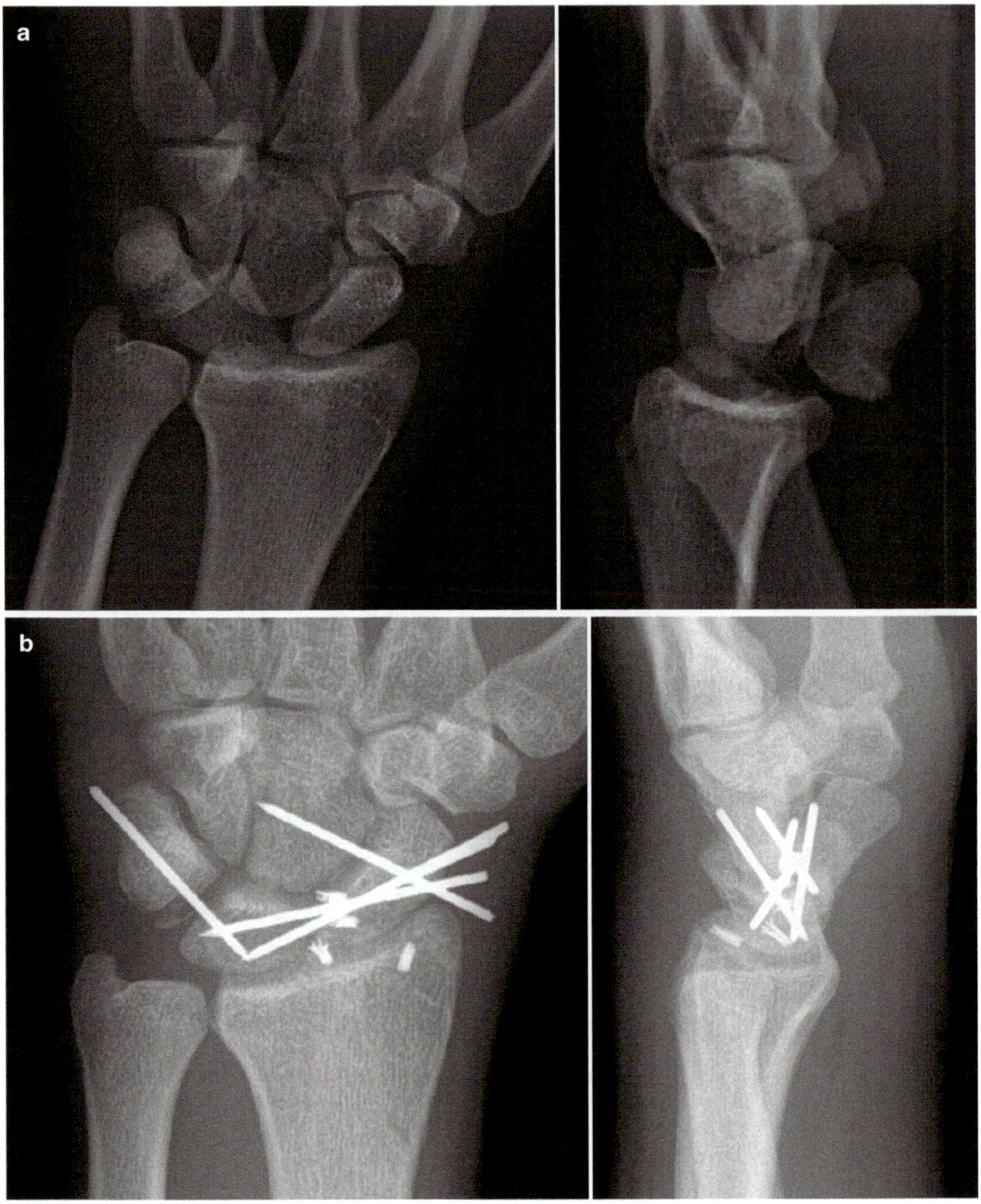

Fig. 18.26 An awkward fall while diving outstretched to catch a line drive resulted in significant wrist pain and ended his game. (**a**) Emergency department radiographs illuminate a Type 4 perilunate dislocation. (**b**) Wrist radiographs after surgical fixation

which sits atop the distal ulna and has important attachments to the radius, the carpus, and the extensor carpi ulnaris (ECU). Injuries to this ligament have been discussed in another chapter, but this discussion will concern this injury in children. The TFCC injury in children and adolescents has been traditionally associated with distal radius fractures in children in some series, but this is not exclusively the case [19, 162]. It is important for the clinician to recognize injury without a history of or associated with an ipsilateral fracture. The average age of children treated for TFCC tears in a few series varies from 13 to 16 [18, 19, 162–164]. Ulnar-peripheral tears (type 1B) are the most common form in adolescents [19, 163–165]. Many athletes recognize the injury when it occurs during a swing or in the field but do not always have enough pain to seek early attention. The athlete seeks attention when it becomes clear that it is both persisting and interfering with their swing or their play.

Pain that is primarily ulnar-sided focused around the soft spot just proximal to the pisiform, between the pisiform and the ulnar styloid. Swelling, bruising, and other externally visual markers of injury are mostly absent, but symptoms like perceived or audible clicks, pain with wrist rotation, and pain when loading their wrist especially in extension and ulnar deviation are mostly present. Checking for tenderness of the ulnar styloid, the triquetrum, and the ulnar midcarpal joint and assessing stability of the lunotriquetral (LT) articulation, the DRUJ, and the ECU are all part of a thorough evaluation of ulnar wrist pain. The 'ulnar foveal sign' describes tenderness in this area and is highly diagnostic for injury to the TFCC (Fig. 18.27) [166]. Other findings on physical exam include ulnar pain with ulnar compression and impingement tests and the "press test" [167]. The contralateral wrist, assuming it is asymptomatic, serves as a terrific template for comparison for questions concerning tenderness and stability. Standard PA and lateral wrist views allow for visualization of the ulnar styloid, the morphology of the lunate and its midcarpal articulation with the hamate, Gilula's midcarpal line for static stability, most partial carpal coalitions involving the LT and capito-hamate

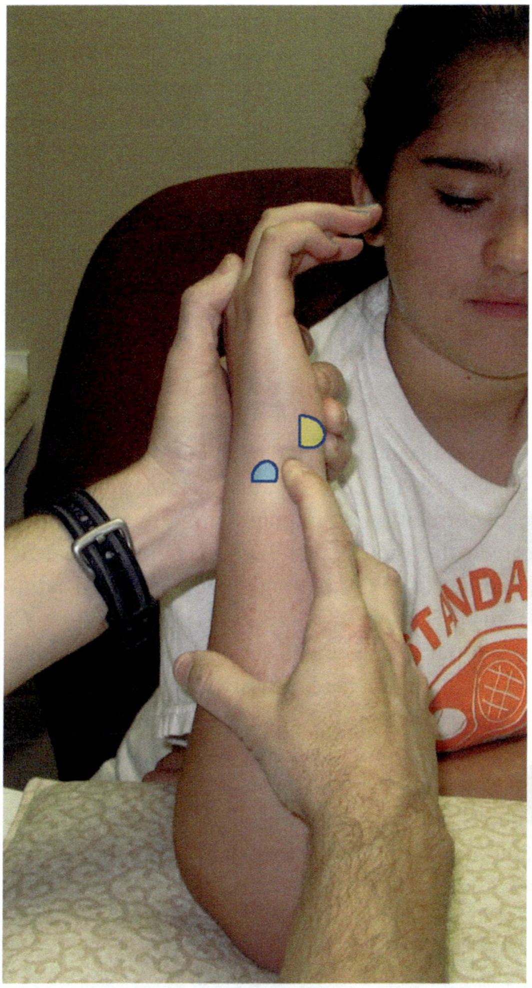

Fig. 18.27 This photograph demonstrates the location of the 'ulnar foveal soft spot.' Tenderness to this area that is also consistent with the epicenter of the athlete's pain is very predictive of TFCC pain. The location of the ulnar styloid and pisiform is illustrated on the photo

(CH) articulations that can present with ulnar pain, static carpal instability patterns (especially LT and volar tilt of the lunate), and static DRUJ variance and alignment [168]. Additional views particularly helpful in the setting of TFCC pain is a pronated clenched fist view which helps to estimate the functional ulnar variance under conditions similar to activity, and pronated laterals can expose a triquetral avulsion fracture [169]. The appearance of a volar-intercalated segmental instability (VISI) is further evaluated with a formal dynamic series looking for excessive LT movement. Advanced imaging is recommended when there is either gross instability or a lack of response of conservative management. Older adolescents, depending upon whether they are in season or being recruited, may opt for early imaging to expedite the workup. MRI is the preferred modality, and an arthrogram is often added to the procedure to enhance the visualization of the TFCC and assess for disruptions but is not the final arbiter regarding treatment given rates of false-negative studies (Fig. 18.28) [162]. A negative MRI does not rule out a TFCC injury in children and adolescents especially when the symptoms and signs are most consistent with this injury [16, 17, 20]. And, just as importantly, clinical correlation with imaging findings are critical given the modest number of people with MRI findings of TFCC pathology but no related symptoms [170].

Initial management of acute injuries includes immobilization and activity restriction for 3–4 weeks, though some authors advocate 6 weeks. A few acute injuries respond well to forearm splinting, but this should be used with caution. The need for a long-arm cast is determined by whether short-arm immobilization with or without interosseous molding to minimize rotation is enough to eliminate pain. Acutely, immobilization is continued for 3–4 weeks. Athletes are sent for physiotherapy to work on a gradual strength and mobility program after the first 3–4 weeks. As pain improves, immobilization transitions to DRUJ support taping. Transition to sport depends upon sufficient strength and sports simulations that demonstrate the athlete can participate without pain. DRUJ support is often continued as athletes transition back to sport (Fig. 18.29). Athletes and their parents should be advised that return to sport even with nonoperative management can take 2–3 months. Athletes who are struggling to progress with therapy can consider receiving a corticosteroid injection. Surgery is indicated for all athletes with either gross instability or those who fail to progress with conservative treatment, and the latter circumstance is probably by far the most common indication. Two studies have attempted to evaluate the natural history of TFCC tears and have found that approximately 60% of people with an acute tear will ultimately recover without the need for surgery [171, 172]. Surgery consists of either repairing or debriding the TFCC, depending upon the specific location of

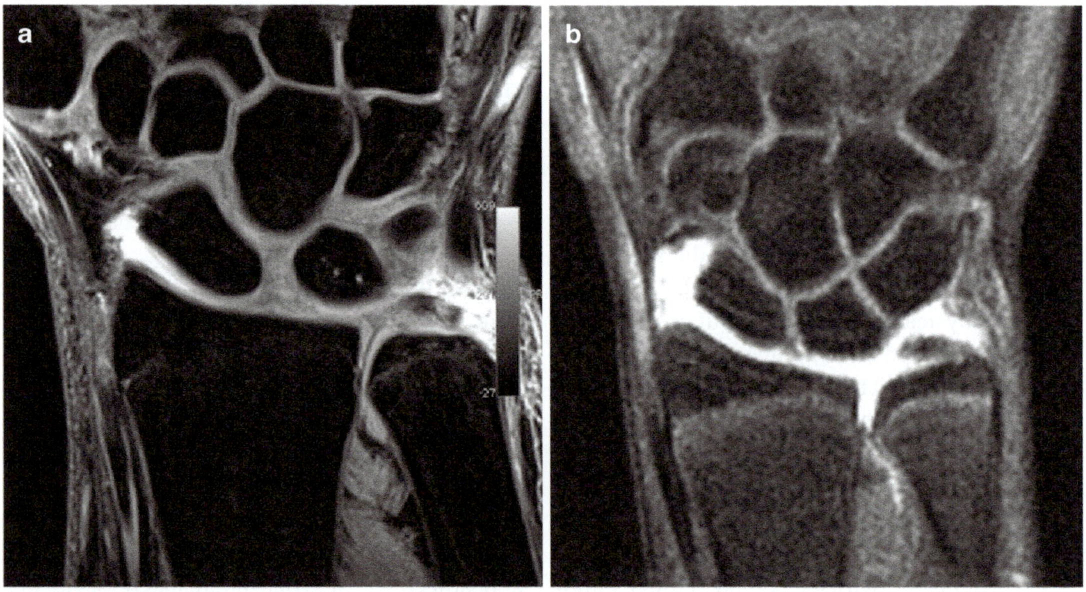

Fig. 18.28 Key images of TFCC injury as visualized with MRI-arthrography. (**a**) Type 1B, ulnar sided, TFCC tear. The articular disc is intact, and this is frequently misinterpreted as normal. (**b**) Type 1D, radial sided, TFCC tear

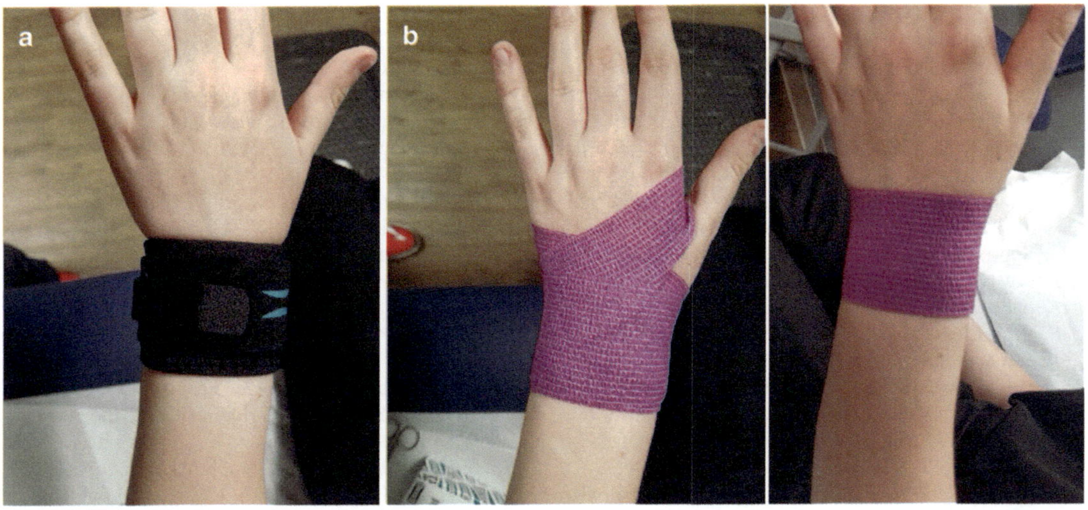

Fig. 18.29 Clinical photographs demonstrating various techniques to tape/wrap the wrist in order to stabilize the DRUJ and unload the TFCC that can be utilized during training and games. (**a**) A DRUJ orthosis. (**b**) Two methods of taping

the injury within the TFCC, and is usually accomplished with arthroscopic techniques. Ulnar shortening osteotomy should be considered in the presence of static ulnar positivity. Young athletes return to sport an average of 3–4 months after surgery [19].

Conclusion

One of the central themes throughout this chapter reflects the age-old adage that 'children are not small adults.' A child's skeletal anatomy has less 'bone,' thicker periosteum, physes, and is growing and enlarging until the transition to skeletal maturity and adult anatomy is completed. Their transitioning and developing musculoskeletal system has implications on joint and bone stability, the types of injuries children sustain and the way these injuries manifest. Radiographic findings change throughout their development which also impact a clinician's ability to detect and assess these injuries. Given the level of stress that children place on their young bodies through high level sports participation, it is critical that those taking care of them be familiar with their specific injuries, how they present, and the best methods of treatment to allow them to return to the field without negative consequences.

References

1. Taylor BL, Attia MW. Sports-related injuries in children. Acad Emerg Med. 2000;7(12):1376–82. https://doi.org/10.1111/j.1553-2712.2000.tb00495.x. DOI: papers3://publication/doi/10.1111/j.1553-2712.2000.tb00495.x.
2. Swenson DM, Henke NM, Collins CL, Fields SK, Comstock RD. Epidemiology of United States High School Sports-Related Fractures, 2008-09 to 2010-11. Am J Sports Med. 2012;40(9):2078–84. https://doi.org/10.1177/0363546512453304. DOI: papers3://publication/doi/10.1177/0363546512453304.
3. Lawson BR, Comstock RD, Smith GA. Baseball-related injuries to children treated in hospital emergency departments in the United States, 1994-2006. Pediatrics. 2009;123(6):e1028–34. https://doi.org/10.1542/peds.2007-3796. DOI: papers3://publication/doi/10.1542/peds.2007-3796.
4. Johnson BK, Brou L, Fields SK, Erkenbeck AN, Comstock RD. Hand and wrist injuries among US High School Athletes: 2005/06-2015/16. Pediatrics. 2017;140(6):e20171255. https://doi.org/10.1542/peds.2017-1255. DOI: papers3://publication/doi/10.1542/peds.2017-1255.
5. Collins CL, Comstock RD. Epidemiological features of high school baseball injuries in the United States, 2005-2007. Pediatrics. 2008;121(6):1181–7. https://

doi.org/10.1542/peds.2007-2572. DOI: papers3://publication/doi/10.1542/peds.2007-2572.
6. Passan J. The arm: inside the billion-dollar mystery of the most valuable commodity in sports. New York: Harper Collins; 2016.
7. Jayanthi NA, LaBella CR, Fischer D, Pasulka J, Dugas LR. Sports-specialized intensive training and the risk of injury in young athletes: a clinical case-control study. Am J Sports Med. 2015;43(4):794–801. https://doi.org/10.1177/0363546514567298. DOI: papers3://publication/doi/10.1177/0363546514567298.
8. Post EG, Trigsted SM, Riekena JW, et al. The association of sport specialization and training volume with injury history in youth athletes. Am J Sports Med. 2017;45(6):1405–12. https://doi.org/10.1177/0363546517690848. DOI: papers3://publication/doi/10.1177/0363546517690848.
9. Bell DR, Post EG, Biese K, Bay C, Valovich MLT. Sport specialization and risk of overuse injuries: a systematic review with meta-analysis. Pediatrics. 2018;142(3):e20180657. https://doi.org/10.1542/peds.2018-0657. DOI: papers3://publication/doi/10.1542/peds.2018-0657.
10. Post EG, Struminger AH, Hibberd EE. Sport specialization is associated with upper-extremity overuse injury in high school baseball players. J Shoulder Elb Surg. 2020;29(9):1775–82. https://doi.org/10.1016/j.jse.2020.01.092. DOI: papers3://publication/doi/10.1016/j.jse.2020.01.092.
11. Arnold AJ, Thigpen CA, Beattie PF, Kissenberth MJ, Tokish JM, Shanley E. Sport specialization and increased injury frequency in youth baseball players: a prospective study. J Athl Train. 2019;54(10):1115–22. https://doi.org/10.4085/1062-6050-349-18. DOI: papers3://publication/doi/10.4085/1062-6050-349-18.
12. Ogden JA, Ganey TM, Light TR, Greene TL, Belsole RJ. Nonepiphyseal ossification and pseudoepiphysis formation. J Pediatr Orthop. 1994;14(1):78–82. https://doi.org/10.1097/01241398-199401000-00016. DOI: papers3://publication/doi/10.1097/01241398-199401000-00016.
13. Ogden JA, Ganey TM, Light TR, Belsole RJ, Greene TL. Ossification and pseudoepiphysis formation in the “nonepiphyseal” end of bones of the hands and feet. Skelet Radiol. 1994;23(1):3–13. DOI: papers3://publication/uuid/FD938A36-F044-43DE-97F1-AA0410486ACE.
14. Limb D, Loughenbury PR. The prevalence of pseudoepiphyses in the metacarpals of the growing hand. J Hand Surg Eur Vol. 2012;37(7):678–81. https://doi.org/10.1177/1753193411436295. DOI: papers3://publication/doi/10.1177/1753193411436295.
15. Kaawach W, Ecklund K, Di Canzio J, Zurakowski D, Waters PM. Normal ranges of scapholunate distance in children 6 to 14 years old. J Pediatr Orthop. 2001;21(4):464–7. DOI: papers3://publication/uuid/6008CB75-4B75-4AF8-9E6F-CD98EE073EC8.
16. Farr S, Grill F, Ganger R, Graf A, Girsch W. Pathomorphologic findings of wrist arthroscopy in children and adolescents with chronic wrist pain. Arthroscopy. 2012;28(11):1634–43. https://doi.org/10.1016/j.arthro.2012.04.152. DOI: papers3://publication/doi/10.1016/j.arthro.2012.04.152.
17. Farr S, Grill F, Girsch W. Wrist arthroscopy in children and adolescents: a single surgeon experience of thirty-four cases. Int Orthop. 2012;36(6):1215–20. https://doi.org/10.1007/s00264-011-1428-y. DOI: papers3://publication/doi/10.1007/s00264-011-1428-y.
18. Farr S, Schüller M, Ganger R, Girsch W. Outcomes after arthroscopic debridement of the triangular fibrocartilage complex in adolescents. J Wrist Surg. 2018;7(1):43–50. https://doi.org/10.1055/s-0037-1604394. DOI: papers3://publication/doi/10.1055/s-0037-1604394.
19. Fishman FG, Barber J, Lourie GM, Peljovich AE. Outcomes of operative treatment of triangular fibrocartilage tears in pediatric and adolescent athletes. J Pediatr Orthop. 2018;38:1–5. https://doi.org/10.1097/BPO.0000000000001243. DOI: papers3://publication/doi/10.1097/BPO.0000000000001243.
20. Ramavath AL, Unnikrishnan PN, George HL, Sathyamoorthy P, Bruce CE. Wrist arthroscopy in children and adolescent with chronic wrist pain: arthroscopic findings compared with MRI. J Pediatr Orthop. 2017;37(5):e321–5. https://doi.org/10.1097/BPO.0000000000000887. DOI: papers3://publication/doi/10.1097/BPO.0000000000000887.
21. Gilsanz V, Ratib O. Hand bone age. Berlin: Springer; 2005.
22. Dua K, O’Hara NN, Shusterman I, Abzug JM. Ossification of the proximal and middle phalangeal condyles: radiographic aid in phalangeal neck fracture reduction. J Pediatr Orthop. 2019;39(3):e222–6. https://doi.org/10.1097/BPO.0000000000001255. DOI: papers3://publication/doi/10.1097/BPO.0000000000001255.
23. Taylor KW, Moore MM, Brian J, Methratta S, Bernard S. Wrist MR imaging in children: effect on clinical diagnosis and management. Clin Imaging. 2017;44:61–5. https://doi.org/10.1016/j.clinimag.2017.04.001. DOI: papers3://publication/doi/10.1016/j.clinimag.2017.04.001.
24. Avenarius DMF, Ording Müller L-S, Eldevik P, Owens CM, Rosendahl K. The paediatric wrist revisited--findings of bony depressions in healthy children on radiographs compared to MRI. Pediatr Radiol. 2012;42(7):791–8. https://doi.org/10.1007/s00247-012-2354-x. DOI: papers3://publication/doi/10.1007/s00247-012-2354-x.
25. Avenarius DFM, Ording Müller L-S, Rosendahl K. Erosion or normal variant? 4-year MRI follow-up of the wrists in healthy children. Pediatr

Radiol. 2016;46(3):322–30. https://doi.org/10.1007/s00247-015-3494-6. DOI: papers3://publication/doi/10.1007/s00247-015-3494-6.
26. Avenarius DFM, Ording Müller L-S, Rosendahl K. Joint fluid, bone marrow edemalike changes, and ganglion cysts in the pediatric wrist: features that may mimic pathologic abnormalities—follow-up of a healthy cohort. Am J Roentgenol. 2017;208(6):1352–7. https://doi.org/10.2214/AJR.16.17263. DOI: papers3://publication/doi/10.2214/AJR.16.17263.
27. Gornitzky AL, Lin IC, Carrigan RB. The diagnostic utility and clinical implications of wrist MRI in the pediatric population. Hand (N Y). 2018;13(2):143–9. https://doi.org/10.1177/1558944717695752. DOI: papers3://publication/doi/10.1177/1558944717695752.
28. Louis DS, Calhoun TP, Garn SM, Carroll RE, Burdi AR. Congenital bipartite scaphoid--fact or fiction? J Bone Joint Surg Am. 1976;58(8):1108–12. DOI: papers3://publication/uuid/5745EF37-E548-4819-BB4A-FC4F88C93E1C.
29. Akahane M, Ono H, Sada M, Saitoh M. Bilateral bipartite lunate: a case report. J Hand Surg Am. 2002;27(2):355–9. https://doi.org/10.1016/S0363-5023(02)80030-2. DOI: papers3://publication/doi/10.1016/S0363-5023(02)80030-2.
30. Yang ZY, Gilula LA, Jönsson K. Os centrale carpi simulating a scaphoid waist fracture. J Hand Surg Br. 1994;19(6):754–6. DOI: papers3://publication/uuid/76B80AFA-D2C8-4EB4-ABCB-2267C2DAD039.
31. Seigerman DA, Matzon JL. Common anomalous muscles encountered during upper extremity surgery. J Hand Surg Am. 2015;40(7):1473-5–quiz 1476. https://doi.org/10.1016/j.jhsa.2015.03.028. DOI: papers3://publication/doi/10.1016/j.jhsa.2015.03.028.
32. Yammine K. The prevalence of extensor digitorum brevis manus and its variants in humans: a systematic review and meta-analysis. Surg Radiol Anat. 2015;37(1):3–9. https://doi.org/10.1007/s00276-014-1312-8. DOI: papers3://publication/doi/10.1007/s00276-014-1312-8.
33. Hastings H, Simmons BP. Hand fractures in children. A statistical analysis. Clin Orthop Relat Res. 1984;(188):120–30. DOI: papers3://publication/uuid/E6FB9C8B-C69E-4E79-8AD4-33CFE19BBE7B.
34. Bohr S, Mammadli T. Early functional treatment of proximal phalanx fractures in children: a case series study. Pediatr Emerg Care. 2021;37(3):e105–9. https://doi.org/10.1097/PEC.0000000000001523. DOI: papers3://publication/doi/10.1097/PEC.0000000000001523.
35. Franz T, Jandali AR, Jung FJ, Leclère FM, von Wartburg U, Hug U. Functional-conservative treatment of extra-articular physeal fractures of the proximal phalanges in children and adolescents. Eur J Pediatr Surg. 2013;23(4):317–21. https://doi.org/10.1055/s-0033-1333636. DOI: papers3://publication/doi/10.1055/s-0033-1333636.
36. Vonlanthen J, Weber DM, Seiler M. Nonarticular base and shaft fractures of children's fingers: are follow-up X-rays needed? Retrospective study of conservatively treated proximal and middle phalangeal fractures. J Pediatr Orthop. 2019;39(9):e657–60. https://doi.org/10.1097/BPO.0000000000001335. DOI: papers3://publication/doi/10.1097/BPO.0000000000001335.
37. Puckett BN, Lui H, Vaquette C, et al. Remodeling potential of phalangeal distal condylar malunions in children. J Hand Surg Am. 2012;37(1):34–41. https://doi.org/10.1016/j.jhsa.2011.09.017. DOI: papers3://publication/doi/10.1016/j.jhsa.2011.09.017.
38. Al-Qattan MM. Fractures of the base of the proximal phalanx in children. Ann Plast Surg. 2019;82(4):399–402. https://doi.org/10.1097/SAP.0000000000001816. DOI: papers3://publication/doi/10.1097/SAP.0000000000001816.
39. Yamagiwa T, Fujioka H, Okuno H, Tomatsuri M, Tanaka J, Yoshiya S. Surgical treatment of stress fracture of the scaphoid of an adolescent gymnast. J Sports Sci Med. 2009;8(4):702–4. DOI: papers3://publication/uuid/B0D2F0FB-6378-4DA3-B0D9-A0066DFD0EB6.
40. Nakamoto JC, Saito M, Cunha AP, Luques IU. Scaphoid stress fracture in gymnastics athlete: a case report. Rev Bras Ortop. 2009;44(6):533–5. https://doi.org/10.1016/S2255-4971(15)30154-3. DOI: papers3://publication/doi/10.1016/S2255-4971(15)30154-3.
41. Nakamoto JC, Saito M, Medina G, Schor B. Scaphoid stress fracture in high-level gymnast: a case report. Case Rep Orthop. 2011;2011(6):492407. https://doi.org/10.1155/2011/492407. DOI: papers3://publication/doi/10.1155/2011/492407.
42. Kohyama S, Kanamori A, Tanaka T, Hara Y, Yamazaki M. Stress fracture of the scaphoid in an elite junior tennis player: a case report and review of the literature. J Med Case Rep. 2016;10(1):8. https://doi.org/10.1186/s13256-015-0785-3. DOI: papers3://publication/doi/10.1186/s13256-015-0785-3.
43. Lutter C, Schweizer A, Hochholzer T, Bayer T, Schöffl V. Pulling harder than the hamate tolerates: evaluation of hamate injuries in rock climbing and bouldering. Wilderness Environ Med. 2016;27(4):492–9. https://doi.org/10.1016/j.wem.2016.09.003. DOI: papers3://publication/doi/10.1016/j.wem.2016.09.003.
44. Mohamed Haflah NH, Mat Nor NF, Abdullah S, Sapuan J. Bilateral scaphoid stress fracture in a platform diver presenting with unilateral symptoms. Singap Med J. 2014;55(10):e159–61. https://doi.org/10.11622/smedj.2014146. DOI: papers3://publication/doi/10.11622/smedj.2014146.
45. Bayer T, Schöffl VR, Lenhart M, Herold T. Epiphyseal stress fractures of finger phalanges in adolescent climbing athletes: a 3.0-Tesla mag-

netic resonance imaging evaluation. Skelet Radiol. 2013;42(11):1521–5. https://doi.org/10.1007/s00256-013-1694-4. DOI: papers3://publication/doi/10.1007/s00256-013-1694-4.
46. Desaldeleer AS, Le Nen D. Bilateral fracture of the base of the middle phalanx in a climber: Literature review and a case report. Orthop Traumatol Surg Res. 2016;102(3):409–11. https://doi.org/10.1016/j.otsr.2016.01.016. DOI: papers3://publication/doi/10.1016/j.otsr.2016.01.016.
47. El-Sheikh Y, Lutter C, Schoeffl I, Schoeffl V, Flohe S. Surgical management of proximal interphalangeal joint repetitive stress epiphyseal fracture nonunion in elite sport climbers. J Hand Surg Am. 2018;43(6):572.e1–5. https://doi.org/10.1016/j.jhsa.2017.10.009. DOI: papers3://publication/doi/10.1016/j.jhsa.2017.10.009.
48. Hochholzer T, Schöffl VR. Epiphyseal fractures of the finger middle joints in young sport climbers. Wilderness Environ Med. 2005;16(3):139–42. DOI: papers3://publication/uuid/A34760BE-4C83-4554-8013-22A09D878AD5.
49. Simmons BP, McKenzie WD. Symptomatic carpal coalition. J Hand Surg Am. 1985;10(2):190–3. DOI: papers3://publication/uuid/25EED267-0C22-4F89-88CA-8F1797C69471.
50. DelaneyTJ,EswarS.Carpalcoalitions.JHandSurgAm. 1992;17(1):28–31. DOI: papers3://publication/uuid/E7393778-619D-4D66-895E-6E7333DA8A7D.
51. Defazio MV, Cousins BJ, Miversuski RA, Cardoso R. Carpal coalition: a review of current knowledge and report of a single institution's experience with asymptomatic intercarpal fusion. Hand (N Y). 2013;8(2):157–63. https://doi.org/10.1007/s11552-013-9498-5. DOI: papers3://publication/doi/10.1007/s11552-013-9498-5.
52. Pruszczynski B, Saller J, Rogers KJ, Holmes L, Ty JM. Incidence of Carpal Coalition in the Pediatric Population. J Pediatr Orthop. 2016;36(8):e106–10. https://doi.org/10.1097/BPO.0000000000000639. DOI: papers3://publication/doi/10.1097/BPO.0000000000000639.
53. van Hoorn BT, Pong T, van Leeuwen WF, Ring D. Carpal coalitions on radiographs: prevalence and association with ordering indication. J Hand Surg Am. 2017;42(5):329–34. https://doi.org/10.1016/j.jhsa.2017.02.002. DOI: papers3://publication/doi/10.1016/j.jhsa.2017.02.002.
54. Ritt MJ, Maas M, Bos KE. Minnaar type 1 symptomatic lunotriquetral coalition: a report of nine patients. J Hand Surg Am. 2001;26(2):261–70. https://doi.org/10.1053/jhsu.2001.21520. DOI: papers3://publication/doi/10.1053/jhsu.2001.21520.
55. Peters S, Colaris JW. Carpal coalition: symptomatic incomplete bony coalition of the capitate and trapezoid--case report. J Hand Surg Am. 2011;36(8):1313–5. https://doi.org/10.1016/j.jhsa.2011.05.011. DOI: papers3://publication/doi/10.1016/j.jhsa.2011.05.011.
56. Dargai F, Kassir R. A painful wrist revealing a hamate-pisiform coalition. J Hand Surg Eur Vol. 2018;43(7):780–2. https://doi.org/10.1177/1753193418773291. DOI: papers3://publication/doi/10.1177/1753193418773291.
57. Lotter O, Amr A, Stahl S, et al. Pseudarthrosis after disruption of an incomplete luno-triquetral coalition: a case report. Ger Med Sci. 2010;8:Doc34. https://doi.org/10.3205/000123. DOI: papers3://publication/doi/10.3205/000123.
58. van Schoonhoven J, Prommersberger KJ, Schmitt R. Traumatic disruption of a fibrocartilage lunate-triquetral coalition--a case report and review of the literature. Hand Surg. 2001;6(1):103–8. https://doi.org/10.1142/s0218810401000497. DOI: papers3://publication/doi/10.1142/s0218810401000497.
59. Zeplin PH, Jakubietz RG, Schmidt K. Symptomatic congenital pisiform hamate coalition. Ann Plast Surg. 2010;65(4):396–7. https://doi.org/10.1097/SAP.0b013e3181d6e30e. DOI: papers3://publication/doi/10.1097/SAP.0b013e3181d6e30e.
60. Nolte I, Mauler F, Sánchez T. Bilateral ulnar-sided wrist pain due to pisiform-hamate coalition. Case Rep Orthop. 2019;2019(4):5891972–3. https://doi.org/10.1155/2019/5891972. DOI: papers3://publication/doi/10.1155/2019/5891972.
61. Ganos DL, Imbriglia JE. Symptomatic congenital coalition of the pisiform and hamate. J Hand Surg Am. 1991;16(4):646–50. DOI: papers3://publication/uuid/9CC0FC36-B2FB-45FD-9B14-3C521615A718.
62. Berkowitz AR, Melone CP, Belsky MR. Pisiform-hamate coalition with ulnar neuropathy. J Hand Surg Am. 1992;17(4):657–62. DOI: papers3://publication/uuid/CC3AD584-91DD-4379-9F8C-3658FDAE682F.
63. Cortese J, Soubeyrand M, Razakamanantsoa L, Bellin M-F, Creze M. Hamate and pisiform coalition: a case report and introduction to the carpal C-sign on lateral radiograph. Skelet Radiol. 2017;46(5):693–9. https://doi.org/10.1007/s00256-017-2593-x. DOI: papers3://publication/doi/10.1007/s00256-017-2593-x.
64. Eustace S, Keogh C, Blake M, Ward RJ, Oder PD, Dimasi M. MR imaging of bone oedema: mechanisms and interpretation. Clin Radiol. 2001;56(1):4–12. https://doi.org/10.1053/crad.2000.0585.
65. Little JT, Klionsky NB, Chaturvedi A, Soral A. Pediatric distal forearm and wrist injury: an imaging review. Radiographics. 2014;34(2):472–90. https://doi.org/10.1148/rg.342135073.
66. Thavarajah D, Syed T, Shah Y, Wetherill M. Does scaphoid bone bruising lead to occult fracture? A prospective study of 50 patients. Injury. 2011;42(11):1303–6. https://doi.org/10.1016/j.injury.2011.02.020.
67. La Hei N, McFadyen I, Brock M, Field J. Scaphoid bone bruising--probably not the precursor of asymptomatic non-union of the scaphoid. J Hand Surg Eur

Vol. 2007;32(3):337–40. https://doi.org/10.1016/J.JHSB.2006.09.018.
68. Berkoff D, Boggess B. Carpal contusions in an elite platform diver. BMJ Case Rep. 2011;2011:bcr0120113691. https://doi.org/10.1136/bcr.01.2011.3691.
69. Lankachandra M, Wells CR, Cheng CJ, Hutchison RL. Complications of distal phalanx fractures in children. J Hand Surg Am. 2017;42(7):574.e1–6. https://doi.org/10.1016/j.jhsa.2017.03.042. DOI: papers3://publication/doi/10.1016/j.jhsa.2017.03.042.
70. Lin JS, Samora JB. Outcomes of splinting in pediatric mallet finger. J Hand Surg Am. 2018;43(11):1041.e1–9. https://doi.org/10.1016/j.jhsa.2018.03.037. DOI: papers3://publication/doi/10.1016/j.jhsa.2018.03.037.
71. Wehbé MA, Schneider LH. Mallet fractures. J Bone Joint Surg Am. 1984;66(5):658–69.
72. Reddy M, Ho CA. Comparison of percutaneous reduction and pin fixation in acute and chronic pediatric mallet fractures. J Pediatr Orthop. 2019;39(3):146–52. https://doi.org/10.1097/BPO.0000000000000896. DOI: papers3://publication/doi/10.1097/BPO.0000000000000896.
73. Guly HR. Fractures of the terminal phalanx presenting as a paronychia. Arch Emerg Med. 1993;10(4):301–5. https://doi.org/10.1136/emj.10.4.301.
74. Chen AT, Conry KT, Gilmore A, Son-Hing JP, Liu RW. Outcomes following operative treatment of adolescent mallet fractures. HSS J. 2018;14(1):83–7. https://doi.org/10.1007/s11420-017-9563-7). DOI: papers3://publication/doi/10.1007/s11420-017-9563-7.
75. Ota T, Itoh S, Matsuyama Y. Comparison of treatment results for mallet finger fractures in children between low-intensity pulsed ultrasound stimulation and Ishiguro's method. Hand (N Y). 2018;13(1):80–5. https://doi.org/10.1177/1558944717692095. DOI: papers3://publication/doi/10.1177/1558944717692095.
76. De Boeck H, Jaeken R. Treatment of chronic mallet finger deformity in children by tenodermodesis. J Pediatr Orthop. 1992;12(3):351–4. https://doi.org/10.1097/01241398-199205000-00013. DOI: papers3://publication/doi/10.1097/01241398-199205000-00013.
77. Kardestuncer T, Bae DS, Waters PM. The results of tenodermodesis for severe chronic mallet finger deformity in children. J Pediatr Orthop. 2008;28(1):81–5. https://doi.org/10.1097/BPO.0b0131815ff31e. DOI: papers3://publication/doi/10.1097/BPO.0b0131815ff31e.
78. Shin EK, Bae DS. Tenodermodesis for chronic mallet finger deformities in children. Tech Hand Upper Extrem Surg. 2007;11(4):262–5. https://doi.org/10.1097/BTH.0b013e31812f5714. DOI: papers3://publication/doi/10.1097/BTH.0b013e31812f5714.
79. Zhang L, Zuo Y-M, Huo Y-X, Wang G-Q, Zhang L. Scar overlapping suture for treating chronic tendinous mallet finger in children. J Orthop Surg Res. 2019;14(1):65. https://doi.org/10.1186/s13018-019-1106-0. DOI: papers3://publication/doi/10.1186/s13018-019-1106-0.
80. Seymour N. Juxta-epiphysial fracture of the terminal phalanx of the finger. J Bone Joint Surg Br. 1966;48(2):347–9. (In eng).
81. Al-Qattan MM. Extra-articular transverse fractures of the base of the distal phalanx (Seymour's fracture) in children and adults. J Hand Surg Br. 2001;26(3):201–6. https://doi.org/10.1054/jhsb.2000.0549.
82. Goodell PB, Bauer A. Problematic pediatric hand and wrist fractures. JBJS Rev. 2016;4(5):1. https://doi.org/10.2106/JBJS.RVW.O.00028. DOI: papers3://publication/doi/10.2106/JBJS.RVW.O.00028.
83. Kiely AL, Nolan GS, Cooper LRL. The optimal management of Seymour fractures in children and adolescents: a systematic review protocol. Syst Rev. 2020;9(1):150–7. https://doi.org/10.1186/s13643-020-01407-5. DOI: papers3://publication/doi/10.1186/s13643-020-01407-5.
84. Krusche-Mandl I, Köttstorfer J, Thalhammer G, Aldrian S, Erhart J, Platzer P. Seymour fractures: retrospective analysis and therapeutic considerations. J Hand Surg Am. 2013;38(2):258–64. https://doi.org/10.1016/j.jhsa.2012.11.015. DOI: papers3://publication/doi/10.1016/j.jhsa.2012.11.015.
85. Lin JS, Popp JE, Balch SJ. Treatment of acute Seymour fractures. J Pediatr Orthop. 2019;39(1):e23–7. https://doi.org/10.1097/BPO.0000000000001275. DOI: papers3://publication/doi/10.1097/BPO.0000000000001275.
86. Rask DMG, Wingfield J, Elrick B, et al. Seymour fractures: a retrospective review of infection rates, treatment and timing of antibiotic administration. Pediatr Emerg Care. 2020; https://doi.org/10.1097/PEC.0000000000002009. DOI: papers3://publication/doi/10.1097/PEC.0000000000002009.
87. Reyes BA, Ho CA. The high risk of infection with delayed treatment of open Seymour fractures: Salter-Harris I/II or Juxta-epiphyseal fractures of the distal phalanx with associated nailbed laceration. J Pediatr Orthop. 2017;37(4):247–53. https://doi.org/10.1097/BPO.0000000000000638. DOI: papers3://publication/doi/10.1097/BPO.0000000000000638.
88. Gibreel W, Charafeddine A, Carlsen BT, Moran SL, Bakri K. Salter-Harris fractures of the distal phalanx: treatment algorithm and surgical outcomes. Plast Reconstr Surg. 2018;142(3):720–9. https://doi.org/10.1097/PRS.0000000000004645. DOI: papers3://publication/doi/10.1097/PRS.0000000000004645.
89. Al-Qattan MM. Phalangeal neck fractures in children: classification and outcome in 66 cases. J Hand Surg Br. 2001;26(2):112–21. https://doi.org/10.1054/jhsb.2000.0506. DOI: papers3://publication/doi/10.1054/jhsb.2000.0506.
90. Dixon GL, Moon NF. Rotational supracondylar fractures of the proximal pha-

lanx in children. Clin Orthop Relat Res. 1972;83:151–6. DOI: papers3://publication/uuid/9D533F2D-1089-4678-812F-A11CF8F31CA0.
91. Park KB, Lee KJ, Kwak YH. Comparison Between Buddy Taping With a Short-Arm Splint and Operative Treatment for Phalangeal Neck Fractures in Children. J Pediatr Orthop. 2016;36(7):736–42. https://doi.org/10.1097/BPO.0000000000000521. DOI: papers3://publication/doi/10.1097/BPO.0000000000000521.
92. Matzon JL, Cornwall R. A stepwise algorithm for surgical treatment of type II displaced pediatric phalangeal neck fractures. J Hand Surg Am. 2014;39(3):467–73. https://doi.org/10.1016/j.jhsa.2013.12.014. DOI: papers3://publication/doi/10.1016/j.jhsa.2013.12.014.
93. Simmons BP, Peters TT. Subcondylar fossa reconstruction for malunion of fractures of the proximal phalanx in children. J Hand Surg Am. 1987;12(6):1079–82. DOI: papers3://publication/uuid/B4B52996-3DF1-4261-A64F-8952088FC32A.
94. Crofoot CD, Saing M, Raphael J. Intrafocal pinning for juxtaarticular phalanx fractures. Tech Hand Upper Extrem Surg. 2005;9(3):164–8. DOI: papers3://publication/uuid/D72F1859-84F1-4126-A7F2-6ABBA81040C7.
95. Karl JW, White NJ, Strauch RJ. Percutaneous reduction and fixation of displaced phalangeal neck fractures in children. J Pediatr Orthop. 2012;32(2):156–61. https://doi.org/10.1097/BPO.0b013e3182423124. DOI: papers3://publication/doi/10.1097/BPO.0b013e3182423124.
96. Radha S, Gould FJ, Harrison JW. Phalangeal neck fractures: the "Push-Pull" technique. Tech Orthop. 2014;29(1):e3–4. DOI: papers3://publication/uuid/E043BE6A-D3D3-4378-A509-B2A177477EFE.
97. Chen K-J, Huang H-K, Wang J-P. Double antegrade intramedullary pinning for proximal phalangeal neck fractures in children. J Hand Surg Eur Vol. 2019;44(3):323–5. https://doi.org/10.1177/1753193418820178. DOI: papers3://publication/doi/10.1177/1753193418820178.
98. Waters PM, Taylor BA, Kuo AY. Percutaneous reduction of incipient malunion of phalangeal neck fractures in children. J Hand Surg Am. 2004;29(4):707–11. https://doi.org/10.1016/j.jhsa.2004.03.007. DOI: papers3://publication/doi/10.1016/j.jhsa.2004.03.007.
99. Al-Qattan MM. Nonunion and avascular necrosis following phalangeal neck fractures in children. J Hand Surg Am. 2010;35(8):1269–74. https://doi.org/10.1016/j.jhsa.2010.03.038. DOI: papers3://publication/doi/10.1016/j.jhsa.2010.03.038.
100. Al-Qattan MM, Al-Zahrani K, Al-Boukai AA. The relative incidence of fractures at the base of the proximal phalanx of the fingers in children. J Hand Surg Eur Vol. 2008;33(4):465–8. https://doi.org/10.1177/1753193408090146. DOI: papers3://publication/doi/10.1177/1753193408090146.
101. Al-Qattan MM, Al-Zahrani K, Al-Boukai AA. The relative incidence of fractures at the base of the proximal phalanx of the thumb in children. J Hand Surg Eur Vol. 2009;34(1):110–4. https://doi.org/10.1177/1753193408092494. DOI: papers3://publication/doi/10.1177/1753193408092494.
102. Valencia J, Leyva F, Gomez-Bajo GJ. Pediatric hand trauma. Clin Orthop Relat Res. 2005;(432):77–86. https://doi.org/10.1097/01.blo.0000155376.88317.b7. DOI: papers3://publication/doi/10.1097/01.blo.0000155376.88317.b7.
103. Adi M, Hidalgo Diaz JJ, Salazar Botero S, et al. Results of conservative treatment of volar plate sprains of the proximal interphalangeal joint with and without avulsion fracture. Hand Surg Rehabil. 2017;36(1):44–7. https://doi.org/10.1016/j.hansur.2016.09.015. DOI: papers3://publication/doi/10.1016/j.hansur.2016.09.015.
104. Giddins GEB. The non-operative management of hand fractures. J Hand Surg Eur Vol. 2015;40(1):33–41. https://doi.org/10.1177/1753193414548170. DOI: papers3://publication/doi/10.1177/1753193414548170.
105. Paschos NK, Abuhemoud K, Gantsos A, Mitsionis GI, Georgoulis AD. Management of proximal interphalangeal joint hyperextension injuries: a randomized controlled trial. J Hand Surg Am. 2014;39(3):449–54. https://doi.org/10.1016/j.jhsa.2013.11.038. DOI: papers3://publication/doi/10.1016/j.jhsa.2013.11.038.
106. Roh YH, Koh Y-D, Go JY, Noh JH, Gong HS, Baek GH. Factors influencing functional outcome of proximal interphalangeal joint collateral ligament injury when treated with buddy strapping and exercise. J Hand Ther. 2018;31(3):295–300. https://doi.org/10.1016/j.jht.2017.02.010. DOI: papers3://publication/doi/10.1016/j.jht.2017.02.010.
107. Sawant N, Kulikov Y, Giddins GEB. Outcome following conservative treatment of metacarpophalangeal collateral ligament avulsion fractures of the finger. J Hand Surg Eur Vol. 2007;32(1):102–4. https://doi.org/10.1016/j.jhsb.2006.06.010. DOI: papers3://publication/doi/10.1016/j.jhsb.2006.06.010.
108. Dinowitz M, Trumble T, Hanel D, Vedder NB, Gilbert M. Failure of cast immobilization for thumb ulnar collateral ligament avulsion fractures. J Hand Surg Am. 1997;22(6):1057–63. https://doi.org/10.1016/S0363-5023(97)80049-4. DOI: papers3://publication/doi/10.1016/S0363-5023(97)80049-4.
109. Kuz JE, Husband JB, Tokar N, McPherson SA. Outcome of avulsion fractures of the ulnar base of the proximal phalanx of the thumb treated nonsurgically. J Hand Surg Am. 1999;24(2):275–82. https://doi.org/10.1053/jhsu.1999.0275. DOI: papers3://publication/doi/10.1053/jhsu.1999.0275.
110. Sorene ED, Goodwin DR. Non-operative treatment of displaced avulsion fractures of the ulnar base of the proximal phalanx of the thumb. Scand J Plast Reconstr Surg Hand Surg.

2003;37(4):225–7. DOI: papers3://publication/uuid/6E9496B6-B3B2-4167-A406-560F5908E7F4.
111. Jørgsholm P, Thomsen N, Besjakov J, Abrahamsson S, Björkman A. MRI shows a high incidence of carpal fractures in children with posttraumatic radial-sided wrist tenderness. Acta Orthop. 2016;87(5):533–7. https://doi.org/10.1080/17453674.2016.1210940. DOI: papers3://publication/doi/10.1080/17453674.2016.1210940.
112. Lempesis V, Rosengren BE, Landin L, Tiderius CJ, Karlsson MK. Hand fracture epidemiology and etiology in children-time trends in Malmö, Sweden, during six decades. J Orthop Surg Res. 2019;14(1):213–0. https://doi.org/10.1186/s13018-019-1248-0. DOI: papers3://publication/doi/10.1186/s13018-019-1248-0.
113. Wood AM, Robertson GA, Rennie L, Caesar BC, Court-Brown CM. The epidemiology of sports-related fractures in adolescents. Injury. 2010;41(8):834–8. https://doi.org/10.1016/j.injury.2010.04.008. DOI: papers3://publication/doi/10.1016/j.injury.2010.04.008.
114. Toh S, Miura H, Arai K, Yasumura M, Wada M, Tsubo K. Scaphoid fractures in children: problems and treatment. J Pediatr Orthop. 2003;23(2):216–21. DOI: papers3://publication/uuid/800CABA8-C7A4-4337-934C-27BE3133FC57.
115. Gholson JJ, Bae DS, Zurakowski D, Waters PM. Scaphoid fractures in children and adolescents: contemporary injury patterns and factors influencing time to union. J Bone Joint Surg Am. 2011;93(13):1210–9. https://doi.org/10.2106/JBJS.J.01729. DOI: papers3://publication/doi/10.2106/JBJS.J.01729.
116. Greene MH, Hadied AM, LaMont RL. Scaphoid fractures in children. J Hand Surg Am. 1984;9(4):536–41. https://doi.org/10.1016/S0363--5023(84)80106-9. DOI: papers3://publication/doi/10.1016/S0363-5023(84)80106-9.
117. Evenski AJ, Adamczyk MJ, Steiner RP, Morscher MA, Riley PM. Clinically suspected scaphoid fractures in children. J Pediatr Orthop. 2009;29(4):352–5. https://doi.org/10.1097/BPO.0b013e3181a5a667. DOI: papers3://publication/doi/10.1097/BPO.0b013e3181a5a667.
118. Ahmed I, Ashton F, Tay WK, Porter D. The pediatric fracture of the scaphoid in patients aged 13 years and under: an epidemiological study. J Pediatr Orthop. 2014;34(2):150–4. https://doi.org/10.1097/BPO.0000000000000102. DOI: papers3://publication/doi/10.1097/BPO.0000000000000102.
119. Elhassan BT, Shin AY. Scaphoid fracture in children. Hand Clin. 2006;22(1):31–41. (In eng). https://doi.org/10.1016/j.hcl.2005.10.004.
120. Carlson EJ, Save AV, Slade JF, Dodds SD. Low-intensity pulsed ultrasound treatment for scaphoid fracture nonunions in adolescents. J Wrist Surg. 2015;4(2):115–20. https://doi.org/10.1055/s--0035-1549276. DOI: papers3://publication/doi/10.1055/s-0035-1549276.
121. Bae DS, Gholson JJ, Zurakowski D, Waters PM. Functional outcomes after treatment of scaphoid fractures in children and adolescents. J Pediatr Orthop. 2016;36(1):13–8. https://doi.org/10.1097/BPO.0000000000000406. DOI: papers3://publication/doi/10.1097/BPO.0000000000000406.
122. Nguyen JC, Nguyen MK, Arkader A, et al. Age-dependent changes in pediatric scaphoid fracture pattern on radiographs. Skelet Radiol. 2020;18(4):462–8. https://doi.org/10.1007/s00256-020-03522-9. DOI: papers3://publication/doi/10.1007/s00256-020-03522-9.
123. Huckstadt T, Klitscher D, Weltzien A, Müller LP, Rommens PM, Schier F. Pediatric fractures of the carpal scaphoid: a retrospective clinical and radiological study. J Pediatr Orthop. 2007;27(4):447–50. https://doi.org/10.1097/01.bpb.0000271309.05924.80. DOI: papers3://publication/doi/10.1097/01.bpb.0000271309.05924.80.
124. Zlotolow DA, Kozin SH. Hand and wrist injuries in the pediatric athlete. Clin Sports Med. 2020;39(2):457–79. https://doi.org/10.1016/j.csm.2020.01.001. DOI: papers3://publication/doi/10.1016/j.csm.2020.01.001.
125. Kohring JM, Curtiss HM, Tyser AR. A scaphoid stress fracture in a female collegiate-level shot-putter and review of the literature. Case Rep Orthop. 2016;2016(6):8098657. https://doi.org/10.1155/2016/8098657. DOI: papers3://publication/doi/10.1155/2016/8098657.
126. Unay K, Gokcen B, Ozkan K, Poyanli O, Eceviz E. Examination tests predictive of bone injury in patients with clinically suspected occult scaphoid fracture. Injury. 2009;40(12):1265–8. (In eng). https://doi.org/10.1016/j.injury.2009.01.140.
127. Suh N, Grewal R. Controversies and best practices for acute scaphoid fracture management. J Hand Surg Eur Vol. 2018;43(1):4–12. (In eng). https://doi.org/10.1177/1753193417735973.
128. Phillips TG, Reibach AM, Slomiany WP. Diagnosis and management of scaphoid fractures. Am Fam Physician. 2004;70(5):879–84. (In eng)
129. Mallee WH, Henny EP, van Dijk CN, Kamminga SP, van Enst WA, Kloen P. Clinical diagnostic evaluation for scaphoid fractures: a systematic review and meta-analysis. J Hand Surg Am. 2014;39(9):1683–1691.e2. (In eng). https://doi.org/10.1016/j.jhsa.2014.06.004.
130. Duckworth AD, Buijze GA, Moran M, et al. Predictors of fracture following suspected injury to the scaphoid. J Bone Joint Surg Br. 2012;94(7):961–8. (In eng). https://doi.org/10.1302/0301-620X.94B7.28704.
131. Toth F, Sebestyen A, Balint L, et al. Positioning of the wrist for scaphoid radiography. Eur J Radiol. 2007;64(1):126–32. https://doi.org/10.1016/j.ejrad.2007.02.008. DOI: papers3://publication/doi/10.1016/j.ejrad.2007.02.008.
132. Cheung GC, Lever CJ, Morris AD. X-ray diagnosis of acute scaphoid fractures. J Hand Surg Br. 2006;31(1):104–9. https://doi.org/10.1016/j.

jhsb.2005.09.001. DOI: papers3://publication/doi/10.1016/j.jhsb.2005.09.001.
133. Jenkins PJ, Slade K, Huntley JS, Robinson CM. A comparative analysis of the accuracy, diagnostic uncertainty and cost of imaging modalities in suspected scaphoid fractures. Injury. 2008;39(7):768–74. https://doi.org/10.1016/j.injury.2008.01.003. DOI: papers3://publication/doi/10.1016/j.injury.2008.01.003.
134. Amrami KK, Frick MA, Matsumoto JM. Imaging for acute and chronic scaphoid FRACTURES. Hand Clin. 2019;35(3):241–57. https://doi.org/10.1016/j.hcl.2019.03.001. DOI: papers3://publication/doi/10.1016/j.hcl.2019.03.001.
135. Lee SK, Desai H, Silver B, Dhaliwal G, Paksima N. Comparison of radiographic stress views for scapholunate dynamic instability in a cadaver model. J Hand Surg Am. 2011;36(7):1149–57. (In eng). https://doi.org/10.1016/j.jhsa.2011.05.009.
136. Mallee W, Doornberg JN, Ring D, van Dijk CN, Maas M, Goslings JC. Comparison of CT and MRI for diagnosis of suspected scaphoid fractures. J Bone Joint Surg Am. 2011;93(1):20–8. https://doi.org/10.2106/JBJS.I.01523. DOI: papers3://publication/doi/10.2106/JBJS.I.01523.
137. Mallee WH, Wang J, Poolman RW, et al. Computed tomography versus magnetic resonance imaging versus bone scintigraphy for clinically suspected scaphoid fractures in patients with negative plain radiographs. Cochrane Database Syst Rev. 2015;90(6):CD010023. https://doi.org/10.1002/14651858.CD010023.pub2. DOI: papers3://publication/doi/10.1002/14651858.CD010023.pub2.
138. Yin Z-G, Zhang J-B, Kan S-L, Wang X-G. Diagnosing suspected scaphoid fractures: a systematic review and meta-analysis. Clin Orthop Relat Res. 2009;468(3):723–34. https://doi.org/10.1007/s11999-009-1081-6. DOI: papers3://publication/doi/10.1007/s11999-009-1081-6.
139. Clementson M, Björkman A, Thomsen NOB. Acute scaphoid fractures: guidelines for diagnosis and treatment. EFORT Open Rev. 2020;5(2):96–103. https://doi.org/10.1302/2058-5241.5.190025. DOI: papers3://publication/doi/10.1302/2058-5241.5.190025.
140. Jørgsholm P, Thomsen NOB, Besjakov J, Abrahamsson S-O, Björkman A. The benefit of magnetic resonance imaging for patients with posttraumatic radial wrist tenderness. J Hand Surg Am. 2013;38(1):29–33. https://doi.org/10.1016/j.jhsa.2012.09.034. DOI: papers3://publication/doi/10.1016/j.jhsa.2012.09.034.
141. Ring D, Lozano-Calderon S. Imaging for suspected scaphoid fracture. J Hand Surg Am. 2008;33(6):954–7. https://doi.org/10.1016/j.jhsa.2008.04.016. DOI: papers3://publication/doi/10.1016/j.jhsa.2008.04.016.
142. Shaterian A, Santos PJF, Lee CJ, Evans GRD, Leis A. Management modalities and outcomes following acute scaphoid fractures in children: a quantitative review and meta-analysis. Hand (N Y). 2019;14(3):305–10. https://doi.org/10.1177/1558944717735948. DOI: papers3://publication/doi/10.1177/1558944717735948.
143. Grewal R, Lutz K, MacDermid JC, Suh N. Proximal pole scaphoid fractures: a computed tomographic assessment of outcomes. J Hand Surg Am. 2016;41(1):54–8. (In eng). https://doi.org/10.1016/j.jhsa.2015.10.013.
144. Chloros GD, Themistocleous GS, Wiesler ER, Benetos IS, Efstathopoulos DG, Soucacos PN. Pediatric scaphoid nonunion. J Hand Surg Am. 2007;32(2):172–6. https://doi.org/10.1016/j.jhsa.2006.11.007. DOI: papers3://publication/doi/10.1016/j.jhsa.2006.11.007.
145. Maxted MJ, Owen R. Two cases of non-union of carpal scaphoid fractures in children. Injury. 1982;13(5):441–3. DOI: papers3://publication/uuid/9537E3CE-085C-4636-8ABD-17B70BC8E101.
146. Onuba O, Ireland J. Two cases of non-union of fractures of the scaphoid in children. Injury. 1983;15(2):109–12. DOI: papers3://publication/uuid/43083762-5CB2-4EF3-8196-6E20F33C6D98.
147. Pick RY, Segal D. Carpal scaphoid fracture and non-union in an eight-year-old child. Report of a case. J Bone Joint Surg Am. 1983;65(8):1188–9. DOI: papers3://publication/uuid/95229277-832F-4309-95F0-BEE9560DD279.
148. Mintzer CM, Waters PM. Surgical treatment of pediatric scaphoid fracture nonunions. J Pediatr Orthop. 1999;19(2):236–9. DOI: papers3://publication/uuid/DC7873E4-E425-4A9C-8B1A-49DD4470DE8C.
149. Oestreich K, Jacomel TUY, Hassan S, Horwitz MD, Lindau TR. Pediatric scaphoid nonunions: a case series, review of the literature, and evidence-based guidelines. J Wrist Surg. 2020;9(1):2–12. https://doi.org/10.1055/s-0039-3401035. DOI: papers3://publication/doi/10.1055/s-0039-3401035.
150. Eckert K, Tröbs RB, Schweiger B, Liedgens P, Radeloff E, Ackermann O. Diagnostically approach to pediatric carpal fractures: a retrospective analysis. Z Orthop Unfall. 2016;154(1):43–9. https://doi.org/10.1055/s-0035-1558078. DOI: papers3://publication/doi/10.1055/s-0035-1558078.
151. Greene WB, Anderson WJ. Simultaneous Fracture of the Scaphoid and Radius in a Child. J Pediatr Orthop. 1982;2(2):191–4. DOI: papers3://publication/uuid/9D744C7D-7F02-4604-B2A2-3F6CBAE89C2C.
152. Foley K, Patel S. Fractures of the scaphoid, capitate and triquetrum in a child: a case report. J Orthop Surg (Hong Kong). 2012;20(1):103–4. https://doi.org/10.1177/230949901202000121. DOI: papers3://publication/doi/10.1177/230949901202000121.
153. Anderson WJ. Simultaneous fracture of the scaphoid and capitate in a child. J Hand Surg Am. 1987;12(2):271–3. DOI: papers3://publication/uuid/A641D1F6-7CCB-45FE-91DE-8972C56BFB72.

154. Sawant M, Miller J. Scaphocapitate syndrome in an adolescent. J Hand Surg Am. 2000;25(6):1096–9. https://doi.org/10.1053/jhsu.2000.18494. DOI: papers3://publication/doi/10.1053/jhsu.2000.18494.
155. Mancini F, De Maio F, Ippolito E. Pisiform bone fracture-dislocation and distal radius physeal fracture in two children. J Pediatr Orthop B. 2005;14(4):303–6. DOI: papers3://publication/uuid/3B5DA74A-32AB-41A3-B3F8-E88A33C056C7.
156. Sallam AA, Briffa N, Mahmoud SS, Imam MA. Normal wrist development in children and adolescents: a geometrical observational analysis based on plain radiographs. J Pediatr Orthop. 2020;40(9):e860–72. https://doi.org/10.1097/BPO.0000000000001584. DOI: papers3://publication/doi/10.1097/BPO.0000000000001584.
157. Joyce EA, Farrell T, McMorrow J, Mulholland D, Browne KM, Snow A. Are adult carpal angle measurements applicable to the pediatric population in the trauma setting? Skelet Radiol. 2018;47(8):1151–6. https://doi.org/10.1007/s00256-018-2905-9. DOI: papers3://publication/doi/10.1007/s00256-018-2905-9.
158. Massicot R, Uzel AP, Céolin JL, Brouard P. Dorsal trans-scaphoid perilunate dislocation in a 9-year-old child. Eur J Pediatr Surg. 2005;15(2):140–3. (In eng). https://doi.org/10.1055/s-2004-821221.
159. Ji JH, Shafi M, Moon CY, Park SE. Trans-scaphoid perilunate dislocation with fractured carpal bones in a child. Chir Main. 2010;29(1):32–5. https://doi.org/10.1016/j.main.2009.10.004. DOI: papers3://publication/doi/10.1016/j.main.2009.10.004.
160. Khan SA, Van Velze M, Pearse A. A rare case of an acute lunate dislocation in a child. BMJ Case Rep. 2017;2017:bcr2017222180. (In eng). https://doi.org/10.1136/bcr-2017-222180.
161. Aad G, Abbott B, Abdallah J, et al. Combined Measurement of the Higgs Boson Mass in pp Collisions at sqrt[s]=7 and 8 TeV with the ATLAS and CMS Experiments. Phys Rev Lett. 2015;114(19):191804. https://doi.org/10.1103/PhysRevLett.114.191803.
162. Terry CL, Waters PM. Triangular fibrocartilage injuries in pediatric and adolescent patients. J Hand Surg Am. 1998;23(4):626–34. https://doi.org/10.1016/S0363-5023(98)80048-8. DOI: papers3://publication/doi/10.1016/S0363-5023(98)80048-8.
163. Wu M, Miller PE, Waters PM, Bae DS. Early results of surgical treatment of triangular fibrocartilage complex tears in children and adolescents. J Hand Surg Am. 2020;45(5):449.e1–9. https://doi.org/10.1016/j.jhsa.2019.06.019. DOI: papers3://publication/doi/10.1016/j.jhsa.2019.06.019.
164. Trehan SK, Schimizzi G, Shen TS, Wall LB, Goldfarb CA. Arthroscopic treatment of triangular fibrocartilage complex injuries in paediatric and adolescent patients. J Hand Surg Eur Vol. 2019;44(6):582–6. https://doi.org/10.1177/1753193418825070. DOI: papers3://publication/doi/10.1177/1753193418825070.
165. Waters PM. Problematic Pediatric Wrist and Hand Injuries. J Pediatr Orthop. 2010;30(2 Supplement):S90–5. DOI: papers3://publication/uuid/FAC45BB0-7816-46EA-A5EE-F4BE9C7882C4.
166. Tay SC, Tomita K, Berger RA. The "ulnar fovea sign" for defining ulnar wrist pain: an analysis of sensitivity and specificity. J Hand Surg Am. 2007;32(4):438–44. https://doi.org/10.1016/j.jhsa.2007.01.022. DOI: papers3://publication/doi/10.1016/j.jhsa.2007.01.022.
167. Lester B, Halbrecht J, Levy IM, Gaudinez R. "Press test" for office diagnosis of triangular fibrocartilage complex tears of the wrist. Ann Plast Surg. 1995;35(1):41–5. (In eng). https://doi.org/10.1097/00000637-199507000-00009.
168. Goldfarb CA, Strauss NL, Wall LB, Calfee RP. Defining ulnar variance in the adolescent wrist: measurement technique and interobserver reliability. J Hand Surg Am. 2011;36(2):272–7. https://doi.org/10.1016/j.jhsa.2010.11.008. DOI: papers3://publication/doi/10.1016/j.jhsa.2010.11.008.
169. Tomaino MM. The importance of the pronated grip x-ray view in evaluating ulnar variance. J Hand Surg Am. 2000;25(2):352–7. https://doi.org/10.1053/jhsu.2000.jhsu25a0352. DOI: papers3://publication/doi/10.1053/jhsu.2000.jhsu25a0352.
170. Bendre HH, Oflazoglu K, van Leeuwen WF, Rakhorst H, Ring D, Chen NC. The prevalence of triangular fibrocartilage complex signal abnormalities on magnetic resonance imaging relative to clinical suspicion of pathology. J Hand Surg Am. 2018;43(9):819–826.e1. https://doi.org/10.1016/j.jhsa.2018.06.117.
171. Park MJ, Jagadish A, Yao J. The rate of triangular fibrocartilage injuries requiring surgical intervention. Orthopedics. 2010;33(11):806. https://doi.org/10.3928/01477447-20100924-03.
172. Lee JK, Hwang J-Y, Lee SY, Kwon BC. What is the natural history of the triangular fibrocartilage complex tear without distal radioulnar joint instability? Clin Orthop Relat Res. 2019;477(2):442–9. https://doi.org/10.1097/CORR.0000000000000533. DOI: papers3://publication/doi/10.1097/CORR.0000000000000533.

The Athletic Trainer's Perspective of Three Common Baseball Injuries

19

George C. Poulis, Michael B. Frostad, and Jeffrey A. Stevenson

The goal of this book has been to cover hand and wrist injuries specific to the sport of baseball. Be it a pitcher, a catcher, an infielder, or an outfielder, along with batting, the hand and wrist are subjected to both acute and chronic trauma. The previous chapters, written by hand surgeons, have covered the injuries from the standpoint of the clinician. Initial history, diagnosis, and treatment, nonsurgical or surgical, have been covered. The goals of the treatment of these injuries, which if missed or under-treated can result in extended time on the Injured List (IL), has been expedient diagnosis and treatment with a plan for early return to play with minimal risk. Crucial to the achievement of this goal is the interaction of the athletic trainer with the physician. The surgeon's first contact with the injured player sets in motion the development of a plan to return the ballplayer to the field safely and productive. Be it surgical or nonsurgical, the athletic trainer's role is key in implementing this algorithm. Some of the chapters have touched on post-injury care, but the emphasis of this chapter is to concentrate on three of the most important injuries to the hand and wrist: hook of the hamate fractures, nail plate and blisters, along with thumb metacarpal phalangeal ulnar collateral ligament injuries. One can read a textbook, but there is no substitute for the experience and guidance of the athletic trainer.

The sport of baseball is very unique. Games are played on a daily basis; so, recovery is the key to getting player through the long season. As you will read in this book, there are many injuries that are specific to the sport of baseball that can easily be related to other sports. All of the injuries listed in this chapter can be of acute or chronic nature, but many of them are acute on chronic. The athletic trainer is faced with many challenges throughout any given season. It has been noticed, overtime, that a common denominator or trait of a quality athletic trainer is the art of forward thinking when it comes to injury management. The athletic trainer is responsible for many athletes and needs to possess the ability to multitask in order to perform the key duties required of him or her. Preventative maintenance and injury prevention are keys to forward thinking. The following injuries commonly occur in the sport of baseball. As previously mentioned, the views discussed in the following chapter are from athletic trainers that are on the front lines dealing with these injuries, on a daily basis in Major League Baseball.

Thumb Ulnar Collateral Ligament (UCL) Tear

The thumb UCL is located at the base of the interphalangeal joint (IP) joint. This injury can cause a tear of the ligament as well as an avulsion

G. C. Poulis (✉) · M. B. Frostad · J. A. Stevenson
Atlanta Braves Baseball Club, Atlanta, GA, USA
e-mail: george.poulis@braves.com; mike.frostad@braves.com; jeff.stevenson@braves.com

G. M. Lourie (ed.), *Hand and Wrist Injuries in Baseball*,
https://doi.org/10.1007/978-3-030-81659-9_19

fracture. Usually, this can be diagnosed by a good clinical exam including history and mechanism of the injury along with and follow-up X-rays and possibly MRI.

Clinical Exam

During examination it is important to take a good history and put together all of the subjective and objective findings. Advanced imaging also is very helpful to put together with the clinical exam. It usually does not take long to arrive at the source of this injury. During the palpation stage of the exam, often there is extreme discomfort and point tenderness noted over the medial aspect of the IP joint along with a slight increase in temperature due to inflammation. Ecchymosis can be visually noted as well but not always present. During the range of motion portion of the exam, abduction of the thumb passively is far more increased when compared to the unaffected side. Pain is noted during this exam, especially at the end range of abduction. Abduction of the thumb actively is decreased as well and usually causes increased discomfort. The manual muscle testing portion of the exam is often limited to abduction, adduction, flexion, and extension of the IP joint. The player is usually very uncomfortable during the clinical exam.

Mechanism

The mechanism of this injury is a radial load, (hyper abduction), of the thumb. This injury, very often, happens, but is not limited to the player sliding headfirst into a base and hyper abducts his thumb as he reaches the base. Other mechanisms can be diving for a ball and jamming the glove hand thumb into the ground and also tagging a runner out with the glove hand all causing a radial load to the IP joint. Usually, it is met with immediate pain and instability.

In one particular case, a player was tagging up from first base and slid headfirst as he advanced and hyper abducted his thumb. He was immediately taken out of the game. Exam revealed and an MRI confirmed an avulsion fracture of the UCL. He was scheduled for surgery and returned to play in 6–8 weeks post internal brace surgery.

Nonsurgical Rehabilitation Approach

In some instances, there is an injury to the thumb which results in a partial tear or sprain to the UCL. It can be considered to play with a torn UCL is the IP joint is stable. In nonoperative cases, it is very important for the athletic trainer to manage the injury daily followed by tape support. Each injury we are faced with has its own challenges. We have used the term "throw the kitchen sink at it," meaning, use every modality and hands-on treatment technique you have in order to keep this player on the field. Ultimately, most of these injuries end up needing to be repaired.

Surgical Rehabilitation Approach

Internal brace seems to be very popular and the chosen surgical option among athletes to repair the UCL versus traditional suture anchor repair. General time frames for return to play after receiving internal bracing technique is approximately 6–8 weeks. The general time frame for return to play following the traditional suture anchor repair is approximately 8–12 weeks. Return to play times vary depending upon the rehabilitation process. It is integral to follow the guidance and advice of the surgeon's rehabilitation protocol which guide the rehabilitation through the protected phases, semi-protected phases, and unprotected phases. Having a plan and simplifying seems to be the most efficient way to manage the rehabilitation process. Simplifying a treatment program is to adhere to four main rehabilitation principles. They are the following: (1) decrease pain, (2) decrease swelling, (3) increase range of motion, and (4) increase strength. Keeping that as our framework for the rehabilitation program will help mainstream the program and keep it interesting as well so it does not become boring or stagnant. Total body conditioning is very important to perform in order to prepare the body for the demands of competition.

Tape Support/Bracing

For both surgical and nonsurgical scenarios, a thumb spica tape support and splinting for protection is very helpful. Either way, tape support and hand protection, especially while running the bases, is a good idea.

Return-to-Play Criteria

Advancement to this phase is highly dependent on the players' strength and range of motion returning to normal. The player needs to be prepared to accept and be exposed to the stresses that will be demanded of them during live competition. All facets of the player's game are required to be performed without any reservations or apprehension. The player must perform all of these activities with confidence and report back to the medical staff the next day with no soreness or return of symptoms. A sports-specific testing protocols should be performed checking all of the boxes based on the position being played. This includes but is not limited to sliding, running, catching, throwing, and diving. After this has been achieved, a simulated game should be setup to put the player in live situations to simulate what they are about to experience once they return to full activity, always keeping in mind that this player will need to. If all the live activities are performed without any issues, then the player can be cleared for all activity.

Overall, the athletic trainer's role takes on a lot of responsibility. Constant conversation with the players during the rehabilitation and treatment process is key in order to mentally keep their minds positive and moving forward daily. This includes incorporating the entire medical staff. The medical staff includes but is not limited to the physical therapists, strength coaches, mental coaches, and nutritionist. Their positional coach also plays a role. The UCL tear is an injury that is something that all of us will experience at one time or another. Bottomline, the internal brace seems to be the most popular surgical technique right now with very little risk of failure when compared to the traditional suture repair.

Hook of Hamate Injury

Hook of hamate fractures are much more common injuries in baseball than in the general population. The majority of these injuries occur in hitters, and almost always involve the bottom hand of the batter. Many baseball players hold the bat with their bottom hand just off the end of the bat. This causes trauma to the hypothenar eminence and the underlying hook of the hamate with the knob of the bat.

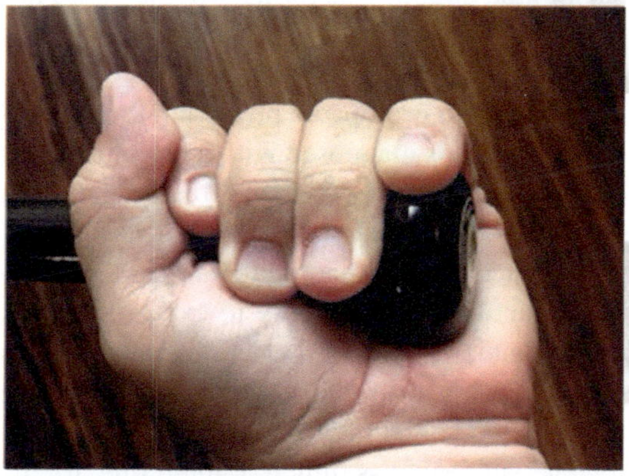

Bat knob over hamate

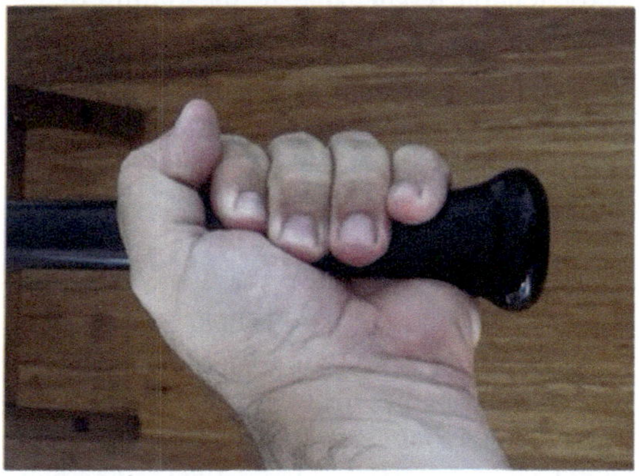

Hand off end of bat

These injuries can occur on one swing when the player feels immediate discomfort over the hook of the hamate, sometimes occurring on a check swing. The player may report having some soreness in that area of their hand prior to the final swing that causes them to shut down their hitting. In one case, I had a player playing in triple A baseball that was continuing to play with some mild hand soreness. We were treating it symptomatically, but he was having a great year and did not want to think about not playing at that time. This player had never had the opportunity to play in Major League Baseball. He thought with the year he was having that he had a real chance to get called up for the first time in his career. It was early August and just a few weeks from teams being able to expand their rosters. After one at bat in a game, this player made the last out of the inning and came back to the dugout wondering why he could not fully flex his fourth and fifth digits. He was removed from the game and evaluated by our hand and wrist orthopedic physician the following day. He was diagnosed with a probable hook of hamate fracture in which the fractured hamate had severed the flexor tendon like a shard of glass. After getting imaging to confirm the diagnosis, he underwent surgery to excise the hook of the hamate with flexor tendon repair. This player made a full recovery in time for spring training the following year. The recovery following surgery was much longer due to the flexor tendon repair. Due to the timing of the injury toward the end of the season, it would not have made a difference for that season. The player was trying to minimize the knowledge of this injury due to his good season, and chance for an MLB call up. However, this case caused me to suspect hamate fractures sooner, and get imaging to rule them out if there was any doubt to prevent a longer recovery time.

The player most often will have discomfort with palpation directly over the hook of the hamate on the palmar side of the hand. This can be done with the hand of the patient facing palm up: placing the interphalangeal joint of the clinician's palpating thumb over the pisiform directed distally toward the base of the index finger. In that position, the hook of the hamate is directly below the palpating thumb. I have had a few cases in which the player did not have discomfort over the hook of the hamate, but had tenderness palpating over the dorsum of the hamate. In most cases if a hook of hamate fracture is suspected, typically we will get a CT scan for diagnosis due to the difficulty of seeing the fracture on X-rays. The pull test is done applying resistance to the fourth and fifth fingers with them in flexion and ulnar deviation. If this causes discomfort, it is positive for a hamate fracture as those tendons pull on the fractured hook of hamate.

The postoperative rehab for the hook of hamate excision is relatively straight forward. The surgery involves removing the fractured piece of the hamate. Due to the fact that there is no tissue being repaired, the rehab consists of wound management, range of motion, strengthening, and return to baseball activities.

The entire rehab process typically requires 6–8 weeks to make a full recovery. Some players return closer to 6 weeks, but they may still have some grip-related complaints for a couple of more weeks. This tends to be especially true with a right-handed hitting catcher, who has had the hamate surgery done on their left hand. The fact that their hand involved in the surgery is the hand they need to catch every pitch. The grip strength stamina may be affected, and not be what they require to catch in a game. In addition, they have the repetitive catching of pitches that can make the hand sore. Most other position players do not deal with these issues because they are catching less baseballs with high velocity, and the glove serves to protect the hand as well.

The wound management phase is allowing the incision to heal without the risk of infection. The wrist will be in a postoperative splint to allow this to occur. When the splint is able to be removed, then we would begin to incorporate some modalities like Hivamat and laser to help to decrease inflammation and promote healing.

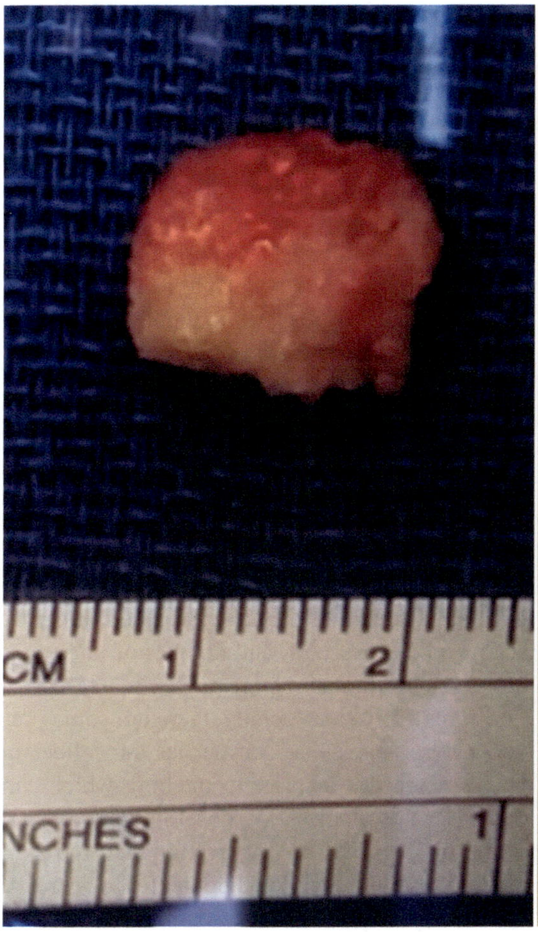

Hamate excised

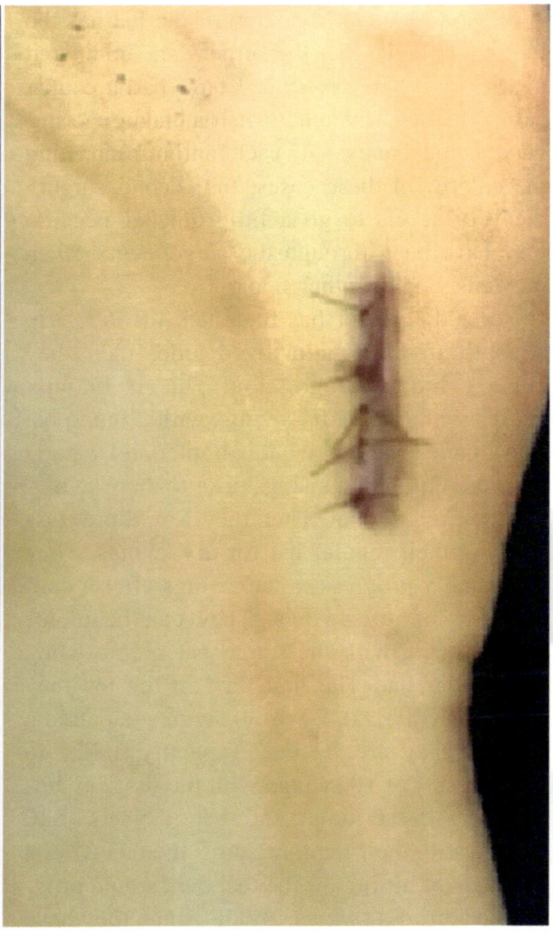

Hamate incision

The next phase is to begin range-of-motion exercises for the fingers, hand, and wrist. This is done to tolerance with most players doing well with this. There are some players who tend to have a little nervy type issues with getting comfortable range of motion in the fourth and fifth digits.

After they have regained range of motion, then they progress to the strengthening phase. This is done with gripping exercises and rice bucket exercises for the wrist and hand. Our goal is for them to have about 80–85% grip strength of their opposite hand to be able to progress to hitting activities. In most players, the surgery hand is going to be their glove hand, if they are same-handed thrower and hitter. In those cases, they can begin throwing earlier with someone catching for them. This allows them to work on getting their throwing arm prepared to return to play sooner. They can begin to catch for themselves while throwing to their tolerance once they have regained some strength. Their baseball glove provides them some protection in this process, and it continues to improve with grip strength. There are some players that are opposite-handed throwers and hitters. In these cases, their throwing arm is the surgically involved hand. They may need to delay throwing a little longer, but in these cases can begin defensive glove work sooner. There are cases with switch hitters having hamate surgery. They have been able to progress their hitting with the surgery hand as the top hand side ahead of the hitting with it on the bottom hand. This is due to when it is the bottom hand, the knob of the bat has the fulcrum directly over the surgery site compared to when it is the top hand. I have had a couple cases in which a switch hitter has undergone surgery on both hands, with each bottom hand being the culprit. In these cases, the second surgery recovery seems to go a little quicker because they have been through the surgery and rehab previously on the other side.

After the player has regained 80–85% grip strength to their uninvolved side, then they begin a hitting progression. This is initially started with taking dry swings with a fungo bat if available. The fungo bat is lighter and is good for these initial first swings prior to them swinging their regular bat. Then they would progress to using their regular bat for dry swings. They can usually progress to tee swings after a couple days of dry swings. They can begin tee swings again with the fungo bat before using the regular bat. The first day on the tee they would usually take 20 to 30 swings depending on how they are feeling. Typically, I like to work in sets of 10 swings with the first day hitting 10 with the fungo, and then two sets of 10 swings with their regular bat off the tee. After a few days of hitting off the tee, they would progress to soft toss swings. By this time, they have reached about 40 swings, initially 20 tee swings followed by 20 soft toss swings. Once they feel comfortable with swinging off the tee and soft toss, they are ready to progress to coach pitched batting practice. The same type of progression is usually done with the first day hitting one round of batting practice. Then they would progress to taking full batting practice. The final steps in preparing to return to playing in games is hitting off some increased game like velocity. This can be done hitting off a pitching machine if that is available or hitting off a pitcher in a live batting practice situation. Both of these will better prepare the player for return to game play. The other thing about the live hitting is the player is more likely to have to perform a check swing. Sometimes a check swing is how the injury initially occurred, so it is nice to check that box prior to them doing it for the first time in a game.

Blister Prevention and Treatment

A blister on the finger, or fingers, of a pitcher's hand can be a debilitating injury that often requires time off from throwing, disrupting a pitcher's normal routine and ability to pitch. Those pitchers that are "heavy sweaters" suffering from hyperhidrosis, as well as those that play in a more humid climate, tend to be more susceptible to developing a blister on the distal aspect of the second or third digit, sometimes both. There are some preventive measures that can be taken to try to decrease the susceptibility of blister formation and minimize the amount of time lost through reactive treatments should a blister arise.

Prevention

Unfortunately, there are external factors that are out of the control of a pitcher: weather/humidity, seams on the baseball, and number of pitches in any given appearance (more pitches increase friction force). But, anecdotally, there are some preventive measures that can be put into effect in between outings or prior to pitching which can decrease the chances of developing a blister. Some pitchers like to try and toughen the skin prior to throwing, while others prefer to decrease the amount that they sweat. It is up to the athletic trainer and the pitcher to determine which method, or combination of methods, are the proper ones to implement in any given case.

Toughening the skin is not something that is easily accomplished, nor does it happen quickly. Daily use of a class IV laser on low power, between 5 and 8 watts for 2 min, over the palmar surface of the distal phalanx of the second and third digit has been used in combination with other measures to help prevent blisters. Laser application can be done multiple times per day, especially in those pitchers that have a history of blisters.

Compounding pharmacies have developed an ointment that is specifically designed to toughen the skin. While they do not divulge exactly what the compound is, some of the main ingredients are tincture of benzoin and hydrocortisone cream, which when applied to the fingers regularly can act to toughen the skin. There is very little scientific data to back up many of the therapeutic methods that are used to toughen the skin, but some pitchers have used pickle juice, rice buckets, or even urine to help prevent blisters on their hand.

Heavy Sweaters

Some pitchers are prone to excessive sweating while in competition, especially those that play in a humid climate. Increased moisture on the hands and fingers increases the risk of blister formation. Trying to keep a pitcher's hands and forearms dry while on the mound is next to impossible with only a rosin bag available to help absorb some of the moisture. Fortunately, there are some products available that can help alleviate most, if not all, of the sweat from reaching the fingers.

Several topical products are being marketed to those who suffer from hyperhidrosis, but the bottom line is that they all contain aluminum chloride, an ingredient found in prescription strength antiperspirants. These products can be in the form of a roll-on antiperspirant stick, a liquid that can be applied using a cotton ball, or as a wipe that is used over the entire forearm and hand. Daily application is recommended to achieve the maximum benefit.

One lesser known product that some pitchers have grown fond of is rosewater and glycerin. Generally, rosewater and glycerin are used to moisturize the skin and face, but in baseball, pitchers use them to help control sweating. Application is through a spray on mist and the rosewater and glycerin are then rubbed over the entire forearm and hand. It is proposed that the glycerin helps to block the pores where it is applied and therefore decreases sweating.

For those pitchers who find that palm sweat is the biggest contributor to their blister formation, there is a technology that has recently been used to control excessive sweating. Tap water iontophoresis, or TWI, can help decrease or eliminate sweating. Studies have shown anywhere from 80% to 91% effectiveness in reduction of palmar sweating [1]. The proposed premise behind TWI is the DC electrical current blocks the synapses to the sweat glands which decreases or eliminates sweat production although this is only one proposed theory. Other theories include hydrogen ion accumulation resulting in decreased pH or ion deposits blocking the sweat glands. Regardless of the mechanism of action, there appears to be some benefit in decreasing palmar hyperhidrosis. Each individual needs to find which settings work best for them through trial and error, but once those settings are discovered they can be maintained. After an initial period of daily use, the user can scale back to 2 or 3 times per week to maintain the benefits of TWI. The iontophoresis units can also be used to decrease hyperhidrosis in the armpits or feet.

What to Do with a Blister

Management of a blister can be a tricky proposition, but if handled appropriately, it can reduce the amount of down time that a pitcher has. Whether the blister roof has torn off or it is still intact will determine immediate blister care. The blister roof offers protection from a potential infection; so, if at all possible, it should be left in place (see Fig. 19.1). To decrease the sensitivity and initiate the healing process, the blister should be drained under sterile conditions only due to risk of infection.

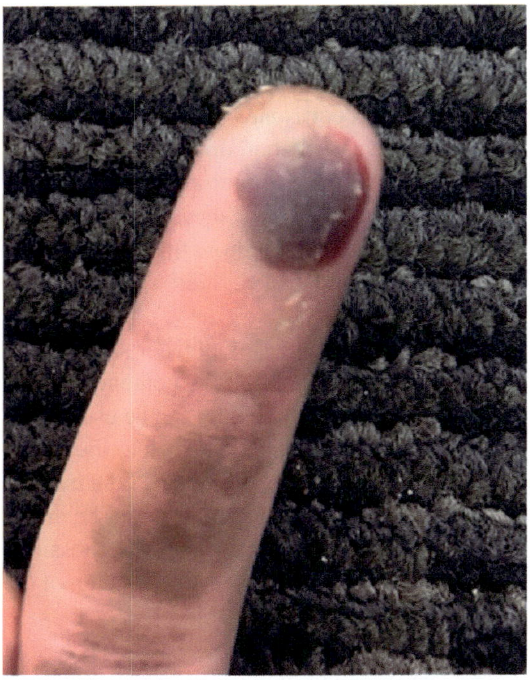

Fig. 19.1 Blister with intact roof

After cleaning the skin with isopropyl alcohol, an 18G or 21G sterile needle can be introduced into a corner of the blister away from where contact with a baseball will be made to drain the serous fluid. A large gauge needle is preferred as oftentimes the hole where the needle entered the blister will close back up allowing serous fluid to accumulate again if the hole is too small. A Betadine and warm water soak (25% Betadine/75% warm water) can help minimize infection and will enter the blister at the hole that was made with the needle. In those cases where the blister is still "hot," ice water can be used instead of warm water.

Laser therapy can also be initiated immediately post-injury and should continue daily. The laser will penetrate through the outer layers of the skin and help to heal the inflamed tissue underneath the roof of the blister. Similar to the settings for blister prevention, the laser can be set at 5–8 watts for 2 min for post-injury treatment but can be adjusted as needed if the blister is irritated by the heat.

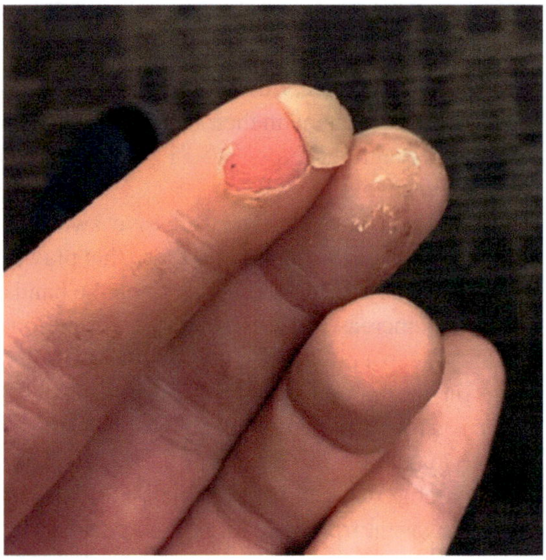

Fig. 19.2 Blister with roof that has been peeled off

In cases where the roof of the blister has come off (see Fig. 19.2), the same Betadine soak and laser treatments can be administered immediately post-injury. The wound should be covered with a cream that promotes the drying and toughening of the skin and then a bandage. Ichthammol ointment, 1% hydrocortisone, tincture of benzoin, and zinc oxide are all good options to use, and in combination with each other also. If the blister roof is still intact, some of these creams can be injected through the same hole that was made to drain the blister and then covered with a bandage overnight.

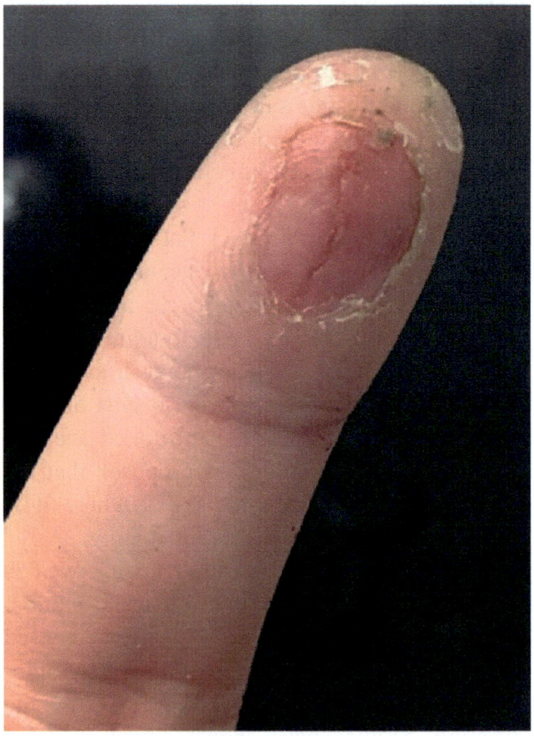

Fig. 19.3 Partially debrided blister

Removal of the roof of the blister should only be attempted once the blister is nontender. After sterile prep, a #15 blade scalpel can be used to cut away the roof of the blister as close to the viable edge as possible (see Fig. 19.3). The goal is to try and make the ridge as smooth as it can be as the pitcher will begin throwing as soon as possible, and any type of ridge can catch on the seam of the baseball and rip the healthy skin.

During the period in which the pitcher is shut down from throwing, it is imperative to continue with shoulder maintenance exercises to minimize the amount of deconditioning that occurs. Return to throwing should only occur once the blister is nontender and good healing has taken place. Care must be taken through the early stages of the throwing progression to ensure the blister does not re-form and throwing mechanics are maintained. Consultation with a pitching coach is encouraged to oversee the return to throwing. As an extra precaution, throwing can be done with a bandage or NewSkin over the blistered area to add protection.

Broken Finger Nail

One other malady that can affect a pitcher's hand is a split, or broken, fingernail (see Fig. 19.4). Generally, the fingernail of the long (middle) finger is at risk of splitting horizontally due to extended contact with the seam of the baseball at ball release. Excessive nail length, even if only a few millimeters, is usually the culprit. In the image below you can see the overall length of the nail is just slightly long and allowed the seam of the baseball to catch the edge and cause a horizontal tear of the nail.

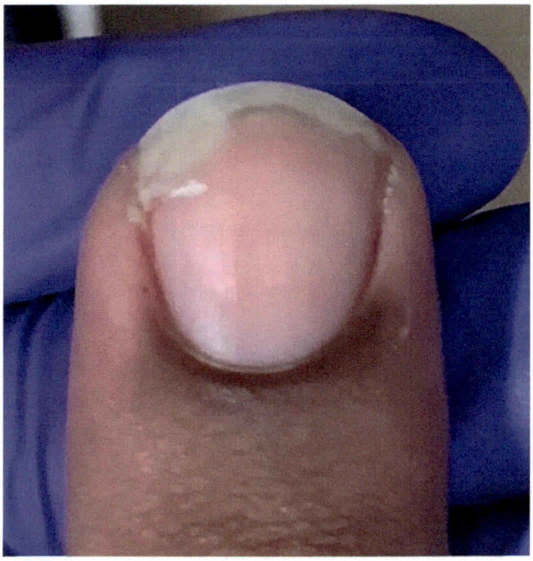

Fig. 19.4 Horizontal split of right long fingernail

Pitchers that split their fingernail during a game should most likely be removed from the game to prevent the split from continuing horizontally across the nail and becoming a larger issue. If caught early enough, these are usually only minimally tender and do not result in further lost time provided that an acrylic nail, which acts as a splint, is applied to allow the pitcher to continue to throw. If an acrylic nail cannot be applied, some athletic trainers have improvised with a silk wrap/nail gel combination or butterfly strips and glue. These options can be used in a pinch but do not provide the support that an acrylic nail does.

Nail care is specific to each individual pitcher and it is ultimately up to them to determine what length of nail works best. The desired length can be influenced by the different types of pitches that they throw. Maintenance should be done multiple times per week. Fingernail clippers should be avoided on the pitching hand and the nail care should be done with an emory board or with a glass nail file. The glass nail file offers a finer grit and is preferred over a disposable emory board as it is more precise. Once the desired length is achieved, then there should be less risk of breaking a nail.

Reference

1. Pariser DM, Ballard A. Iontophoresis for palmar and plantar hyperhidrosis. Dermatol Clin. 2014;32(4):491–4. https://doi.org/10.1016/j.det.2014.06.009.

Index

G. M. Lourie (ed.), *Hand and Wrist Injuries in Baseball*,
https://doi.org/10.1007/978-3-030-81659-9

GPSR Compliance

The European Union's (EU) General Product Safety Regulation (GPSR) is a set of rules that requires consumer products to be safe and our obligations to ensure this.

If you have any concerns about our products, you can contact us on ProductSafety@springernature.com

In case Publisher is established outside the EU, the EU authorized representative is:

Springer Nature Customer Service Center GmbH
Europaplatz 3
69115 Heidelberg, Germany

Batch number: 10732809

Printed by Printforce, the Netherlands